# Self-Expandable Stents
# in the Gastrointestinal Tract

Richard Kozarek  •  Todd Baron
Ho-Young Song
Editors

# Self-Expandable Stents in the Gastrointestinal Tract

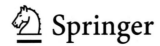 Springer

*Editors*

Richard Kozarek
Digestive Disease Institute
Virginia Mason Medical Center
  and University of Washington
Seattle, WA 98111, USA

Todd Baron
Division of Gastroenterology
  and Hepatology
Mayo Clinic College of Medicine
Rochester, MN 55905, USA

Ho-Young Song
Department of Radiology
Asan Medical Center
388-1 Pungnap-2 Dong
Songpa-Gu, Seoul 138-736
Korea, Republic of (South Korea)

ISBN 978-1-4614-3745-1        ISBN 978-1-4614-3746-8 (eBook)
DOI 10.1007/978-1-4614-3746-8
Springer New York Heidelberg Dordrecht London

Library of Congress Control Number: 2012940930

Printed on acid-free paper

Springer is part of Springer Science+Business Media (www.springer.com)

# Preface

Historically, nonsurgical reconstitution of the gut lumen was limited to the placement of rigid tubes in unresectable esophageal cancer. Initially fashioned out of boxwood or ivory, they were fixed into place by suture tied to a handlebar mustache or looped around the ears. Later they were fashioned out of a compound used by British dentist, Charles T. Stent (1807–1885), who initially developed it to create dental impressions. These conduits ultimately were called *stents,* a term that first appeared in the medical literature in 1952.

Rigid biliary prostheses (stents) were first placed surgically in the mid-1950s, and the first percutaneous placement was described by Molnar and Stockum approximately two decades later. A mere 5 years later, in 1979, Reynders-Fredrix and Soehendra described the first endoscopic placement of a 7 Fr plastic stent in the biliary tree, although it took almost another decade to routinely place small diameter prostheses into the pancreas and to produce endoscopes with a channel size large enough to place 10–11.5 Fr stents.

Self-expandable metal stents (SEMS), placed through a small diameter delivery system and which conform to the body's angulations, have allowed additional anatomical areas to be bypassed, decreased risks associated with placement of relatively large diameter plastic tubes through natural orifices, and have expanded our ability to palliate and effectively treat a wide variety of GI disorders, benign as well as malignant. Their development and application has been nothing short of revolutionary in the treatment of malignant, and to a lesser extent, noncancerous stenoses and acute and chronic GI tract leaks and perforations.

This is the context of our text, *Self-Expandable Stents in the Gastrointestinal Tract*. It brings together the world's experts in stent design and placement, including polyethylene (plastic) prostheses, and a variety of expandable stents (metal, silicone, and absorbable/polylactide). It also brings together the disciplines with the greatest experience in their use in the GI tract: therapeutic endoscopists and interventional radiologists.

This book covered the state of the art in a rapidly changing technology. Despite this evolution, however, and the fact that the FDA and its equivalent in other countries, defines ultimate product availability, basic physics and the design of expandable prostheses are crucial in defining current and future devices and their applications. Although defined historically and anatomically throughout the text, this distinction is artificial and is limited by anatomic access, either percutaneously or by the current use of natural orifices (mouth and anus). The ability to deliver these prostheses by endoscopic ultrasound to straddle the inner and outer wall of the GI tract has revolutionized our ability to drain extraluminal fluid collections and perform anastomoses to include gastrojejunostomy, chole-cystoduodenostomy, and other anastomoses from the stomach or duodenum into the intra- or extrahepatic biliary tree. Add the application of these stents through laparoscopic portals or transgastric or transcolonic neolumens in the setting of NOTES and one can begin to see the yet unrealized potential of this technology.

It is with enthusiasm and the humility of knowing, that by the time of this text's publication, that there will be continued evolution in SEMS technology and placement techniques, that the editors proffer *Self-Expandable Stents in the Gastrointestinal Tract.*

Seattle, WA, USA                                    Richard A. Kozarek, M.D
Rochester, MN, USA                                          Todd Baron, M.D
Seoul, Republic of Korea                              Ho-Young Song, M.D

# Acknowledgments

We acknowledge Jane Babione for her invaluable assistance in manuscript preparation and editing, Anne Marie Howe for clinical practice support, and our families for their patience and support during the editing of this text.

# Contents

# Contributors

**Todd Baron** Department of Medicine, Mayo Clinic, Rochester, MN, USA

**Maarten W. van den Berg** Department of Gastroenterology and Hepatology, Academic Medical Center, University of Amsterdam, Amsterdam, AZ, The Netherlands

**Kenneth F. Binmoeller** Paul May and Frank Stein Interventional Endoscopy Center, California Pacific Medical Center, San Francisco, CA, USA

**Antonella De Ceglie** Department of Gastroenterology and Digestive Endoscopy, Cancer Institute Giovanni Paolo II, Bari, Italy

**Il Ju Choi** Center for Gastric Cancer, National Cancer Center, Goyang, Republic of Korea

**Massimo Conio** Department of Gastroenterology and Digestive Endoscopy, General Hospital Sanremo, Sanremo (IM), Italy

**John T. Cunningham** Department of Internal Medicine, Section of Gastroenterology and Hepatology, University of Arizona, Tucson, AZ, USA

**Daniel de Paula Pessoa Ferreira** Instituto Clinico Humanitas, Rozzano, Milan, Lombardia, Italy

**Martin L. Freeman** Division of Gastroenterology, Hepatology and Nutrition, University of Minnesota, Minneapolis, MN, USA

**Jesús García-Cano** Department of Digestive Diseases, Hospital Virgen de la Luz, Cuenca, Spain

**Jeanin E. van Hooft** Department of Gastroenterology and Hepatology, Academic Medical Center, University of Amsterdam, Amsterdam, AZ, The Netherlands

**Shayan Irani** Departments of Gastroenterology and Hepatology, and Colorectal Cancer, Digestive Disease Institute, Virginia Mason Medical Center, Seattle, WA, USA

**Chan Gyoo Kim** Center for Gastric Cancer, National Cancer Center, Goyang, Republic of Korea

**Jin Hyoung Kim** Radiology Department, Asan Medical Center, Seoul, Republic of Korea

**Tae Il Kim**  Division of Gastroenterology, Department of Internal Medicine, Institute of Gastroenterology, Severance Hospital, Yonsei University College of Medicine, Seodaemun-gu, Seoul, Republic of Korea

**Richard A. Kozarek**  Digestive Disease Institute, Virginia Mason Medical Center and University of Washington, Seattle, WA, USA

**Hans-Ulrich Laasch**  Department of Radiology, The Christie NHS Foundation Trust, Manchester, UK

**Dong Ki Lee**  Department of Internal Medicine, Gangnam Severance Hospital, Yonsei University, Gangnam-gu, Seoul, Republic of Korea

**Joseph W. Leung**  Department of Gastroenterology, VA Northern California Health Care System, Davis School of Medicine, Sacramento VA Medical Center, University of California, Mather, CA, USA

**Wesley Leung**  Center for Endoscopic Research and Therapeutics, Section of Gastroenterology, Department of Medicine, The University of Chicago Medical Center, Chicago, IL, USA

**Mohan Ramchandani**  Gastroenterology Department, Asian Institute of Gastroenterology, Hyderabad, AP, India

**D. Nageshwar Reddy**  Gastroenterology Department, Asian Institute of Gastroenterology, Hyderabad, AP, India

**Alessandro Repici**  Digestive Endoscopy Unit, IRCCS Istituto Clinico Humanitas, Rozzano (Milano), Italy

**Andrew S. Ross**  Digestive Disease Institute, Virginia Mason Medical Center and University of Washington, Seattle, WA, USA

**Mariano Gonzalez-Haba Ruiz**  Center for Endoscopic Research and Therapeutics, Section of Gastroenterology, Department of Medicine, The University of Chicago Medical Center, Chicago, IL, USA

**Peter D. Siersema**  Department of Gastroenterology and Hepatology, University Medical Center Utrecht, Utrecht, The Netherlands

**Ho-Young Song**  Department of Radiology, Asan Medical Center, University of Ulsan College of Medicine, Seoul, Republic of Korea

**Mustafa A. Tiewala**  Division of Gastroenterology, Hennepin County Medical Center, Minneapolis, MN, USA

**Irving Waxman**  Center for Endoscopic Research and Therapeutics, Section of Gastroenterology, Department of Medicine, The University of Chicago Medical Center, Chicago, IL, USA

**Chang Jin Yoon**  Department of Radiology, Seoul National University Bundang Hospital, Seongnam, Republic of Korea

# Part 1

# History of GI Tract Stenting

# History of GI Stenting: Rigid Prostheses in the Esophagus

### Shayan Irani and Richard A. Kozarek

The major function of the esophagus is to serve as a conduit to the passage of a food bolus from the mouth to the stomach. Mechanical obstruction of the esophagus usually produces symptoms late in the disease process, usually when the luminal diameter is less than 13 mm or at least 50% narrowed [1]. The majority of esophageal cancer patients have unresectable disease at presentation. Even after curative therapy, about 20% of patients develop dysphagia from recurrent strictures. Therefore, palliative therapy has been, and will continue to remain, an important part of the management of esophageal malignancy [2].

There have been several modalities used to palliate esophageal obstruction. Surgery carried a high morbidity and mortality and quickly fell to the wayside once less invasive options became available. Dilation of malignant esophageal strictures was associated with the lack of durability, required multiple procedures, and carried a significant perforation rate. Gastrostomy tube placement provided the ability for nutritional support but did nothing to improve quality of life

or ability to eat or to swallow one's secretions. Radiation and chemotherapy are effective in relief of dysphagia, but with a delay in improvement ranging from weeks to months, are not universally tolerated, and have complications [3]. Neolumen creation with Nd-YAG laser is effective in patients with short, exophytic lesions but requires frequent interventions and is not suitable for treatment of long tortuous strictures and does not allow closure of fistulas. Photodynamic therapy was shown to be as effective as Nd-YAG laser in relieving malignant dysphagia due to esophageal cancer with a lower perforation rate than Nd-YAG laser [4]. These modalities were used as an alternative to esophageal stents which continued to evolve and are now the palliative modality of choice due to their ability to provide instant, long-lasting relief from dysphagia with minimal morbidity and negligible mortality [2, 5].

## Era Prior to the First Successful Esophageal Stent

Prior to the first successful placement of an esophageal stent across a malignant stricture, surgery was the only option for patients with esophageal cancer. The four types of surgeries performed up until 1884 were outlined in an article by Dr. Samuel Gross, surgeon at Jefferson College, Philadelphia: (1) Esophagectomy with a curative intent was initially considered only for lesions in the upper esophagus. (2) Internal

S. Irani, M.B.B.S., M.D. (✉)
Departments of Gastroenterology and Hepatology, and Colorectal Cancer, Digestive Disease Institute, Virginia Mason Medical Center, 1100 9th Ave., MS: C3-GAS, Seattle, WA 98101, USA
e-mail: shayan.irani@vmmc.org

R.A. Kozarek, M.D.
Digestive Disease Institute, Virginia Mason Medical Center and University of Washington, 1100 9th Ave., C3-GAS, Seattle, WA 98111, USA

R. Kozarek et al. (eds.), *Self-Expandable Stents in the Gastrointestinal Tract*,
DOI 10.1007/978-1-4614-3746-8_1, © Springer Science+Business Media New York 2013

esophagotomy (internal division of the carcinomatous stricture). This was performed in one patient and required repeated dilation to maintain patency. (3) Esophagostomy (establishment of a permanent fistula in the neck for the introduction of food). The mortality within the first 17 days was unacceptably high at 81% and with no advantage over gastrostomy. It was quickly abandoned along with internal esophagostomy. (4) Surgical gastrostomy carried a 29% associated mortality [6].

Endoesophageal intubation now known as nasogastric or orogastric (external-internal) tube placement was initially used in the mid-1800s for the palliation of esophageal cancer. Drs. Krishaber (four cases), Croft (two cases), and Durham (one case) recommended the use of a long esophageal tube, made of gum-elastic or black caoutchouc (natural rubber) passed through the nose or mouth, to be used as a feeding tube. These tubes had a prolonged patency and had no immediate or procedure-related mortality. However, they did not provide relief of dysphagia and the control of one's secretions and were uncomfortable [7, 8].

As early as 1845, James Leroy d'Etoilles (1798–1860), a French surgeon, was the first to toy with the idea of making a short internal esophageal tube, which was made from decalcified ivory to tunnel through a malignant growth. His attempts as well as similar attempts by a British surgeon, Sir Morrell Mackenzie, to use such tubes failed [7].

## The First Successful Esophageal Stent

In 1885, Sir Charters James Symonds (1852–1932), a Canadian-born surgeon working at Guy's Hospital in London, was the first to record the successful use of a short, rigid, esophageal tube to internally stent a malignant stricture. The tube was 6 in. long made of No. 10 esophageal tubing that was fixed to a boxwood funnel by German silver wire. Later he used a funnel made of silver and ivory instead of boxwood but finally settled on a tube and funnel made from the same gum-elastic material (Fig. 1.1). After

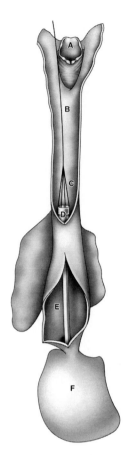

**Fig. 1.1** Sir Charters Symonds' esophageal tube in situ. (**a**) Larynx. (**b**) Esophagus laid open. (**c**) Silk thread by which tube is held in position. (**d**) Wide upper end of the tube above the stricture. (**e**) Narrow lower part of the tube below the stricture. (**f**) Gastric cardia

stricture dilation, the 6-in. tube was passed over a conical bougie or by a special introducer made of copper wire. To overcome the problem of migration, a proximal funnel was used in addition to the attachment of a silk suture to the proximal end of the tube, which was brought out of the mouth and attached to the patient's ear. With the tube in place, patients were allowed to ingest liquids. Every 10 days or so, the tube would be removed for cleaning, and the patient was permitted to eat solid food for a short period of time until the tube was replaced, occasionally with a larger diameter tube. This tube not only provided adequate nutrition and palliation but also improved quality of life [8].

## The Post-Symonds Era

Until this point, tubes had been inserted blindly. In 1914, M. Guisez, a French surgeon suggested esophageal stenting over an introducer. A De Pezzer-like catheter was used which was 6 cm long and ended blindly. Side holes were in place to allow passage of fluid. It was stretched thin over an introducer, making it easier to navigate through the stricture. Once in position, the introducer was withdrawn and the catheter was gripped by the stricture. Guisez made full use of the esophagoscope and bougies and reported low complication rates [9].

In 1924, Sir Henry Souttar continued the trend for direct endoscopic visualization prior to tube/stent placement [10]. Souttar had a background in engineering from Oxford before taking up medicine at London Hospital. He designed a stent made of a tightly coiled metal spring from a 1-mm wire with 25 turns per inch. This coiled metallic stent, originally made of German silver and later stainless steel, was placed using a special introducer (Fig. 1.2). The stent was rigid enough to be

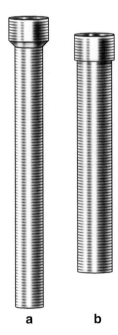

**a**          **b**

**Fig. 1.2** (**a, b**) The Souttar tube. The original type made of German silver and the subsequent model made of stainless steel

pushed through the esophagus without collapsing, yet had the flexibility to bend and elongate through a tortuous stricture. A proximal lip, 2 mm wider than the body of the prosthesis, was present and sometimes reinforced with an even wider funnel made of rubber [10, 11]. Results were satisfactory in the 100 personal cases he reported. However, two problems remained: false passage and spontaneous migration. To reduce the risk of a false passage/perforation, J. H. Resamo (Argentina) modified Souttar's technique using a guide to direct the stents, and in his hands, the mortality rate from intubation was 0.5% [5].

After World War II, there was a resurgence in esophageal surgery and at the same time a rise in the use of stents to palliate esophageal cancer. In 1949, A. L. Brown, an American physician, recommended the use of a tube made of silver with a distal flange. He inserted the tube surgically through a slit opened below the esophageal obstructing lesion. Under direct visualization, the stent was advanced proximally (retrograde). A suture was then placed around the esophagus below the distal flange to prevent migration into the stomach, while the flange prevented proximal migration [12]. The use of silver was abandoned for more flexible synthetic materials after a review showed plastic to be superior to metal and rubber [13].

In 1952, M. Ravitch and T. Bahnson inserted a plastic prosthesis (variant of the Souttar tube) over an obturator intraoperatively when an unresectable esophageal cancer was encountered [14]. Similarly, in 1954, S. Mackler and R. Mayer introduced an indwelling tube through a longitudinal incision in the esophagus 2 in. above the lesion at the time of thoracic exploration when resection was not possible. Mortality using this approach was around 32% [15]. In the same year, Coyas in Greece in collaboration with Triboulet-Piton in France introduced a plastic tube to palliate esophageal cancer under direct endoscopic visualization. The stent lacked a funnel but had parallel rings to grip the tumor and metal rings at the end to make it radiopaque [16]. In the same year, Kropff described a funnel-shaped polyethylene tube introduced through a cervical esophagotomy [17].

There was even an alternative approach in which the combination of resection and stent placement was attempted. In 1952, Berman reported his experience of replacing the midesophagus of 20 dogs with plastic tubes through a thoracoabdominal approach, which translated to resection of the lesion with reattachment of the defect with the stent. In 1956, this was followed by a thorough review of esophageal cancer and rationale to abandon this combined approach. This was due to the poor prognosis of esophageal cancer, the high morbidity and mortality of any esophageal surgery, and the inability for complete resection of malignancy [18, 19].

One of the more ingenious prostheses produced during this time was a tube designed by Sachs in 1958 [20]. The prosthesis was designed in the form of a hollow screw machined from a nylon rod for per oral insertion without the need for preinsertion dilation. The thread of the screw had a horizontal shoulder perpendicular to the axis of the tube, which prevented proximal migration. The inner diameter of the screw was 8 mm and was inserted by screwing it through the lesion using a driver that fit snugly in knurls at the proximal end of the prosthesis. The stent was placed successfully in four patients (Fig. 1.3) [21].

## The Push and Pull Technique of Placing Esophageal Stents

The aforementioned esophageal prostheses were placed by the *push* technique alone, initially blindly, and then under endoscopic visualization. In 1956, Mousseau and Barbin, two French surgeons, reported a new method of permanent intubation/stenting of the esophagus using the *push and pull* technique. Their stent consisted of a circular, neoplex tube with a catheter-like portion at the distal end and a funnel at the proximal end. After passing the catheter transorally blindly into the proximal stomach, a high gastrostomy was performed and the lower end of the catheter portion was grasped and pulled distally until the proximal stent funnel engaged the stricture. The excess lower end of the catheter was then cut in the stomach and the prosthesis remained in place.

The authors claimed that this method had a lower false passage and perforation rate, given the guidance provided by the pull from the stomach ensuring its luminal placement (Fig. 1.4) [22].

## The Celestin Tube

In 1959, Celestin reported an improvement/modification of the Mousseau-Barbin tube. This new tube was made from natural polythene, was oval in its various diameters (as opposed to circular), and carried a thin barrel-shaped funnel (as opposed to the more conventional V-shaped funnel). The author claimed that the oval lumen of the tube would be more desirable in view of the natural shape of the lumen of the esophagus in situ. The barrel shape to the proximal end was also supposed to provide a more secure fitting as well as potentially reduce the risk of obstruction by a ring of proximal edematous hypertrophic tissue. The prosthesis consisted of two parts, a solid pilot bougie attached by a suture to the endoesophageal tube/stent (25 cm long, 10 mm diameter, and 1 mm thick) (Fig. 1.4). The bougie was introduced under direct visualization, often preceded by dilation of the stricture. Through a high gastrostomy, the lower end of the bougie was grasped and the stent pulled securely into place. In the event that the stent was not well gripped by the stricture, the lower end of the stent was sutured in place in the stomach. This allowed patients to tolerate a solid diet with careful mastication and frequent sips of water or carbonated beverages [7]. Celestin later modified his tube to be made of latex rubber and enmeshed a nylon spiral into it with a radiopaque strip (Fig. 1.5).

## Era of Plastic and Latex Endoprosthesis

After the introduction of the Celestin tube, plastic (polyvinyl/Tygon) became the predominant material of which esophageal stents were manufactured, and direct endoscopic insertion became the standard insertion technique. In 1976, Tytgat et al. of the Amsterdam group standardized the

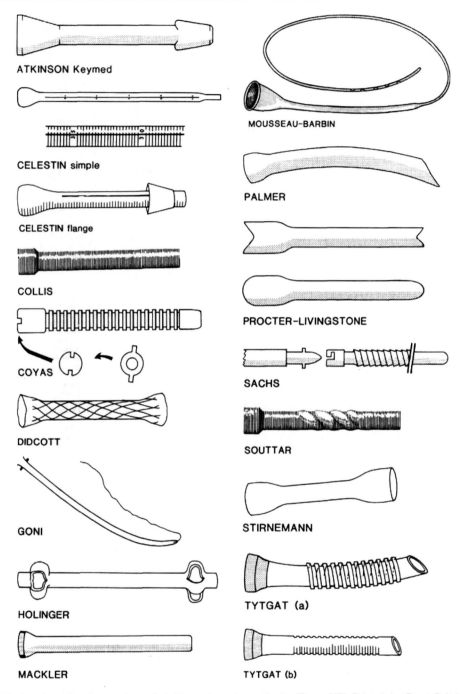

**Fig. 1.3** A schematic of a variety of rigid esophageal prosthesis (From [67] Printed in Great Britain, with permission)

endoscopic insertion of plastic endoprosthesis. Measurement of the exact length of the stricture and use of external radiopaque markers for fluoroscopic guidance were felt to be imperative prior to stent placement [23]. The stricture was dilated to a diameter that was a few millimeters larger than the external diameter of the stent (usually 16–20 mm). An over the wire dilator was

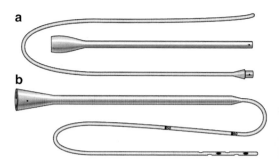

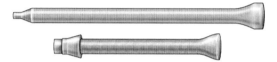

**Fig. 1.4** (**a**) The original Celestin tube. (**b**) Mousseau-Barbin tube

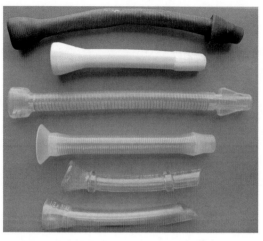

**Fig. 1.5** The commercially manufactured Medoc-Celestin tube (Medoc, Tetbury, UK), with and without a distal flange

**Fig. 1.6** The common commercially available prosthesis: from *top to bottom*: Celestin tube (distal flange), Atkinson's tube, Eska-Buess prosthesis, Wilson-Cook prosthesis (low profile), homemade Tygon stent with and without ridges

used which was originally Eder-Peustow and later Savary. Stents were passed over an insertion device which was usually a Savary dilator (30–33 Fr), although an Atkinson introducer (Olympus America) or an endoscope shaft could also be used. The stent was advanced into place using a pusher tube such as a Dumon introducer (Wilson-Cook, Inc., Winston Salem, NC) under fluoroscopic guidance [24]. A barium esophagram was usually obtained to ensure adequate positioning.

The most common plastic endoprosthesis used was homemade from polyvinyl (Tygon) tubing. The tubing was cut to sufficient length to exceed the length of the tumor by about 6–7 cm. This allowed for a 2–3 cm proximal flange and about a 2–4 cm extension beyond the distal end of the tumor to prevent later occlusion by tumor overgrowth. The proximal flange was created by heating the Tygon tubing in hot mineral oil and then pressing it on an inverted laboratory glass funnel or an anoscope obturator. The distal end was beveled to facilitate passage through the tumor. Both ends of the stent were smoothed with a file to reduce mucosal damage. A second tube (pusher tube) was cut to sufficient length so as to extend from the orad tumor margin to about 8–10 cm beyond the incisor teeth. Both the pusher tube and the prosthesis were then placed over a dilator

(Savary or Hurst) and inserted under fluoroscopic guidance [25].

The common commercially available prostheses were the Medoc-Celestin tube (Medoc, Tetbury, UK), Proctor-Livingstone tube (Latex Products, Johannesburg), Wilson-Cook prosthesis (Wilson Cook), Key-Med Atkinson stent (Olympus America, USA), and Eska-Buess stent (Eska, Germany) (Fig. 1.6). The Medoc-Celestin tube was made of latex reinforced with a nylon spiral, available in lengths of 12.5, 15, and 21 cm, with an outer diameter of 15 mm and inner diameter of 12 mm. The Proctor-Livingstone tube was also an armored latex tube with an internal diameter of 12 mm and outer diameter of 18 mm and a proximal 3 cm long flare of 25 mm diameter. It was available in lengths of 10, 15, and 19 cm [26]. The Wilson-Cook prosthesis was made of silicone with a stainless steel spiral spine, an outer diameter of 16 mm, inner diameter of 12 mm, and lengths ranging from 4.4 to 16.4 cm. The Key-Med Atkinson prosthesis was made of silicone with a central nylon spiral, ranging in length from 14 to 19 cm, an outer diameter of 16 mm, and inner diameter of 14 mm. The Eska-Buess prosthesis was made of silicone with a stainless steel spiral, with hooks in the proximal flange to allow grasping the stent for repositioning or retrieval, if needed [2].

**Table 1.1** Plastic/rubber esophageal prosthesis: review of selected series

| Author/year (Ref #) | Prosthesis | Number of patients | Technical success (%)[a] | Complications (%)[b] | Deaths (%)[c] |
|---|---|---|---|---|---|
| O'Connor/1963 [25] | Tygon | 388 | 97 | 17 | 0.6 |
| Hegarty/1977 [26] | Proctor-Livingstone | 181 | 98 | NR | 17 |
| Angorn/1979 [27] | Proctor-Livingstone | 652 | 97 | 9 | 8 |
| den Hartog/1979 [28] | Tygon | 200 | 97 | 57 | 7 |
| Tytgat/1980 [29] | Tygon | 297 | 97 | 47 | 1 |
| Ogilvie/1982 [30] | Celestin and silicone | 121 | 98 | 50 | 7 |
| Buset/1987 [32] | Tygon | 116 | 95 | 32 | 4 |
| Gasparri/1987 [32] | Medoc, Atkinson, Celestin, Harring | 248 | 100 | 21 | 7 |
| Cotton/1988 [33] | Proctor-Livingstone | 250 | 76 | NR | 27 |

*NR* not reported

[a]Technical success was defined as the successful placement of the prosthesis

[b]Complications included short- and long-term, fatal and nonfatal complications

[c]Deaths included both procedure-related and delayed deaths as a direct complication of the stent

The larger case series using plastic and latex prostheses to palliate malignant esophageal strictures are listed in Table 1.1 [25–33]. In addition to the nine series reported, multiple other smaller series using one or a combination of prostheses resulted in similar outcomes [34–43]. The cumulative experience of palliation of malignant dysphagia in 2,951 patients with a plastic or latex prosthesis was associated with mean technical success rates of 94% (range 75–100%) and complication rates of 23% (3–60%). The differences in complication rates were attributed to the retrospective nature of most studies. Some authors included immediate complications and others only included perforations as complications. Studies that included long-term complications had mean complication rates of 45–50%. Perforation rates ranged from 2% to 12%. Mean procedure-related mortality was 8% (0.5–27%). With such high perforation and complication rates and associated mortality due to the need for aggressive dilation of strictures prior to placement of rigid stents, there was a search for a less cumbersome and safer stent to palliate malignant dysphagia.

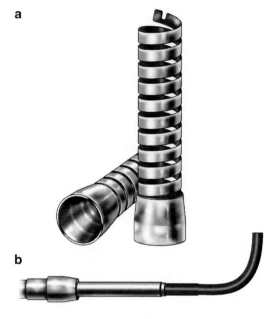

**Fig. 1.7** (**a**) The Frimberger expanding spiral stent. (**b**) The spiral stent wound around a pediatric gastroscope

## Era of Self-Expandable Metal Stents

Frimberger appears to be the first to have developed the concept of placing a self-expandable metal stent (SEMS) in the gastrointestinal tract. Although the Souttar tube was a metal stent made

of a coiled spring, it required the stricture to be dilated to 1–2 mm larger than the size of the prosthesis that needed to be placed (10 mm). The Frimberger stent was a metal spiral coil with an initial diameter of 13–15 mm (Fig. 1.7). With a special fixation tube and a thread, the spiral was wound tightly around a pediatric gastroscope. The prosthesis was advanced into the stricture and then released by the fixation tube. It was held in place by the radial expansion of the stent as well as by tumor pressing into the spaces between the windings. Frimberger reported his experience in 10 patients in whom stents were successfully placed [44]. There were no deaths, but three distal migrations occurred. It took nearly a decade before modern manufacturing methods and new stent designs allowed the development of clinically applicable SEMS. The basic principle of the Frimberger stent was embodied in the EsophaCoil stent.

In the early 1990s, there were many retrospective and prospective case series on self-expandable metal stents but it was the seminal randomized controlled trial by Knyrim et al. in 1993 that provided evidence that led to the replacement of rigid prostheses with SEMS for the palliation of malignant dysphagia. In this study, the uncovered Wallstent was the SEMS used. Complications, particularly stent-insertion-related complications, were significantly higher in the rigid prosthesis group. Although initial costs were higher in the SEMS group, lower hospitalization rates and mortality resulted in overall cost-effectiveness [45]. Later in 1996, DePalma et al. published the second randomized controlled study comparing a rigid plastic prosthesis (Wilson-Cook prosthesis) to an uncovered SEMS (Ultraflex, Boston Scientific). In this small study of 39 patients, technical success rates and improvement in dysphagia scores were similar, but early complications (21% vs. 0%) and mortality (16% vs. 0%) were significantly higher in the plastic prosthesis group [46].

The first commercially produced self-expandable metal stent was the Wallstent, made of stainless steel and manufactured originally by Schneider Inc. (Switzerland). The stent and delivery systems were essentially the same as endovascular Wallstents, already in production in the late 1980s. In addition, SEMS had already been shown to have better patency rates in the biliary tree compared to plastic stents [47–49]. The first SEMS to be inserted in the esophagus was by Domschke in Germany. He inserted two 20 mm endovascular Wallstents in patients with inoperable esophageal cancer with relief of dysphagia for 4 months [50]. Some of the disadvantages or the endovascular stents were also seen including

the relatively short lengths, absence of a proximal flare, and the exposed wire filaments at the ends, which caused mucosal injury and endoscope damage [51, 52]. The main limiting factor however was tumor ingrowth through the stent interstices with subsequent obstruction. This led to termination of a multicenter European study. Attempts to fully cover this stent with a synthetic material were also unsuccessful. Due to the above problems, an American model of the Wallstent with a partial silicone covering and a tulip-shaped proximal end was designed. This prototype stent had a bulky insertion delivery system (13 mm diameter), making delivery difficult [53]. A partially covered version of this stent was later produced and found to be effective [54, 55].

The second type of esophageal SEMS to be manufactured was the Gianturco Z-stent. This was also a stainless steel metal stent designed in the United States by interventional radiologists, Gianturco and Rösh. This stent had interconnected consecutive Z-shaped segments, was not braided, and thus did not foreshorten during deployment. A polyurethane covering was applied to prevent tumor ingrowth. The European version of this stent had two rows of external, lateral projecting barbs to reduce migration. The Song stent was essentially a Z-stent without antimigration barbs [56–58].

The third SEMS to be developed was the Ultraflex stent, developed by Boston Scientific (Natick, MA, USA). It was the first stent to be made of nitinol, a shape-retaining nickel and titanium alloy. The first-generation Ultraflex stent was completely uncovered and encountered the same problem of tumor ingrowth, as other uncovered SEMS [59–61]. In addition to the advantages of nitinol as a material, the stent being more flexible, the delivery system was also small enough to allow easy deployment. Subsequently, a partially covered Ultraflex stent was developed and is still being used in many parts of the world. A disadvantage of this stent is the high degree of foreshortening (25–40%) that occurs during deployment, which makes precise stent placement difficult. There were also reports of poor stent expansion, requiring dilation in up to a third of patients [51].

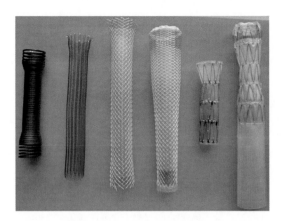

**Fig. 1.8** Self-expandable metal stents (SEMS) no longer routinely manufactured or marketed in the United States. From *left to right*: EsophaCoil (Medtronic/Instent), uncovered Ultraflex (Boston Scientific), partially covered Wallstent (Boston Scientific), partially covered Flamingo Wallstent (Boston Scientific), fully covered Z-stent (Cook Inc.)

The EsophaCoil stent was the second SEMS to be made from nitinol, with a similar design to the spiral coil stent of Frimberger. Developed in Israel in 1994, by Goldin and colleagues, they reported successful deployment in four patients [62]. This stent was designed to overcome the disadvantages of previously designed uncovered stents, i.e., tumor ingrowth and tissue injury due to sharp exposed stent ends. This flat wire coil spring stent was wrapped tightly on an introducing catheter 9 mm in diameter and deployed by pulling a wire holding the distal and proximal ends. Once released, the stent foreshortened by 50% from the ends toward the center. This stent not only foreshortened more than any other stent, it also had the strongest and most rapid radial expansile force (Fig. 1.8).

With the large-scale production of the above-mentioned stents, and where upfront costs were not an issue, SEMS quickly replaced plastic prosthesis as the method of choice to palliate esophageal cancer. Thus, the SEMS revolution began, an era that has not ended. Of the previously mentioned SEMS, all but the uncovered Ultraflex have been discontinued in most markets for different reasons, mostly due to improvement in stent designs. In a nonrandomized, uncontrolled study in 82 patients, Schmassmann et al. compared the uncovered Wallstent with the Ultraflex stent

(Boston Scientific Inc.). The Wallstent was associated with higher stent-related mortality (16% vs. 0%), higher rate of early complications (32% vs. 8%), and severe persistent chest pain (23% vs. 0%) compared to the Ultraflex stent [63]. At least some of these differences were attributed to the sharp uncovered stainless steel ends of the Wallstent. Given these differences, the Wallstent is no longer manufactured. Another version of the esophageal Wallstent was the Flamingo Wallstent marketed in Europe for use in distal esophageal malignant strictures. It had a tapered design to theoretically reduce migration with a proximal flare (30 or 24 mm) and a gradual distal taper (20 or 16 mm). In two separate, prospective, randomized controlled trials comparing it to the Gianturco Z-stent (Cook Inc.) and Ultraflex stent (Boston Scientific Inc.), there were no differences in outcomes for palliation of dysphagia, migration rates, or complication rates [64, 65]. Due to the higher cost of the Flamingo Wallstent and reports of higher rates of chest pain (given the proximal flare of 30 mm), this stent was never marketed in the United States. The EsophaCoil stent was the first to be withdrawn from the market. In addition to the 50% foreshortening, making accurate placement difficult, the very high expansile force led to sudden full expansion of the stent at deployment, often resulting in severe chest pain [3, 66]. The most recent stent to be withdrawn from the US market was the esophageal Z-stent (Cook Medical Endoscopy) and was replaced by the Evolution stent by the same company.

## Summary

Esophageal stents have come a long way since their origin in the late nineteenth century, from decalcified ivory, to boxwood and German silver, to rigid plastic and latex, to stainless steel, and now to the most commonly used stent material, nitinol. There been an explosion in stent design with many manufacturers joining the SEMS revolution. Indications for esophageal stents have recently come to include benign conditions. Lately, self-expandable plastic stents and biodegradable stents have been manufactured, studied, and are finding a niche in the treatment of benign esophageal conditions. Drug-eluting stents are on the horizon. The future looks bright for the continued role of esophageal stents in the management of various esophageal disorders, especially in the palliation of malignant dysphagia.

# References

1. Peura DA, Johnson L. Treatment of esophageal obstruction. In: Castel DO, Johnson LF, editors. Esophageal function in health and disease. New York: Elsevier Biomedical; 1982. p. 372. Book 17.
2. Mohan VK, Kozarek RA. Placement of conventional and expandable stents for malignant esophageal stenoses. Tech Gastrointest Endosc. 2001;3:166–75.
3. Naso P, Bonanno G, Aprile G, et al. EsophaCoil for palliation of dysphagia in unresectable oesophageal carcinoma: short- and long-term results. Dig Liver Dis. 2001;33:653–8.
4. Lightdale CJ, Heier SK, Marcon NE, et al. Photodynamic therapy with porfimer sodium versus thermal ablation therapy with Nd:YAG laser for palliation of esophageal cancer: a multicenter randomized trial. Gastrointest Endosc. 1995;42:507–12.
5. Lux G, Groitl H, Eli C. Tumor stenoses of the upper gastrointestinal tract – therapeutic alternatives to laser therapy. Endoscopy. 1986;18(Suppl 1):37–43.
6. Gross SW. Gastrostomy, oesophagostomy, internal oesophagotomy, combined oesophagotomy, oesophagectomy, and retrograde divulsion in the treatment of stricture of the oesophagus. Am J Med Sci. 1884; 88:58–69.
7. Celestin LR. Permanent intubation in inoperable cancer of the oseophagus and cardia. A new tube. Ann R Coll Surg Engl. 1959;25:165–70.
8. Symonds CJ. The treatment of malignant stricture of the oesophagus by tubage or permanent catheterism. Br Med Journal 1887; 1(1373):870–873.
9. Guisez J. De l'intubation caoutchoutee oesophagienne. Presse Med. 1914;22:85–7.
10. Souttar AHS. A method of intubating the oesophagus for malignant stricture. BMJ. 1924;1:782–3.
11. Earlam R. Souttar tubes for esophageal carcinoma. Surg Gastroenterol. 1979;13:15–20.
12. Resano JH. Treatment of cancer of the esophagus. Bull Soc Int Chir. 1975;6:311.
13. Ingraham FD, Alexander Jr E, Matson DD. Synthetic plastic materials in surgery. N Engl J Med. 1947; 236(11):402–7.
14. Ravitch MM, Bahnson HT, Johns TN. Carcinoma of the esophagus: a consideration of curative and palliative procedures. J Thorac Surg. 1952;24:256–70.
15. Mackler SA, Mayer RM. Palliation of esophageal obstruction due to carcinoma with a permanent intraluminal tube. J Thorac Surg. 1954;28:431–43.
16. Coyas A. Palliative intubation in carcinoma of oesophagus. Lancet. 1955;269(6891):647–9.
17. Kropff G. Esophageal intubation with plastic tube followed by radium therapy in treatment of cancer of the esophagus. Mem Acad Chir (Paris). 1943;80(23–24):628–34. French.
18. Bermane F. The Experimental replacement of portions of the esophagus by a plastic tube. Ann Surg. 1952;135:337.
19. Bermane F. Plastic prosthesis in carcinoma of the esophagus. Surg Clin North Am. 1956;36:883.
20. Parker CH, Peura DA. Palliative treatment of esophageal caracinoma using esophageal dilation and prosthesis. Gastroenterol Clin North Am. 1991;20: 717–29.
21. Sachs L. A plastic prosthesis for palliating carcinoma of the esophagus. Surgery. 1959;45:377–88.
22. Mousseau M, Leforestier J, Barbin J, et al. Place de l'intubation a derneure dans le traitement palliatif du cancer de l'eosophage. Arch Mal App Digest. 1956; 45:208.
23. Tytgat GN, den Hartog Jager FC, Haverkamp HJ. Positioning of a plastic prosthesis under fiber endoscopic control in the palliative treatment of cardioesophageal cancer. Endoscopy. 1976;8:180–5.
24. Irani S, Kozarek R. Esophageal stents: past, present, and future. In: Siersema P, editor. Techniques in Gastrointestinal Endoscopy. Philadelphia: Saunders-Elsevier; 2011. p. 178–90.
25. Oconnor T, Watson R, Lepley Jr D, et al. Esophageal prosthesis for palliative intubation. Further evaluation of 378 patients. Arch Surg. 1963;87:275–8.
26. Hegarty MM, Angorn IB, Bryer JV, et al. Pulsion intubation for palliation of carcinoma of the oesophagus. Br J Surg. 1977;64:160–5.
27. Angorn IB, Hegarty MM. Palliative pulsion intubation in oesophageal carcinoma. Ann R Coll Surg Engl. 1979;61:212–4.
28. den Hartog Jager FC, Bartelsman JF, Haverkamp HJ, Tytgat GN. Palliative treatment of impaired esophageal and gastric food transit by means of an endoscopically-positioned prosthesis. Ned Tijdschr Geneeskd. 1980;124(52):2213–8. Dutch.
29. Tytgat GN, den Hartog Jager FC, Bartelsman JF. Endoscopic prosthesis for advanced esophageal cancer. Endoscopy. 1986;18(Suppl 3):32–9.
30. Ogilvie AL, Dronfield MW, Ferguson R, et al. Palliative intubation of oesophagogastric neoplasms at fibreoptic endoscopy. Gut. 1982;23:1060–7.
31. Buset M, des Marez B, Baize M, et al. Palliative endoscopic management of obstructive esophagogastric cancer: laser or prosthesis? Gastrointest Endosc. 1987;33:357–61.
32. Gasparri G, Casalegno PA, Camandona M, et al. Endoscopic insertion of 248 prostheses in inoperable carcinoma of the esophagus and cardia: short-term and long-term results. Gastrointest Endosc. 1987;33:354–6.
33. Cotton MH, Sammon AM. Carcinoma of the oesophagus in Transkei: treatment by intubation. Thorax. 1989;44:42–7.

34. Atkinson M, Ferguson R, Ogilvie AL. Management of malignant dysphagia by intubation at endoscopy. J R Soc Med. 1979;72:894–7.

35. Palmer ED. Peroral prosthesis for the management of incurable esophageal carcinoma. Am J Gastroenterol. 1973;59:487–98.

36. Peura DA, Heit HA, Johnson LF, et al. Esophageal prosthesis in cancer. Am J Dig Dis. 1978;23:796–800.

37. Jones DB, Davies PS, Smith PM. Endoscopic insertion of palliative oesophageal tubes in oesophagogastric neoplasms. Br J Surg. 1981;68:197–8.

38. Seifert E, Reinhard A, Lütke A, et al. Palliative treatment of inoperable patients with carcinoma of the cardia region. Gastrointest Endosc. 1983;29:6–7.

39. Lux G, Groitl H, Riemann JF, et al. Tumor stenosis of the upper gastrointestinal tract – non-surgical therapy by bridging tubes. Endoscopy. 1983;15(Suppl 1):207–12.

40. Valbuena J. Endoscopic palliative treatment of esophageal and cardial cancer: a new antireflux prosthesis. A study of 40 cases. Cancer. 1984;53:993–8.

41. Chavy AL, Rougier M, Pieddeloup C, et al. Esophageal prosthesis for neoplastic stenosis. A prognostic study of 77 cases. Cancer. 1986;57:1426–31.

42. McIntyre AS, Morris DL, Sloan RL, et al. Palliative therapy of malignant esophageal stricture with the bipolar tumor probe and prosthetic tube. Gastrointest Endosc. 1989;35:531–5.

43. Kratz JM, Reed CE, Crawford FA, et al. A comparison of endoesophageal tubes. Improved results with the Atkinson tube. J Thorac Cardiovasc Surg. 1989;97:19–23.

44. Frimberger E. Expanding spiral – a new type of prosthesis for the palliative treatment of malignant esophageal stenoses. Endoscopy. 1983;15(Suppl 1):213–4.

45. Knyrim K, Wagner HJ, Bethge N, et al. A controlled trial of an expansile metal stent for palliation of esophageal obstruction due to inoperable cancer. N Engl J Med. 1993;329:1302–7.

46. De Palma GD, di Matteo E, Romano G, et al. Plastic prosthesis versus expandable metal stents for palliation of inoperable esophageal thoracic carcinoma: a controlled prospective study. Gastrointest Endosc. 1996;43:478–82.

47. Coons HG. Self-expanding stainless steel biliary stents. Radiology. 1989;170:979–83.

48. Huibregtse K, Carr-Locke DL, Cremer M, et al. Biliary stent occlusion – a problem solved with self-expanding metal stents? European Wallstent Study Group. Endoscopy. 1992;24:391–4.

49. Davids PH, Groen AK, Rauws EA, et al. Randomised trial of self-expanding metal stents versus polyethylene stents for distal malignant biliary obstruction. Lancet. 1993;340(8834–8835):1488–92.

50. Domschke W, Foerster EC, Matek W, et al. Self-expanding mesh stent for esophageal cancer stenosis. Endoscopy. 1992;22:134–6.

51. Ell C, May A. Self-expanding stents for palliation of stenosing tumors of the esophagus and cardia: a critical review. Endoscopy. 1997;29:392–8.

52. Bethge N, Knyrim K, Wagner HJ, et al. Self-expanding metal stents for palliation of malignant esophageal obstruction – a pilot study of eight patients. Endoscopy. 1992;24:411–5.

53. Nelson DB, Axelrad AM, Fleischer DE, et al. Silicone-covered Wallstent prototypes for palliation of malignant esophageal obstruction and digestive-respiratory fistulas. Gastrointest Endosc. 1997;45:31–7.

54. Born P, Neuhaus H, Rösch T, et al. Initial experience with a new, partially covered Wallstent for malignant biliary obstruction. Endoscopy. 1996;28:699–702.

55. Wagner HJ, Knyrim K, Bethge N, et al. The palliative therapy of malignant esophageal obstruction with self-expanding metal endoprostheses. Dtsch Med Wochenschr. 1992;117:248–55. German.

56. Schaer J, Katon RM, Ivancev K, et al. Treatment of malignant esophageal obstruction with silicone-coated metallic self-expanding stents. Gastrointest Endosc. 1994;38:7–11.

57. Song HY, Do YS, Han YM, et al. Covered, expandable esophageal metallic stent tubes: experiences in 119 patients. Radiology. 1994;193:689–95.

58. Wu WC, Katon RM, Saxon RR, et al. Silicone-covered self-expanding metallic stents for the palliation of malignant esophageal obstruction and esophagorespiratory fistulas: experience in 32 patients and a review of the literature. Gastrointest Endosc. 1994;40:22–33.

59. Cwikiel W, Stridbeck H, Tranberg KG, et al. Malignant esophageal strictures: treatment with a self-expanding nitinol stent. Radiology. 1993;187:661–5.

60. Grund KE, Storek D, Becker HD. Highly flexible self-expanding meshed metal stents for palliation of malignant esophagogastric obstruction. Endoscopy. 1995;27:486–94.

61. De Palma GD, Galloro G, Sivero L, et al. Self-expanding metal stents for palliation of inoperable carcinoma of the esophagus and gastroesophageal junction. Am J Gastroenterol. 1995;90:2140–2.

62. Goldin E, Beyar M, Safra T, et al. A new self-expandable, nickel-titanium coil stent for esophageal obstruction: a preliminary report. Gastrointest Endosc. 1994;40:64–8.

63. Schmassmann A, Meyenberger C, Knuchel J, et al. Self-expanding metal stents in malignant esophageal obstruction: a comparison between two stent types. Am J Gastroenterol. 1997;92:400–6.

64. Sabharwal T, Hamady MS, Chui S, et al. A randomised prospective comparison of the Flamingo Wallstent and Ultraflex stent for palliation of dysphagia associated with lower third oesophageal carcinoma. Gut. 2003;52:922–6.

65. Siersema PD, Hop WC, van Blankenstein M, van Tilburg AJ, et al. A comparison of 3 types of covered metal stents for the palliation of patients with dysphagia caused by esophagogastric carcinoma: a prospective, randomized study. Gastrointest Endosc. 2001;54:145–53.

66. Mayoral W, Fleischer DE. The EsophaCoil stent for malignant esophageal obstruction. Gastrointest Endosc Clin N Am. 1999;9:423–30.

67. Richard Earlam, Cunha-Melo JR. Malignant oesophageal strictures: a review of techniques for palliative intubation. Br J Surg. 1982;69:61–8.

# History of Bile Duct Stenting: Rigid Prostheses

Joseph W. Leung

## Biliary Obstruction: The Need for Drainage

Malignant obstructive jaundice caused by tumor obstruction at the head of pancreas, peri-ampullary area, bile duct or gall bladder, and hilar lymphadenopathy carries considerable morbidity and mortality (Fig. 2.1a, b). Biliary obstruction can lead to severe itching, and prolonged obstruction leads to impaired immune (both humoral and cellular) defense mechanisms predisposing the patient to increased risk of infection, endotoxemia, coagulopathy, impaired vascular response with acute renal failure, bleeding, wound sepsis, and impaired wound healing [1–13].

Various imaging modalities have evolved over time to define the exact level and nature of bile duct obstruction. In addition, the advent of needle aspiration and biopsy allows nonoperative tissue sampling to help discern the underlying cause of malignant biliary obstruction. Surgery is the only hope of cure for many of these patients, but for those with unresectable lesions, direct cholangiography via ERCP [14] and percutaneous transhepatic access [15] provides imaging as well as

J.W. Leung, M.D., F.R.C.P., F.A.C.P., M.A.C.G.,
F.A.S.G.E. (✉)
Department of Gastroenterology, VA Northern California
Health Care System, Davis School of Medicine,
Sacramento VA Medical Center, University of California,
10535 Hospital Way, Mather, CA 95655, USA
e-mail: jwleung@ucdavis.edu

access to the biliary system for decompression and palliative drainage.

Over the past several decades, we have seen the evolution and development of different biliary stent technologies with improved plastic stents and stent deployment systems as well as the introduction of self-expandable metal stents (SEMS). This chapter will discuss the development of plastic biliary stents for the management of bile duct obstruction. As noted above, stents were originally developed for the palliative treatment of malignant obstructive jaundice. Currently, indications for the use of plastic biliary stents have widened to include the treatment of patients with numerous benign biliary processes, such as large bile duct stones and benign bile duct strictures.

## The Evolution of Techniques for Bile Duct Drainage

### Surgical Drainage for Malignant Obstructive Jaundice

Until the late 1970s, surgical bypass including cholecystojejunostomy and choledocho- and hepaticojejunostomy was the mainstay for bile duct decompression in patients with unresectable head of pancreas cancers or cholangiocarcinomas. Patients treated with surgical bypass tended to have a longer survival compared to those with only exploratory laparotomy [16, 17]. For patients with duodenal involvement, a gastric bypass operation was also performed to prevent gastric

R. Kozarek et al. (eds.), *Self-Expandable Stents in the Gastrointestinal Tract*,
DOI 10.1007/978-1-4614-3746-8_2, © Springer Science+Business Media New York 2013

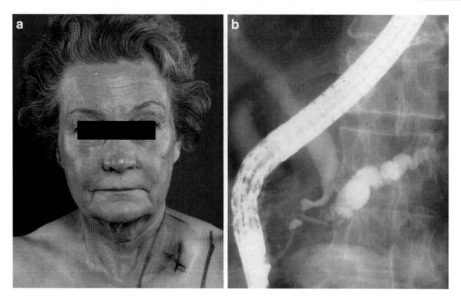

**Fig. 2.1** (**a**) A patient with malignant obstructive jaundice and lymph node metastasis. (**b**) Cholangiogram showing double duct stricture sign with obstruction of the pancreatic duct and distal bile duct from head of pancreas cancer

outlet obstruction (a double bypass procedure). However, even surgical palliation carried a significantly high morbidity and mortality in the presence of obstructive jaundice [18, 19], and alternative drainage methods were sought to improve clinical outcomes.

## Percutaneous Transhepatic Biliary Drainage

Percutaneous transhepatic cholangiography (PTC) became popular with the introduction of the thin flexible 22-gauge needle (Chiba needle) by Okuda in 1974 [20]. The percutaneous approach to the intrahepatic biliary system improved the safety and efficiency of fluoroscopic visualization of dilated bile ducts with success rates of 90%. Further modification of the PTC technique with catheter placement changed this from a diagnostic to a therapeutic procedure by allowing the insertion of a simple external drainage catheter [21, 22]. However, prolonged external drainage led to significant bile loss and electrolyte imbalance. Hoevels [23] and Nakayama [24] successfully negotiated a guide-wire and catheter across a bile duct stricture (now

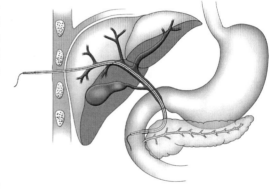

**Fig. 2.2** Schematic diagram for percutaneous transhepatic biliary drainage (PTBD)

called percutaneous transhepatic biliary drainage or PTBD) to provide combined external and internal drainage of bile into the duodenum (Fig. 2.2). Ring [25] and Ferrucci [26] further improved this technique and reported a success rate of 95% [27]. The main advantage of PTBD was to minimize the external loss of bile; flushing the catheter via an external connector helped prevent blockage of the drainage catheter. Exchange of the blocked catheter could also be performed over a guidewire. Long-term complications related to bacterial contamination included sepsis, and intrahepatic abscesses formation, and local skin irritation by the catheter and bile seepage [28, 29]. Despite the initial success, subsequent use of PTBD for preoperative biliary drainage did not show improvement in postsurgical outcome compared to surgery alone [30, 31].

Pereira [32] and Burcharth [33] described a percutaneous internal drainage method by the insertion of a prosthesis through a tumor obstruction, thus allowing antegrade flow of bile into the duodenum. These 6–7-Fr tubes blocked soon after placement leading to cholangitis and recurrent jaundice. Larger diameter stents were subsequently placed to prevent early stent occlusion [23]. However, bleeding, hematoma formation, and tumor seeding at the puncture site [34, 35] as well as the inability to remove a blocked prosthesis have limited the application of this drainage method. Soon after reports of percutaneous transhepatic biliary drainage (PTBD), endoscopic retrograde biliary drainage (ERBD) with placement of biliary endoprostheses using a side-viewing duodenoscope using endoscopic retrograde cholangiopancreatography (ERCP) was reported and offered a better alternative for nonoperative palliation of malignant obstructive jaundice [36].

## Endoscopic Retrograde Biliary Drainage

Although first described in 1969, ERCP only became popular after introduction of side-viewing duodenoscopes in 1970 [37]. It is now an established treatment for patients with many pancreaticobiliary diseases. The advent of duodenoscopy and biopsy allows for direct examination of the papilla to rule out ampullary lesions, endoscopic (tumor) papillotomy, and improved drainage and allows for access to bile duct obstruction and strictures for therapeutic intervention.

Early Teflon-coated steel guidewires were stiff, kinked easily, and made manipulation difficult. The ability to traverse biliary obstruction was further improved with the use of flexible tip guidewires to negotiate strictures. Even with flexible guidewires, manipulation through angulated or hilar biliary strictures remains challenging. Prior to the advent of internal endoscopically

placed stents, nasobiliary drainage tubes offered a reasonable alternative to percutaneous biliary tubes. Nasobiliary catheters can be inserted over a guidewire above an obstruction to provide biliary decompression and subsequent noninvasive cholangiographic access. Placement of these devices involves pushing the nasobiliary tube over the wire, removing the duodenoscope, and rerouting the tube through the nose. The tube may be connected to a drainage bag to provide decompression of the obstructed biliary system if so desired [38, 39]. Like percutaneous catheters, nasobiliary drains cause external loss of bile and may be dislodged accidentally.

Soehendra and Reynders-Frederix [36] working in Hamburg, Germany, described the first case of endoscopic insertion of a biliary endoprosthesis for drainage of malignant obstructive jaundice. They fashioned a single-pigtail endoprosthesis using the cut end of an angiography catheter. The procedure was technically successful, but ultimately, the stent migrated upstream. Cotton [40], working in London, reported the use of an endoprosthesis made with a double-pigtail design to prevent upward migration. Huibregtse and Tytgat [41] from Amsterdam described the creation of side flaps in the wall of a straight endoprosthesis instead of pigtails to prevent migration. Cremer from Brussels introduced a different endoprosthesis design with a snake-shaped proximal tip and a distal C-loop in the duodenum to prevent migration (Fig. 2.3).

Because the working channel diameters of the first duodenoscopes were small, early biliary endoprostheses were only 8-Fr tubes. Cholangitis and stent occlusion occurred at high rates [42]. With the introduction of larger (3.2 mm) channel duodenoscopes, placement of larger (10 Fr) endoprosthesis was possible [43, 44]. One plastic stent – the Tannenbaum stent [45] (Fig. 2.4) – maintained an intact inner surface with anchoring side flaps cut out from the wall of the stent without damaging the lumen to insure a smooth bile flow. It was initially reported to reduce the risk of bacterial attachment as compared with the conventional stents and to minimize the risk of stent occlusion.

Over time, other concepts have been tried to reduce stent occlusion. Endoprostheses with

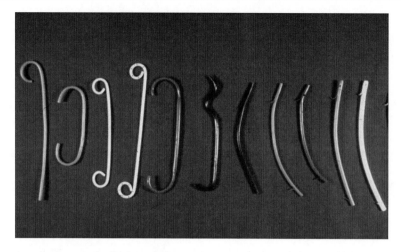

**Fig. 2.3** A display of different types of plastic stents available in the mid-1980s with single-pigtail, double-pigtail, straight with flaps, and curved stents

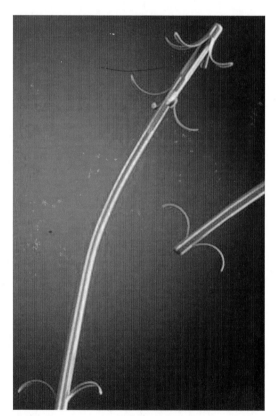

**Fig. 2.4** Tannenbaum stent with multiple side flaps for anchorage

with side flaps and small side holes along the shaft, endoprosthesis with multiple side flaps and curves created to resist migration, and in addition, different plastic materials were incorporated including Teflon, polyethylene (PTFE), polyurethane, and other plastic polymers. These materials varied considerably in their physical properties including wall thickness, rigidity, and the *melting* temperature which affected their ability to be molded into different shapes or curves. There was no consensus or standard in endoprostheses design at the time of early development which made comparison of study results difficult [46]. This clinical hodgepodge prompted a retrospective review of endoscopic biliary drainage at the Middlesex Hospital. The lack of clarity of that study led to subsequent laboratory work in search of an *ideal* biliary endoprosthesis [47, 48].

## Design of the Cotton-Leung Stent

Early pigtail designs had very small side holes at either end of the stent that limited bile drainage; this concept was abandoned early in the design process and replaced with a straight tube. Similarly, the small end hole at the tapered tip of a Cremer endoprosthesis, which also restricted bile flow, was removed. Despite pigtail ends and anchoring flaps, the single-pigtail endoprosthesis

different designs have been investigated. Pigtail stents with small side holes placed over the pigtail portion of the prosthesis, straight endoprosthesis

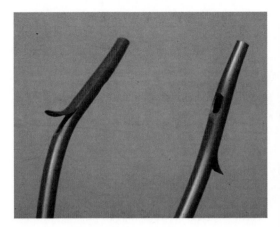

**Fig. 2.5** Original design of Cotton-Leung stent showing proximal tapered tip, side flap, and side hole for drainage

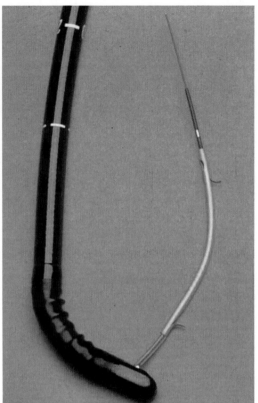

**Fig. 2.6** Setup of stenting system with large channel duodenoscope and stenting unit consisting of a 0.035 guidewire, a 6-Fr guiding catheter and a 10-Fr (PTFE) CL stent, and a 10-Fr Teflon pusher

and the early Amsterdam endoprosthesis were prone to migration because of the straight shaft. The proximal tip of the Amsterdam endoprosthesis tended to get stuck at the lower level of a tight or angulated bile duct stricture because of the gap between the guidewire and the stent lumen (a shoulder effect), which created resistance to passage of the endoprosthesis. The curved ends of a double-pigtail endoprosthesis also made it difficult to push over a guidewire or through a tight stricture because of the bending effect on the guidewire.

The unique feature of the Cotton-Leung stent (Cook Endoscopy, Winston-Salem, NC) is the proximal coaxial tapered tip design, which minimizes the potential gap between the guidewire and the inner guide catheter and the proximal tapered tip of the stent, thus offering a good fit to facilitate passage of the stent through tight or angulated bile duct strictures [48] (Figs. 2.5 and 2.6). In vitro flow studies demonstrated that drainage through a tube (inserted through a stricture) depended on the diameter of the end hole (Table 2.1) (Fig. 2.7). A tapered proximal tip reduced the flow through the stent [48, 49]. To overcome this problem, we created a 5-mm side hole at the proximal end of the tube to optimize flow through the stent. Without completely cutting and removing the plastic, we created a side flap design very similar to that of the Amsterdam endoprosthesis. This side flap offered resistance

**Table 2.1** The effect of changing configuration of tube on flow rates (ml/min)

| French size | 8 | 10 |
|---|---|---|
| Internal diameter (mm) | 1.75 | 2.2 |
| Control straight tube | 115 | 288 |
| Proximal flap and large side hole | 111 | 277 |
| Sharp proximal tapered tip | 103 | 239 |
| Less proximal tapered tip + side hole | 110 | 263 |
| Proximal tapered tip + side hole + flap | 110 | 261 |
| Complete Cotton-Leung stent | 110 | 258 |

to the downward migration of the stent but could be collapsed if it were being pushed against the bile duct wall or a tumor, which closed off the opening and reduced flow. To avoid this potential problem, we created another 5-mm side hole (without flap) on the reverse side of the proximal shaft between the end hole and the side flap to

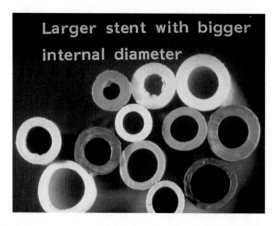

**Fig. 2.7** Picture showing cross section of plastic tubes with different diameter and wall thickness; drainage is dependent on the inner diameter

**Table 2.2** Comparison of mean flow rates (ml/min) through stents of different caliber and configurations

| French size | 8 | 10 |
|---|---|---|
| Internal diameter (mm) | 1.75 | 2.2 |
| Control tube | 121 | 305 |
| Single-pigtail stent | 95 | 188 |
| Double-pigtail stent | 89 | 133 (sharp taper) |
| | | 187 (less taper) |
| Straight Cotton-Leung stent | 110 | 246 |

ensure optimal drainage of an obstructed system. In addition, the proximal tip of the stent extended for about 1.5 cm above the proximal side flap to allow the side hole on the reverse side to be made without weakening the stent and to prevent buckling of the stent in the deployed position. In order to prevent upward stent migration, we created another 5-mm side flap on the same side over the distal end of the stent about 1 cm from the distal tip of the stent. This side flap, which opened up almost at a right angle to the shaft to provide maximum resistance to prevent upward stent migration, was meant to be positioned at the level of the papilla in the final deployed position (Fig. 2.5). The side hole at the distal flap also allowed continuous drainage from the stent in the event of downward stent migration should the distal end hole become blocked by the opposite duodenal wall (a problem that could affect straight stents without a distal side hole). Assuming a perfect stent deployment and no subsequent stent migration, the distal side (flap) hole would be placed close to the pancreatic orifice, thus avoiding any local pressure effect on the pancreatic opening. (NB: We have not observed a significant increase in poststenting pancreatitis when a single 10-Fr stent was used without performing a biliary sphincterotomy). It is worth noting that a partially collapsed distal side flap might not be

effective in preventing upward migration in the presence of a large papillotomy.

There is a small risk of duodenal irritation, ulcer formation, and rarely even perforation if downward stent migration occurs and the distal end of the stent impacts against the opposite duodenal wall [43]. In order to avoid this complication, we placed the distal tip of the stent just 1 cm beyond the distal flap. We also created a C-curve at the midshaft of the stent to conform to the shape of the bile duct. The idea was that in the deployed position, the curvature of the stent followed the contour of the bile duct, thus also providing a springlike action holding the stent in place, further reducing the risk of stent migration. We purposely did not place side holes in the shaft of the stent (which traversed the tumor) between the side flaps to avoid the theoretical risk of tumor ingrowth. In subsequent laboratory flow studies, the final Cotton-Leung stent design provided more effective drainage than double-pigtail endoprostheses (Table 2.2).

There was a less commonly used design specifically catered to provide drainage of the left hepatic system in patients with hilar obstruction where bilateral stent placement was desirable. This design was never manufactured as a regular item, but the goal was to avoid kinking of the stent at the proximal flap when the usual design was deployed in the left hepatic duct. A modification of the design (left hepatic duct or LHD stent) was created by removing the proximal side flap and shaping a 15-cm-long stent into an S-shape configuration instead of the usual C-shape. This allowed the proximal limb to be placed inside the left hepatic system and the angulations of the stent served to prevent stent migration (Fig. 2.8).

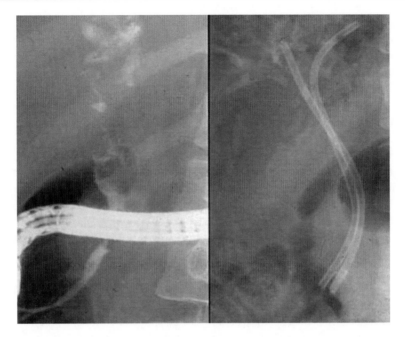

**Fig. 2.8** Cholangiogram showing common hepatic duct stricture (*left*) and bilateral *right* and *left* hepatic duct stents (*right*)

## Why Cotton-Leung Stents Are Made of Polyethylene

In the early 1980s, homemade stents were popular and were often tailor-made for the individual patient. Therefore, it was crucial to find a material that could be easily shaped, manipulated, or cut by hand. After experimenting with different plastic materials, polyethylene was chosen over Teflon or polyurethane. Polyethylene (PTFE) was chosen because of its lower *melting* temperature (87°C) – a temperature at which the material became soft and malleable, compared to the much higher temperature required to soften Teflon (Product guide, Wilson-Cook, Winston-Salem, NC). A polyethylene stent could be shaped and molded easily using boiling water or steam and subsequently set by holding it and immersing it in cold (sterile) water. PTFE was also softer than Teflon, making the creation of side holes and cutting side flaps much easier. To date, manufacturers have developed more complex plastic materials that are softer and have memory to retain their shape. Although a softer material is less traumatic to tissue, there is a higher tendency

for the stent to kink. In addition, soft material does not transmit the pushing force well and therefore may buckle when being pushed against resistance such as a tight stricture, making deployment more difficult without prior dilation of the stricture. On the other hand, stiffer materials are less malleable, and the stents are more prone to migration.

## Selection of Stent Length

By definition, the length of a straight stent was defined as the distance between the proximal and distal anchoring flaps. In order to accommodate obstruction at different levels, stents were made available in different lengths between 5 cm for distal CBD obstruction to 15 cm for hilar obstructions. Ideally, the proximal flap of a deployed stent should extend about 1 cm above the upper level of the stricture or tumor obstruction (to accommodate tumor growth), while the distal flap should be remain at the level of the papilla. In the event of a downward stent migration, only 2 cm of the stent could protrude from the papilla into the duodenum in theory. However, this was true only if a significantly tight stricture was holding the stent in position and might not apply when the stent was placed for stones or when the stricture had been dilated. In general, an 8-cm stent would be suitable for obstruction at the level of the common bile duct, either caused by a stricture or large CBD stones. Stents were also available in various diameters: 7, 8.5, 10, and 11.5 Fr. The larger stents provided a higher flow, and there was a difference observed in the reported stent patency rates between the 10- and 12-Fr stents [50]. There was also a difference in wall thickness resulting in comparable internal diameters between the 10- and 11.5-Fr stents. Since larger 11.5-Fr stents were more difficult to remove through the 4.2-mm therapeutic endoscope channel because of the thicker wall, we preferred to use 10-Fr stents because they could be easily removed. Some would argue that a 7- or 8.5-Fr stent would provide sufficient drainage to empty the biliary system and they could be more easily placed, but my concern is that the smaller lumen was too prone to blockage by sludge and biofilm formation.

## Position of the Stent: Why Leave the Distal Tip in the Duodenum?

Over the years, there have been many discussions as to the best/proper position for the distal end of the stent, i.e., should the distal end be placed within the bile duct to avoid ascending infections and stent blockage, or should the tip protrude into the duodenum to maximize the ease of removal when exchange was necessary. Our experience suggested that ease of removal was more important; therefore, the original design of the Cotton-Leung stent provided for placement of the distal tip in the duodenum with the distal flap preventing upward migration. The 1-cm distal tip allowed the stent to be captured easily with a snare and removed through the endoscope channel. Although total internal placement might minimize ascending reflux and infection, placement of the stent above the papilla was equivalent to upward migration and it was well-recognized that

retrieval of an upwardly migrated stent could be very challenging, and the risks outweighed any potential benefits in our minds.

## The Stent Introducer System

The early stent introducer system for the Cotton-Leung stent (Wilson-Cook, Winston-Salem, NC) consisted of a three-layer coaxial system – a regular Teflon-coated 0.035″ guidewire, a 6-Fr Teflon guiding catheter with radiopaque markers (placed 7 cm apart), and a 10-Fr Teflon pusher. Stent placement was performed in a systematic manner with initial manipulation of the guidewire across the stricture followed by inserting the guiding catheter over the guidewire. The markers on the guiding catheter helped in the selection of a stent of suitable length which was then loaded onto the guiding catheter. The stent was advanced over the guiding catheter and positioned across the stricture using the pusher. When the stent was deemed to be in the proper position, the pusher was used to hold the stent in position and the guidewire and guiding catheter were removed to deploy the stent. This method of stent deployment required multiple coordinated exchanges with risk of losing control from a lack of coordination between assistant and operator resulting in placement failure. This design was later improved to a double-layer system using a Luer lock mechanism to combine the guiding catheter and the pusher into the simplified "One Action Stent Introducer System" (OASIS, Cook Medical, Winston-Salem, NC), which was launched in the early 1990s (Fig. 2.9a, b). To date, all of the plastic stent deployment systems (from different manufacturers) utilize a similar concept of interlocking the inner guiding catheter and the pusher using with a Luer lock mechanism to minimize the number of exchanges and to facilitate stent deployment.

## Stent Length Measurement

As discussed before, the length of the stent is defined as the separation between the anchoring

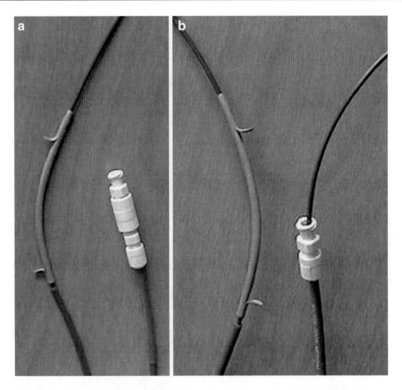

**Fig. 2.9** (**a**) OASIS stenting system combined the guide catheter and pusher into one unit using a Luer lock mechanism. (**b**) Stent deployment is effected by separating the Luer lock and pulling back on the inner catheter to release the stent

flaps for straight stents and the separation between the pigtailed ends for the double-pigtail stents. Obviously, the vertical separation could be less if the stent was bent to conform to the shape of the bile duct. Using the old stent system, the length of the stent could be estimated by referencing the radiopaque markers on the inner guiding catheter (which are 7 cm apart). Alternatively, the length of the stent could be measured by using the scope diameter as a guide (1.3 cm for the therapeutic endoscope). If the measurement was obtained directly from a radiograph, a correction for the magnification (usually 30%) was necessary. Another method was to measure the distance traveled by the guidewire outside the endoscope at the accessory port when the tip of the guidewire was pulled back (within the catheter/accessory) from the upper level of the obstruction to the level of the papilla (as seen endoscopically through the catheter).

With a combined guiding catheter and pusher system such as the OASIS, a suitable length stent had to be chosen and loaded onto the deployment system before advancing the delivery system over the guidewire (as described above). The radiopaque marker(s) on the inner catheter (e.g., set 5 cm apart in the OASIS system) could be used to aid positioning of the guiding catheter for proper stent deployment. The stent was then advanced over the guiding catheter and deployed by unlocking the guiding catheter from the pusher. For patients in whom the stent was placed to provide drainage but without an obvious stricture, e.g., large obstructing CBD stones, a bile leak, or to insure drainage from a small papillotomy complicated by postpapillotomy bleeding, an 8-cm long stent could suffice.

## Guidewire Selection for Stent Placement

Early stent systems included a Teflon-coated steel wire which was stiff and kinked easily, thus increasing the resistance to the passage of the guiding catheter and other accessories (dilating or brushing devices). For the past 15 years, Teflon-coated memory (nitinol) guidewires with a flexible hydrophilic tip have been available to facilitate negotiation of strictures and deployment of stents. Guidewires come in different diameters ranging from 0.018″ to 0.021″ to 0.025″ and 0.035″. The thicker guidewires were stiffer and allowed better application of the pushing force, whereas smaller, e.g., 0.025″, guidewires were more flexible and could be shaped (i.e., creating curves at the tip of the guidewire) to allow bending and loop formation to help negotiate tight or angulated strictures. For stenting of the left hepatic system, a stiffer or stronger guidewire was necessary because of the angulations and to provide a more stable system while pushing the stent. If a soft guidewire was used to negotiate the stricture, then exchange to a stiffer guidewire might be needed to facilitate subsequent stent placement.

It is important to note that proper positioning of the guidewire is necessary for successful stent placement. A steady or secure position of the guidewire requires coordination between the endoscopist and the assistant during the exchange process. The introduction of guidewires with different colored stripes or even numbers helps with endoscopic observation and monitoring of the position of the guidewire during the exchange process. In order to secure the position of the guidewire, other novel ideas have been tried including the *Peel-Away* catheter, which allows the catheter to be split in half around the guidewire without having to move the guidewire once it is inserted in position. Insertion of a single biliary stent across a common bile duct stricture is feasible with any type of guidewire.

## Short-Wire Technology for Stent Placement: Rapid Exchange, Fusion, and V-Scope

Concerns over control of the guidewire during the exchange process and a desire to give the endoscopist better control over the guidewire and

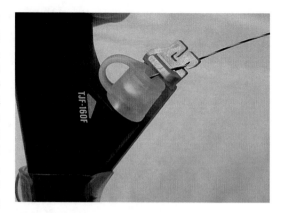

**Fig. 2.10** Wire locking device for the RX system

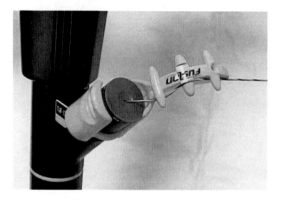

**Fig. 2.11** Wire locking device for the Fusion system

deployment of accessories have led to the introduction of different short-wire technology platforms, notably the Rapid Exchange system (RX, Boston Scientific, Natick, MA) and the Fusion system (Cook Endoscopy, Winston-Salem, NC). The use of a wire locking device strapped to the endoscope (RX) (Fig. 2.10) or as a modified biopsy valve with a set of plastic *teeth* (Fusion) serves to anchor the guidewire (Fig. 2.11) during exchange and to minimize the risk of losing guidewire position.

Only a short segment of the accessory passes over the guidewire, making manipulation of accessories and exchange much easier and more controlled. On the other hand, the V-system (Olympus Tokyo, Japan) incorporates a modified elevator that provides additional elevation and a V-notch that serves to grip and hold a much shorter guidewire during insertion and removal

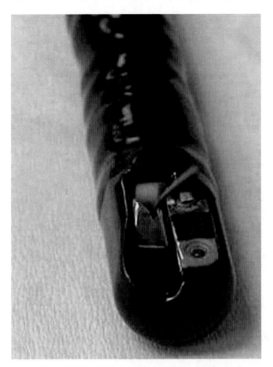

**Fig. 2.12** The V-scope system with a small notch created on the elevator mechanism

of the accessory over the guidewire (Fig. 2.12). This allows short wires to be used with traditional long-wire (nonmonorail) accessories. With the V-scope, the only time the elevator loses its grip on the guidewire is when the accessory is passing over the elevator mechanism. This can easily be compensated for with proper endoscope positioning. Locking the guidewire to the endoscope with whichever mechanism serves to stabilize the guidewire during exchanges, but it also means that the endoscope position has to be stable; otherwise, the guidewire can easily be dislodged from the bile duct with excessive endoscope movement or manipulation.

One advantage of the new Fusion OASIS design (Cook Endoscopy, Winston-Salem, NC) is the incorporation of a side port close to the tip (2.5 cm) of the guiding catheter which allows the guidewire to be freed above the stricture or obstruction in the bile duct (Fig. 2.13a, b). This concept of intraductal release (or exchange, IDR, or IDE) of the guidewire has proven to be useful in facilitating the placement of multiple stents

across a bile duct stricture especially for the management of benign strictures, without having to reattempt cannulation or negotiation of the guidewire across the stricture (Fig. 2.14a–c). With this setup, prior to final stent deployment, the guidewire must be separated from the guiding catheter using the intraductal release feature before the guiding catheter is pulled back to deploy the stent. The guidewire is left inside the bile duct across the stricture, and a second stent can be delivered over the same guidewire, thereby decreasing procedure time.

## Complications of Biliary Stenting

Complications and risks of biliary stenting are those inherent to the ERCP procedure and papillotomy which include postpapillotomy bleeding and perforation and post-ERCP pancreatitis. The most common complication of biliary stenting is occlusion from bacterial contamination with subsequent biofilm and biliary sludge formation [51–53] (Fig. 2.15a, b). Observational studies have shown that even though the bile is considered to be sterile, transient bacteriobilia from enteric bacteria that migrate from the portal circulation into the bile duct radicals is relatively common [54]. The Kupffer cells that line the hepatic sinusoids generally limit the migration of these organisms. Any residual bacteria which reach the biliary system are then attacked by immunoglobulin A (IgA) secreted by the bile duct epithelium and trapping by the mucus secreted in bile and the downward flow of bile into the small bowel. However, the presence of a foreign body such a stone or an indwelling device (stent or NB tube) will provide a surface for the attachment of the bacteria leading to infected biofilm [54, 55]. In addition, an indwelling stent with the tip in the duodenum will lead to ascending infection and contamination of the biliary system and sludge formation. Clinical manifestations of a blocked stent include recurrent jaundice, with or without cholangitis.

A series of laboratory studies have examined ways to prevent bacterial attachment and sludge

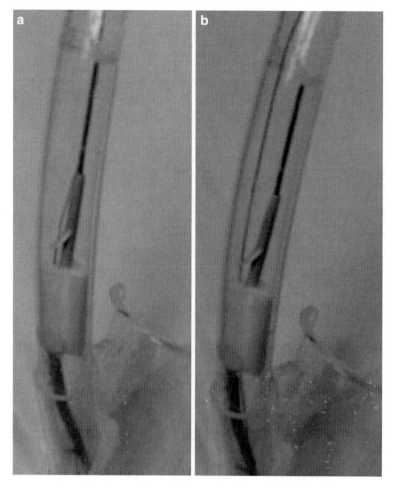

**Fig. 2.13** (**a**) Stent introduced through an artificial bile duct with a simulated stricture using the Fusion OASIS system. The stent is caught between the guidewire and the guiding catheter. (**b**) Intraductal release of the guidewire above the simulated stricture allows the stent to be deployed while maintaining the guidewire above the stricture to minimize the need for repeat cannulation if a second stent is to be deployed

formation, but the overall results have not been impressive [56–58].

The use of different plastic polymers, changing stent design by eliminating the side holes and creating side flaps that do not cut through the lumen to maintain a laminar flow [45] and anchorage, the use of hydrophilic materials which are more slippery and may even be useful for antibiotic loading to provide antibacterial effects [59], as well as surface modification using different polymers have been used to overcome this problem. A more recent design change involves the use of plastic stent with an antireflux valve to minimize ascending infection [60].

Although temporary reduction of bacterial attachment has been reported, prolonged exposure of the stent to bile still leads to bacterial biofilm formation. Biodegradable expandable nonmetallic *plastic* stents may hold promise in the future [61], and future exploratory research may involve the use of nanotechnology to modify the stent surface as well as the possibility of using external stimulation or energy to alter the surface properties of the stent material to prevent

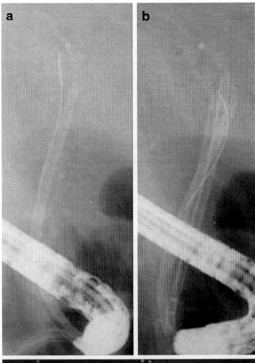

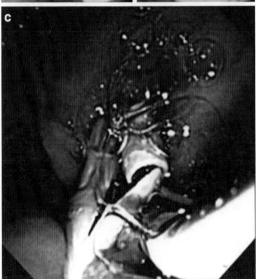

**Fig. 2.14** (a) Radiography showing guidewire is released from the guiding catheter to facilitate stent deployment. (b) Multiple plastic stents have been deployed using the Fusion OASIS system, and the radiograph showed three stents side by side with the guidewire alongside the stents. (c) Endoscopic view of multiple biliary stenting (c, Reprinted with permission from SLACK, Incorporated: Leung J, Lo S. Curbside Consultation in Endoscopy: 49 Clinical Questions. Thorofare, NJ, Slack Incorporated; 2009)

or minimize bacterial attachment. However, currently, the most effective method to prevent stent blockage is still elective stent exchange on a regular basis as well as antibiotic therapy if the patient develops symptoms of cholangitis (Fig. 2.16). The observation that bacterial adherence can occur on different plastic surfaces raises the concern that this phenomenon can also occur on the plastic membrane of the covered self-expandable metal stent (SEMS). However, with the much larger lumen, the effect of bacterial attachment and blockage may be less obvious for covered SEMS.

## Stent Retrieval Systems

Stent blockage by biliary sludge necessitates the removal of the blocked stent and replacement with a new one to insure drainage of the obstructed bile duct. With the distal tip of the stent in the duodenum, it can be grasped with a polypectomy snare and pulled out of the bile duct. It is important to avoid grasping too much of the distal tip of the stent to avoid unnecessary resistance when the stent is buckled when pulled into the scope channel. Grasping the stent at the level of the flap can potentially break the stent, as this is the weakest part of the stent. To avoid the risk of losing access through the bile duct stricture when the stent is pulled, different methods have been tried [62] including initially inserting a guidewire through the blocked stent and engaging the distal end of the stent using the Soehendra stent retriever (Cook Endoscopy, Winston-Salem, NC) which has a screw tip that is used to hold on to the stent and then exchanging the stent retriever over the guidewire. There is a risk of pushing the stent into or further proximally in the bile duct while engaging the distal end of the stent. Another method is to use a mini-snare over the guidewire to engage the distal end of the stent and subsequently exchanging it over the guidewire. However, in the majority of cases, access through the stricture is possible immediately after non-wire-guided stent removal without using special devices using either a catheter or a wire-guided papillotome.

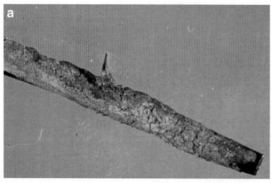

**Fig. 2.15** (**a**) A blocked biliary stent covered with thick *yellowish* sludge on the outside of the stent. (**b**) Scanning electron micrography of a blocked biliary stent showing the microcolonies of rod-shaped bacteria on the surface of the stent – typical appearance of a bacterial biofilm

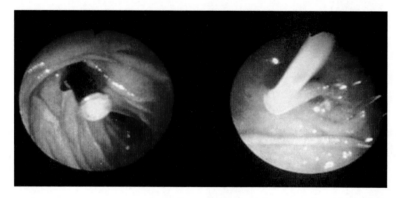

**Fig. 2.16** Cholangitis secondary to blocked biliary stent (*left*) and exchanged stent-draining pus (*right*) (Reprinted with permission from SLACK, Incorporated: Leung J, Lo S. Curbside Consultation in Endoscopy: 49 Clinical Questions. Thorofare, NJ, Slack Incorporated; 2009)

## Removal of a Migrated Stent

Downward or distal stent migration is possible if the stent does not conform to the shape of the bile duct. Rarely, perforation of the duodenum caused by the distal end of the stent can occur. Removal of a migrated stent can be achieved by advancing the scope further into the second/third part of the duodenum to engage the stent with a snare. Alternatively, it may be necessary to grasp the stent with rat-tooth forceps and *deliver* the stent back into the bile duct in order to engage the distal end of the stent. Upward migration of the stent can also occur, especially in patients with a prior papillotomy where the distal flap failed to hold the stent in position. Attempts can be made to engage the stent with a snare, basket, or grasping forceps inside the bile duct and pulling the stent back into the duodenum and removing it with a snare as described. If the engaged stent is difficult to be pulled into the endoscope, the engaged stent and endoscope can be removed as a whole. A stone extraction balloon can be inflated alongside the migrated stent and pulled back to create sufficient friction against the stent in the hope of dragging the stent into the duodenum. A papillotomy is usually necessary to facilitate retraction of an upwardly migrated stent. If grasping the stent inside the bile duct proves to be difficult, a guidewire can be inserted initially through the stent and advancing a small stone extraction balloon or a wire-guided papillotome into the distal end of the stent. The stent can then be removed by insufflating the balloon or tightening the papillotome cutting wire within the distal end of the stent [63].

## Shaping the Stent

Because of the varying shape of the bile ducts (and as a personal preference), it may be necessary to alter the C-curve on the stent to conform to the curvature of the bile duct. Also, the side flaps may sometimes be collapsed when the stent is removed from the sterile package. It is easy to use hot water from a kettle (contained in a plastic kidney tray) to open the flaps and shape the stent and then set it in sterile cold water.

## Application of Plastic Stents in Biliary Diseases

Plastic stents were first introduced for palliative drainage of malignant biliary obstruction. Successful application of endoscopic stent placement in patients with benign bile duct strictures has since been reported. This drainage method has also been applied to the management of patients with acute suppurative cholangitis secondary to bile duct stones [64]. Pilot data as well as subsequent RCT demonstrated a significant benefit with urgent endoscopic biliary drainage when papillotomy and stent placement (or nasobiliary catheter) are used compared with emergency surgery for acute cholangitis as well as a significant reduction in morbidity and mortality [64, 65] (Figs. 2.17 and 2.18). Spontaneous disintegration of the bile duct stones has been observed with stent placement (in combination with oral stone dissolution agents) [66] and with stent placement alone in patients with large bile duct stones [67].

## Conclusion

Over the past three decades since the introduction of the Cotton-Leung stent, many new stent designs and materials have been developed and tested. Expandable metal stents have played an important role in patients with unresectable malignancies. Despite these changes, the original Cotton-Leung stent has remained one of the most popular endoscopic biliary stents throughout the world.

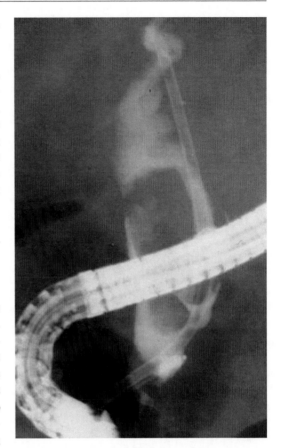

**Fig. 2.17** Cholangiogram showing stenting for large obstructing bile duct stone

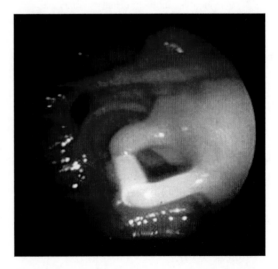

**Fig. 2.18** Stent-draining pus in acute suppurative cholangitis (Reprinted with permission from SLACK, Incorporated: Leung J, Lo S. Curbside Consultation in Endoscopy: 49 Clinical Questions. Thorofare, NJ, Slack Incorporated; 2009)

# References

1. Dooley JS. Pathophysiology of jaundice: effect on the rest of the body. The practical management of obstructive jaundice. BSG Teaching Day, London; 1983.
2. Dawson JL. The incidence of postoperative renal failure in obstructive jaundice. Br J Surg. 1965; 52:663–5.
3. Dawson JL. Acute post-operative renal failure in obstructive jaundice. Ann R Coll Surg Engl. 1968;42:163–81.
4. Bayer I, Ellis H. Jaundice and wound healing: an experimental study. Br J Surg. 1976;63:392–6.
5. Irvin TT, Vassilakis JS, Chattopadhyay DK, Greaney MG. Abdominal wound healing in jaundice patients. Br J Surg. 1978;65:521–2.
6. Kunz F, Constantini R, Semenitz E, et al. The production of disseminated intravascular coagulation (DIC) by spaced injections of endotoxin in non-pregnant rats. Throm Res. 1977;12:119–30.
7. Nolan JP. Endotoxin reticuloendothelial function and liver injury. Hepatology. 1981;1:458–65.
8. Bomzon L, Kew MC. Renal blood flow in experimental obstructive jaundice. In: Epstein M, editor. The Kidney in liver disease. Philadelphia: Elsevier; 1983. p. 313.
9. Hunt DR, Allison MEM, Prentice CRM, Blumgart LH. Endotoxemia, disturbance of coagulation and obstructive jaundice. Am J Surg. 1982;144:325–9.
10. Kelly DA, Tuddenham EGD. Hemostatic problem in liver disease. Gut. 1986;27:339–49.
11. Feduska NJ, Dent TL, Lindenauer SM. Results of palliative operation for carcinoma of the pancreas. Arch Surg. 1971;103:330–4.
12. Mortimer PR, Mackie DB, Haynes S. Ampicillin levels in human bile in the presence of biliary tract diseases. Br Med J. 1969;3:88–9.
13. Keighley MRB, Lister DM, Jacob SI, Giles GR. Hazards of surgical treatment due to microorganism in the bile. Surgery. 1974;75:578–83.
14. Cotton PB. ERCP progress report. Gut. 1977;18:316–41.
15. Burcharth F, Christiansen LA, Efsen F, et al. Percutaneous transhepatic cholangiography in diagnostic evaluation of 160 jaundiced patients. Am J Surg. 1977;1(33):559–61.
16. Rodgers CM, Adams JT, Schwartz SI. Carcinoma of the extrahepatic bile ducts. Surgery. 1981;90:596–601.
17. Sarr MG, Cameron JL. Surgical management of unresectable carcinoma of the pancreas. Surgery. 1982;91:123–33.
18. Bufkin WJ, Smith PE, Krementz FT. Evaluation of palliative operation for carcinoma of the pancreas. Arch Surg. 1967;94:240–2.
19. Porter EA. Carcinoma of the pancreas. NZ Med J. 1970;71:288–92.
20. Okuda K. Thin needle percutaneous transhepatic cholangiography – historical review. Endoscopy. 1980;12:2–7.
21. Burcharth F, Nielbo N. Percutaneous cholangiography with selective catheterization of the common bile duct. Am J Roentgenol. 1976;127:409–12.
22. Tylen V, Hoevels J, Vang J. Percutaneous transhepatic cholangiography with external drainage of obstructive biliary lesions. Surg Gynecol Obstet. 1977;144:13–8.
23. Hoevels J, Lunderquist A, Owman T, Ihse I. A large bore Teflon endoprosthesis with side holes for non-operative decompression of the biliary duct in malignant obstructive jaundice. Gastrointest Radiol. 1980;5:361–6.
24. Nakayama T, Ikeda A, Okuda K. Percutaneous transhepatic drainage of the biliary tract. Gastroenterol. 1978;74:554–9.
25. Ring EJ, Oleaga JA, Freiman DB. Therapeutic application of catheter cholangiography. Radiology. 1978;128:333–8.
26. Ferrucci JT, Mueller PR, Harbin WP. Percutaneous transhepatic biliary drainage. Technique, results and applications. Radiology. 1980;135:1–13.
27. Ferrucci JT, Mueller PR. Interventional radiology of the biliary tract. Gastroenterol. 1982;83:974–85.
28. Pennington L, Kauffman S, Cameron J. Intrahepatic abscess as a complication of long term percutaneous internal biliary drainage. Surgery. 1982;91:642–5.
29. Carrasco CH, Zornoza J, Bechtel WJ. Malignant biliary obstruction: complication of percutaneous biliary drainage. Radiology. 1984;152:343–6.
30. Hatfield ARW, Terblanche J, Fataar S, et al. Preoperative external biliary drainage in obstructive jaundice. Lancet. 1982;2:896–9.
31. Speer AG, Cotton PB, Russell RCG, Mason RR, et al. Randomised trial of endoscopic versus percutaneous stent insertion in malignant obstructive jaundice. Lancet. 1987;2:57–62.
32. Pereira RV, Rheingold OJ, Hutson D, et al. Relief of malignant obstructive jaundice by percutaneous insertion of a permanent prosthesis in the biliary tree. Ann Intern Med. 1978;89:589–93.
33. Burcharth F. A new endoprosthesis for non-operative insertion of the biliary tract in malignant obstructive jaundice. Surg Gynecol Obstet. 1978;146:76–8.
34. Kim WS, Barth KH, Zuiner M. Seeding of pancreatic carcinoma along the transhepatic catheter tract. Radiology. 1982;143:427–8.
35. Shorvon PJ, Leung J, Corcoran MO, et al. Cutaneous seeding of malignant tumours after insertion of percutaneous prosthesis for obstructive jaundice. Br J Surg. 1984;71:694–5.
36. Soehendra N, Reynders-Frederix V. Palliative bile duct drainage – a new endoscopic method of introducing a transpapillary drain. Endoscopy. 1980;12:8–11.
37. Oi I, Kobayashi S, Kondo T. Endoscopic pancreatic cholangiography. Endoscopy. 1970;2:103–5.
38. Cotton PB, Burney PG, Masson RR. Transnasal bile duct catheterization after endoscopic sphincterotomy – method for biliary drainage, perfusion and sequential cholangiography. Gut. 1979;20:285–7.

39. Leung J, Cotton PB. Endoscopic nasobiliary drainage in biliary and pancreatic disease. Am J Gastroenterol. 1991;86:389–94.

40. Cotton PB. Duodenoscopic placement of biliary prosthesis to relief malignant obstructive jaundice. Br J Surg. 1982;69:501–3.

41. Huibregtse K, Haverkamp J, Tytgat GN. Transpapillary positioning of a large 3.2 mm biliary endoprosthesis. Endoscopy. 1981;13:217–9.

42. Speer A, Leung J, Yin TP, Cotton PB. 10 French gauge straight biliary stent perform significantly better than 8 French gauge pigtail stents. Gastrointest Endosc. 1985;31:140.

43. Huibregtse K, Tytgat GN. Palliative treatment of obstructive jaundice by transpapillary introduction of large bore bile duct endoprosthesis. Gut. 1982;23:371–5.

44. Siegel JH. Improved biliary decompression with large caliber endoscopic prosthesis. Gastrointest Endosc. 1984;30:21–3.

45. Binmoeller KF, Seitz U, Seifert H, et al. The Tannenbaum stent: a new plastic biliary stent without side holes. Am J Gastroenterol. 1995;90:1764–8.

46. Huibregtse K, Tytgat GN. Transpapillary introduced large caliber biliary endoprosthesis in malignant bile duct obstruction. In: Salmon P, editor. Advances in gastrointestinal endoscopy. London: Chapman & Hall; 1983.

47. Leung J, Emery R, Cotton PB, et al. Management of malignant obstructive jaundice at the Middlesex hospital. Br J Surg. 1983;70:584–6.

48. Leung J. Endoscopy and malignant obstructive jaundice. M.D. thesis, The Chinese University of Hong Kong, 1986.

49. Leung J, Del Favero G, Cotton PB. Endoscopic biliary prosthesis – a comparison of material. Gastrointest Endosc. 1985;31:93–5.

50. Siegel JH, Pullano W, Kodsi B, et al. Optimal palliation of malignant bile duct obstruction: experience with endoscopic 12 French prostheses. Endoscopy. 1988;20:137–41.

51. Leung J, Banez VP. Clogging of biliary stents: mechanisms and possible solutions. Dig Endosc. 1990;2:97–104.

52. Leung J, Ling TKW, Kung JLS, Vallance-Owen J. The role of bacteria in the blockage of biliary stents. Gastrointest Endosc. 1988;34:19–22.

53. Leung J, Sung JY, Costerton JW. Bacteriological and electron microscopy examination of brown pigment stones. J Clin Microbiol. 1989;27:915–21.

54. Sung JY, Leung JWC, Olson ME. Demonstration of transient bacteriobilia by foreign body implantation in the feline biliary tract. Dig Dis Sci. 1991;36:943–8.

55. Sung JY, Shaffer EA, Olson ME, et al. Bacterial invasion of the biliary system by way of the portal-venous system. Hepatology. 1991;14:313–7.

56. Libby E, Leung JWC. Prevention of biliary stent clogging: a clinical review. Am J Gastroenterol. 1996;91:1301–8.

57. Leung JW, Libby ED, Morck DW, et al. Is prophylactic ciprofloxacin effective in delaying biliary stent blockage? Gastrointest Endosc. 2000;51:175–82.

58. Leung JW, Liu YL, Desta TD, et al. In vitro evaluation of antibiotic prophylaxis in the prevention of biliary stent blockage. Gastrointest Endosc. 2000;51:296–303.

59. Leung JW, Liu YL, Cheung SW, et al. Effect of antibiotic-loaded hydrophilic stent in the prevention of bacterial adherence: a study of the charge, discharge, and recharge concept using ciprofloxacin. Gastrointest Endosc. 2001;53:431–7.

60. Dua K, Reddy N, Rao V, et al. Impact of reducing duodenobiliary reflux on biliary stent patency: an in vitro evaluation and a prospective randomized clinical trial that used a biliary stent with an antireflux valve. Gastrointest Endosc. 2007;65:819–28.

61. Meng B, Wang J, Zhu N, et al. Study of biodegradable and self-expandable PLLA helical biliary stent in vivo and in vitro. J Mater Sci Mater Med. 2006;17:611–7.

62. Chaurasia OP, Rauws EA, Fockens P, Huibregtse K. Endoscopic techniques for retrieval of proximally migrated biliary stents: the Amsterdam experience. Gastrointest Endosc. 1999;50:780–5.

63. Tarnasky PR, Cotton PB, Baillie J, et al. Proximal migration of biliary stents: attempted endoscopic retrieval in forty-one patients. Gastrointest Endosc. 1995;42:513–20.

64. Leung J, Chung SCS, Sung JY, et al. Urgent endoscopic drainage for acute suppurative cholangitis. Lancet. 1989;1:1307–9.

65. Lai EC, Mok FP, Tan ES, et al. Endoscopic biliary drainage for severe acute cholangitis. N Engl J Med. 1992;326:1582–6.

66. Johnson GK, Geenen JE, Venu RP, et al. Treatment of non-extractable common bile duct stones with combination ursodeoxycholic acid plus endoprostheses. Gastrointest Endosc. 1993;39:528–31.

67. Chan ACW, Ng EKW, Chung SCS, et al. Common bile duct stones become smaller after endoscopic biliary stenting. Endoscopy. 1998;30:356–9.

# Part 2

# History of SEMS/SEPS Development and Current Design

# History of Self-Expandable Metal and Self-Expandable Plastic Stent Development

**3**

Ho-Young Song, Jin Hyoung Kim, and Chang Jin Yoon

## Esophageal Stents

### Background

Sir Charters Symonds, a British surgeon, is believed to be the first physician to use indwelling tubes in 1885 [1]. The tubes were made of boxwood, ivory, or gum elastic. Strings were used to maintain the tube's position with one end of the string attached to the stent and the other end to the patient's moustache or strapped behind the ear. Subsequently, different kinds of rigid tubes without need for external fixation, such as the Celestin tube and the Wilson-Cook tube, were developed [2, 3]. However, it was quite difficult to place these rigid, fixed diameter tubes within a narrowed esophageal lumen because of their large outer diameter delivery systems of 25 mm.

H.-Y. Song, M.D. (✉)
Department of Radiology, Asan Medical Center,
University of Ulsan College of Medicine,
388-1, Poongnap-2dong Songpa-gu, Seoul 138-736,
Republic of Korea
e-mail: hysong@amc.seoul.kr

J.H. Kim, M.D.
Radiology Department, Asan Medical Center,
Seoul, Republic of Korea

C.J. Yoon, M.D., Ph.D.
Department of Radiology, Seoul National University
Bundang Hospital, Seongnam, Republic of Korea

## Development of Self-Expandable Esophageal Stents

### First Generation: Bare SEMS

In 1990, Domschke et al. placed a 20-mm, bare (uncovered) wire self-expandable esophageal stent (SEMS) in a patient with extensive esophageal cancer [4]. Local anesthesia of the pharynx was achieved using aerosolized lidocaine. Since then, different kinds of uncovered SEMS have been used for palliative treatment of patients with malignant esophageal strictures [5–9]. Though the overall technical success rates for placement of these uncovered SEMS were 96–100%, progressive tumor ingrowth through the openings between the wire filaments (interstices) causes recurrent dysphagia. In addition, uncovered SEMS are not effective for the treatment of esophagorespiratory fistulas.

### Second Generation: Covered SEMS

In 1991, Song et al. were the first to describe placement of covered esophageal SEMS [10]. In this report, Z-stents with two anti-migration barbs loaded onto a 12-mm introducer tube were placed in seven patients with unresectable malignant esophageal strictures using topical anesthesia. The subsequent introduction of different types of fully and partially covered SEMS ushered in a new era in esophageal stent placement [10–18]. Song et al. placed fully covered Z-stents without anchoring barbs in 119 patients with malignant and benign strictures using a 13-mm polyethylene introducer [11]. Esophageal perforation occurred

R. Kozarek et al. (eds.), *Self-Expandable Stents in the Gastrointestinal Tract*,
DOI 10.1007/978-1-4614-3746-8_3, © Springer Science+Business Media New York 2013

in 0% of patients in whom SEMS were placed and in 11% in those who received conventional rigid tubes (Table 3.1). Covered SEMS sealed esophagorespiratory fistula [12–16]. However, overall stent migration occurred in 10% and in nearly one-third when placed across the gastroesophageal junction (GEJ) [11].

### Third Generation: Retrievable SEMS and Self-Expandable Plastic Stent

To allow removability, Song et al. designed a retrievable fully covered SEMS [19] (Fig. 3.1). Two drawstrings were attached to the upper, inner margin of each stent (Fig. 3.2). A dilator and 13-French sheath allowed introduction of a hook wire (Fig. 3.3), and the stents were grasped and retrieved under fluoroscopic guidance alone. Using this stent and removal technique, Yoon et al. removed all but 1 of 119 SEMS [20].

Subsequently, retrievable stents were used for patients with benign esophageal strictures [21, 22]. Kim et al. used retrievable SEMS, including polytetrafluoroethylene (PTFE)-covered stents in 55 patients with benign esophageal strictures

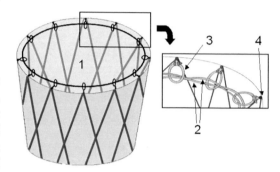

**Fig. 3.2** Diagrams show drawstrings attached to the upper inner margin of the stent. 1 = central lumen, 2 = drawstrings, 3 = nylon loop, 4 = upper margin of the wire

**Table 3.1** Complication rates of expandable metallic stents versus those of conventional nonexpandable tubes

|  | Nonexpandable tubes | | Expandable metallic stents |
| --- | --- | --- | --- |
|  | Ogilvie et al. [2] | Liakakos et al. [3] | Song et al. [11] |
| Number of patients | 118 | 105 | 119 |
| Number of tubes or stents | 135 | 116 | 136 |
| Initial perforation (%) | 11 | 10 | 0 |
| Bleeding (%) | 3 | 0 | 3 |
| Migration (%) | 12 | 4 | 10 |
| Blockage (%) | | | |
| Food impaction | 19 | 5 | 2 |
| Tumor overgrowth | 5 | 22 | 7 |

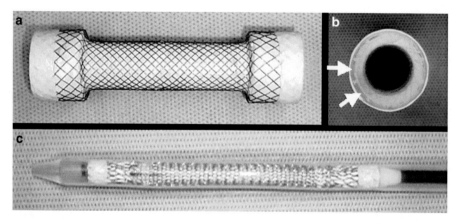

**Fig. 3.1** (**a**) Lateral view of a PTFE-covered retrievable nitinol stent, (**b**) a top view of the stent showing drawstrings (*arrows*), and (**c**) a stent delivery system (guiding olive tip, compressed stent, sheath, pusher catheter)

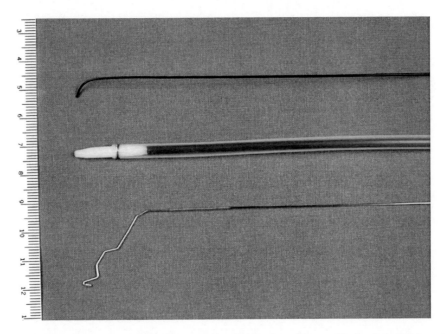

**Fig. 3.3** Photograph shows a stent removal set, a guide wire (*top*), a dilator with sheath (*middle*), and a hook (*bottom*)

refractory to balloon dilation [22]. Stents were electively removed 2 months after placement. During a mean follow-up of 38 months (range 1–105 months) after stent removal, the maintained patency rates at 1, 3, and 6 months were 58%, 43%, and 38%, respectively; patency rates at 1, 2, and 4 years were 33%, 26%, and 21%, respectively.

In the late 1990s, a novel thin-walled expandable prototype silicone airway stent (PolyFlex stent, Willy Rüsch AG, Kernen, Germany) was used in humans. Its subsequent application for esophageal use for palliation of malignant dysphagia and fistula was fueled by a lower cost than SEMS [23–27], though this advantage has not persisted. The PolyFlex is a totally covered SEPS made of polyester netting surrounded by silicone. It was quickly realized from the pulmonary literature that esophageal SEPS removal was feasible. They are easily removed endoscopically 4–8 weeks after placement by grasping them at the proximal end with rat-tooth forceps and withdrawing with or without fluoroscopic assistance [25]. Disadvantages of SEPS over SEMS are the large diameter and less flexible stent delivery sys-

tem that does no adapt well to angulated stenoses [27]. In addition, the stent must be loaded onto the delivery system prior to deployment.

Conio et al. performed a prospective controlled trial to compare a SEPS (PolyFlex, Boston Scientific, Natick, MA) with a partially covered SEMS (Ultraflex, Boston Scientific) in 101 patients with unresectable esophageal carcinoma [27]. No difference was seen in degree of palliation of dysphagia between the SEPS and SEMS. However, significantly more complications, especially late stent migration, were observed in the SEPS group.

### Fourth Generation: Antireflux SEMS

Gastroesophageal reflux (GER) occurs in patients who have a stent placed across the GEJ. Symptoms can be relieved by taking antacids, by sleeping with the head of the bed raised by approximately 30°, and by avoidance of eating large meals before lying down. GER can be prevented by the use of antireflux stents [28–30]. Laasch et al. compared the effectiveness of an antireflux stent with that of a standard, open stent in patients with SEMS that crossed the GEJ [30]. Twenty-four of

25 patients (96%) with open stents had reflux symptoms, compared to only 3 of 25 patients (12%) with the antireflux stent.

## Fifth Generation: Radiation-Emitting SEMS

To combine the advantages of SEMS in the immediate relief of dysphagia with the antitumor effects of brachytherapy, an esophageal stent loaded with Iodine-125 seeds was developed [31]. Outcomes were compared in patients with advanced esophageal cancer that underwent placement of the radiation-emitting stent (27 patients) to those in whom a standard, covered stent was placed (26 patients). Median patient survival in the radiation-emitting stent group was 7 months (mean 8.3 months), while the median survival in the standard, covered SEMS group was 4 months (mean 3.5 months) [32].

## Sixth Generation: Biodegradable or Drug-Releasing SEMS

To solve the problems of stricture recurrence after covered SEMS removal and to prevent granulation tissue formation at the end of a SEMS, biodegradable stents, drugs, and drug-releasing stents have been studied [33–35]. Repici et al. placed a self-expandable biodegradable stent in 21 patients with refractory benign esophageal strictures [33]. Stent migration occurred in two patients (9.5%) at 4 and 7 weeks following stent placement. A 3-month endoscopic examination showed the stents to be almost completely fragmented in all of the remaining patients.

# Gastroduodenal Stents

## Background

Patients with gastric outlet obstruction experience intractable nausea, vomiting, and anorexia, which in turn may cause electrolyte imbalance, dehydration, and malnutrition. Although gastrojejunostomy with or without gastrectomy has been the traditional method of palliative treatment, many patients are unfit for surgery. Moreover, surgery carries a significant rate of morbidity and mortality and is associated with prolonged hospital stay [36].

# Development of Self-Expandable Gastroduodenal Stents

## First Generation: Covered SEMS

In 1991, Song et al. placed the first metallic gastric stent in a patient with a gastric outlet obstruction caused by recurrent gastric cancer [10]. An 18-mm diameter, covered Z-stent with two anchoring barbs was placed transorally using a 12-mm diameter delivery system.

At that time, peroral placement of a covered SEMS into the gastric outlet or duodenum in a patient without prior bypass surgery was not possible because the 12-mm delivery system was too large and rigid. In 1993, Song et al. placed an 18-mm, covered SEMS without anchoring barbs for palliation of malignant gastric outlet obstruction from inoperable gastric cancer [37]. The stent was mounted on a 13-mm delivery system and placed through a surgical gastrostomy which was created using local anesthesia. The patient was able to eat a regular diet until his death 120 days following stent placement due to diffuse metastasis.

## Second Generation: Uncovered SEMS

In 1992, Kozarek et al. endoscopically placed uncovered esophageal SEMS for palliation of malignant small-bowel obstruction in two patients [38]. In both patients, a SEMS was placed in a jejunal limb – one in the efferent limb and the other in the afferent limb. In 1995, Strecker et al. published the first report of a transoral, duodenal stent placement in a patient without prior surgically altered anatomy [39]. An 18-mm diameter uncovered nitinol stent was placed in a patient with malignant duodenal obstruction caused by extrinsic compression from recurrent colon cancer. Subsequently, a variety of different kinds of uncovered SEMS have been used for palliation of malignant gastroduodenal obstruction [40–43].

## Third Generation: Retrievable SEMS

In 2000, Jung et al. published the first report of transoral placement of a fully covered, retrievable

SEMS into the gastric outlet and duodenum in patients without prior surgery [44]. Polyurethane-covered, nitinol stents were placed in 19 patients with gastroduodenal obstruction. Since then, transoral placement of covered SEMS outside the USA has been used for nonsurgical palliation of malignant gastroduodenal obstruction performed either under fluoroscopic guidance alone or under endoscopic guidance with or without fluoroscopic assistance [45–48]. Stent migration rates of covered stents are approximately 30% and for uncovered stents 3–6%. Stent migration of covered SEMS is offset by the elimination of recurrent obstruction due to tumor ingrowth through the wire filaments (interstices) of uncovered

SEMS which occurs in 26–50% of patients. The prevention of ingrowth occurs as long as the covering remains intact (Table 3.2). Unfortunately, various covering materials may degrade leading to tumor ingrowth [48]. Materials such as polyurethane, polyethylene, and silicone rubber covering have been used, and chemical degradation of these polymers may occur after exposure to highly acidic gastric fluid or to certain hydrolytic enzymes (Fig. 3.4).

## Fourth Generation: Dual SEMS

To overcome the problems of migration of covered SEMS and tumor ingrowth of uncovered SEMS, Song et al. designed a dual gastroduodenal

**Table 3.2** Complication rates of bare SEMS and covered SEMS

| Types of stents | Adler [36]<br>Bare stent | Nassif [38]<br>Bare stent | Park [41]<br>Covered stent | Jung [39]<br>Covered stent |
|---|---|---|---|---|
| Number of patients | 36 | 63 | 24 | 19 |
| Stent diameter (mm) | 20–22 | 18–22 | 16–18 | 16 |
| Technical success (%) | 100 | 95 | 75 | 95 |
| Clinical success (%) | 86 | 92 | 67 | 94 |
| Migration (%) | 3 | 6 | 28 | 28 |
| Ingrowth (%) | 3 | 19 | 0 | 0 |
| Mean survival (weeks) | 12 | 10 | 18 | 8 |

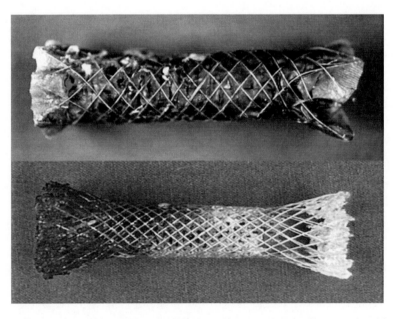

**Fig. 3.4** Photograph shows degraded covering polyurethane membrane, two covered stents removed from the stomach 1 month (*top*) and 3 months (*bottom*) after stent placement

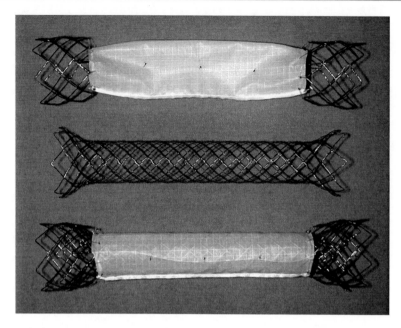

**Fig. 3.5** Photograph shows an outer partially covered stent (*top*), an inner bare nitinol stent (*middle*), and an assembled dual expandable nitinol stent (*bottom*)

stent consisting of two stents: an outer partially covered stent and an inner uncovered nitinol stent [49] (Fig. 3.5). The outer stent has proximal and distal uncovered 28-mm-diameter flanges, while the 18-mm-diameter midportion has a nylon or PTFE covering. The inner uncovered nitinol stent is 18 mm in diameter, also with flared end of 28 mm. The outer stent is placed first, and the inner stent is then placed coaxially inside the outer stent using a 3.8-mm delivery system. The experience using this stent was published in 2007 [50]. SEMS was placed in 213 patients for palliation of malignant, gastroduodenal obstruction. Clinical success rate was 94% and overall complication rate was 21% with a migration rate of only 4%.

## Colorectal Stents

### Background

Malignant colonic obstruction is the most common cause of emergent colon surgery [51–53]. However, emergency surgery for patients with acute malignant colonic obstruction is associated with high rates of morbidity and mortality of 40–50% and 10–20%, respectively [53]. In addition, patients with total or near-total colonic obstruction and a potentially resectable tumor often cannot undergo a one-stage resection and immediate reanastomosis because stool within the unprepared proximal colon leads to breakdown of the anastomosis. Therefore, the initial surgery involves resection of the primary tumor and creation of a colostomy followed by reanastomosis during a second surgery [54].

## Development of Self-Expandable Colorectal Stents

In 1990, Dohmoto et al. first described endoscopic placement of a self-expandable metallic stent for palliative treatment of malignant large-bowel obstruction [55]. In 1993 and 1994, Keen et al. and Tejero et al. each described a case where SEMS was successfully placed as a bridge to surgery [56, 57]. Since then, SEMS placement has been increasingly used as a minimally invasive option for relieving malignant colon obstruction for both palliation and as a bridge to surgery [58–64].

As dedicated colonic stents had not yet been developed, biliary, esophageal, and tracheobronchial stents were initially utilized and placed either endo-scopically or using interventional radiologic tech-niques to treat malignant obstruction of the left colon [55, 57, 65–70]. The enteral Wallstent was subse-quently introduced and was a larger version (18- and 20-mm diameter) of the biliary and tracheobronchial Wallstents, composed of stainless steel but with the advantage of having small diameter (10Fr) and long-length delivery systems. The delivery system allowed through the scope passage and deployment to treat lesions as far as the endoscope could be passed (including the distal terminal ileum).

In 1998, Tack et al. introduced an uncovered self-expandable metal stent for palliation of rec-tosigmoid carcinoma [71]. The stent had a fun-nel-shaped flare at each end. The nitinol stent resisted radial compression and conformed to the bends and curves of the colorectal anatomy with-out collapsing [71]. They found that placement of uncovered self-expandable nitinol stents was technically feasible and effective in the palliation of malignant rectosigmoid obstruction.

Similar to other areas within the gastrointesti-nal tract, tumor ingrowth through the interstices of uncovered colonic SEMS may result in reob-struction [72, 73]. In 2002, Choo et al. in 1998 and Kang et al. designed a covered colonic SEMS to prevent tumor ingrowth [74, 75]. A flexible polyurethane stent composed of stainless steel or nitinol was used. As expected, no tumor ingrowth occurred when used for palliation of malignant colonic obstruction [74, 75]. In addition, covered SEMS can be used to close colonic fistula, though fully covered stents have migration rates of up to 50% [74–76].

In 2007, Song et al. [61] designed a dual stent to take advantage of the qualities of uncovered and covered stents. This dual stent was similar to the one designed by the same group for gastrodu-odenal obstruction [49] and consisted of two nitinol SEMS: an outer, partially covered, stent and an inner, uncovered stent. The stents were placed using only fluoroscopic guidance. Stent migration occurred in 3%, and there were no cases of tumor ingrowth. However, perforation occurred in 11%. It was believed that this rela-tively high perforation rate was caused by the large stent diameter, particularly by the 38-mm, uncovered flared ends [61].

In 2007 and 2008, Repici et al. published results using two newly designed uncovered stents for colorectal use: the Ultraflex and WallFlex colonic stents [77, 78]. These stents were made of nitinol wire, and either the proxi-mal end or both ends were flared and placed endoscopically. The diameters of these stents, of 22–25 mm at the mid-body, were larger than the predecessor enteral Wallstent to allow more com-plete and lasting relief of obstruction [77, 78]. High technical and clinical success rates were achieved with low rates of complications such as tumor ingrowth, perforation, and stent migration.

In 2010, Park et al. introduced a newly devel-oped, covered ComVi stent designed to protect against tumor ingrowth by incorporating a PTFE membrane and to prevent stent migration by posi-tioning the PTFE membrane between two layers of stent meshwork [79]. Compared with the uncovered WallFlex stent, the covered ComVi stent had low rates of tumor ingrowth but a higher rate of stent migration compared [79]. The self-expandable metallic stents currently commer-cially available for colorectal use are listed in Table 3.3 [51].

## Biliary Stents

### Background

Stents for biliary drainage were first used by Burcharth and Pereiras et al. in 1978 [80, 81]. These rigid plastic stents were intended to ensure antegrade bile flow without the disadvantages of external drainage such as the need for regular catheter flushing and dressing, possible bile leak-age, infection and pain at the catheter entry site, and lifestyle restrictions. However, the limited inner diameter of the plastic stents resulted in stent occlusion from the development of bacterial biofilm [82]. Attempts to prolong patency with administration of chronic antibiotic therapy, ursodeoxycholic acid, changes in the type of polymer used, or coating the inner lining with a variety of agents so as to preclude bacterial colo-nization all proved unsuccessful [83]. It was with this background that expandable metallic stents were first used in the biliary system to overcome

**Table 3.3** Currently marketed self-expandable metal stents (SEMS) and self-expandable plastic stents (SEPS)

| Stent | Manufacturer | Material | Lengths (cm) | Diameter (mm) (flare-shaft/flanges) | Covering | Braided |
|---|---|---|---|---|---|---|
| **Currently marketed in the United States** | | | | | | |
| Ultraflex | Boston Scientific | Nitinol | 10/12/15 | 18/23 23/28 | PC | Y |
| Wallflex | Boston Scientific | Nitinol | 10/12/15 | 18/23 18/25 23/28 | PC/FC | Y |
| Esophageal-Z | Cook Inc. | Stainless steel | 8/10/ 12/14 | 18/25 | Antireflux (Dua) | N |
| Evolution | Cook Inc. | Nitinol | 8/10/12.5/15 | 18/23 20/25 | PC/FC | Y |
| Alimaxx-ES | Merit Endotek ™ | Nitinol | 7/10/12 | 12/14/16/ 18/22 | FC | N |
| Polyflex | Boston Scientific | Polyester | 9/12/15 | 16/20 18/23 21/28 | FC | Y |
| Niti-S (single or double) | Taewoong Medical, Seoul, Korea | Nitinol | 6/9/12/ 15 | 16/24 18/26 20/28 | PC/FC +/− antireflux | Y |
| Bonastent | Standard Sci Tech, Seoul, Korea | Nitinol | 6/8/10/12/15 | 18/23 20/25 22/27 | PC/FC +/− antireflux | Y |
| **Currently marketed in Europe and Asia Only** | | | | | | |
| Ella Esophageal stent family | ELLA-CS, Czech Rep. | Stainless steel and nitinol | 9–21 | 20/25 20/36 | UC/PC/FC | Y/N |
| Choo | M.I Tech, Seoul, Korea | Nitinol | 6–17 | 18 | PC/FC +/− antireflux | Y |
| Song | Stentech, Seoul, Korea | Nitinol | 5–18 | 16 18 | UC/PC/FC Double stent | Y |
| Ella-BD | ELLA-CS, Czech Rep. | Polypdi-axanon | 6/8/10/13.5 | 18/23 20/25 23/28 25/31 | FC | Y |
| Ella-Danis | ELLA-CS, Czech Rep. | Nitinol | 13.5 | 25 | FC | Y |

the limited internal diameter of rigid plastic stents and to prolong patency.

## Development of Self-Expandable Biliary Stents

### First Generation: Gianturco Z-Stent and Wallstent

The first SEMS designed for the biliary system was the Gianturco Z-stent (Cook, Bloomington, IN, USA), which was first used in 1985 [84]. The Gianturco Z-stent was made of stainless steel wire bent into a zigzag (Z) pattern with connected ends. It was compressed and introduced through a Teflon sheath of 8–12 French depending on the wire caliber and the diameter of the stent. The Gianturco Z-stent had a high expansile force that could be adjusted by changing the caliber of the wire, the length of the stent, and the number and angle of the bends. Although these stents have been used primarily in large blood vessels.

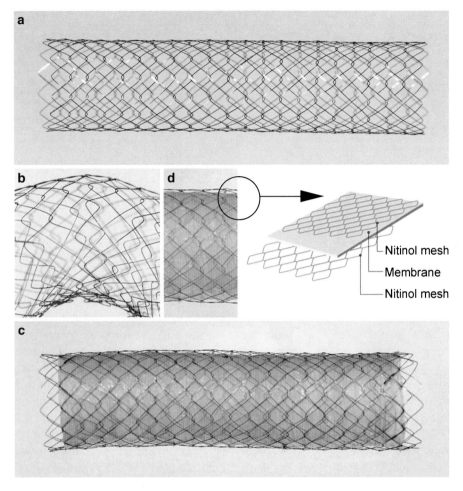

**Fig. 3.6** Photographs of Gianturco Z-stents. Original Gianturco stainless steel stent (**a**), modified Gianturco stent (**b**), modified Gianturco stent with *skirt* (**c**), and double-modified Gianturco stent (**d**) (From Sung et al. [83] with permission)

Rosch et al. modified the original Z-stent by suturing its bent *eyes* using a monofilament in order to prevent overexpansion [85, 86]. This modification facilitated percutaneous use in the biliary system. Carraso et al. introduced the modified Z-stents in animal experiments and proved their feasibility for use in extrahepatic bile ducts [87]. In 1989, the first clinical use of an expandable metallic stent in the biliary system was accomplished by Dr. Harold Coons (Fig. 3.6) who reported successful stent placement in right-sided biliary strictures from a left-duct access using the modified Z-stents [88]. Since then, many pioneering investigators have applied this type of stent in the treatment of both benign and malignant biliary diseases [89–91]. Although Gianturco Z-stents were useful for treatment of benign biliary obstruction, follow-up data showed they are less suitable for treating malignant lesions because the large spaces between the metal struts facilitated tumor ingrowth [92–94].

The Wallstent (Schneider, Bulach, Switzerland), developed by an engineer, Hans Wallsten, consists of 16–20 alloy spring filaments of medical-grade stainless steel woven into a tubular, braid configuration. The cross-points of the filaments are not soldered; the stent is highly self-expansile and flexible in its longitudinal axis [95].

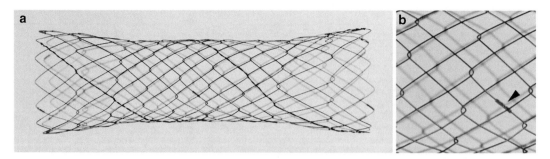

**Fig. 3.7** Photographs of T-configuration biliary stents for hilar obstruction. Kim stent with a large central mesh (**a**) and T-configuration with a Kim stent and a vertical stent (**b**) (From Huibregtse et al. [96], with permission)

During deployment, the stent shortens by approximately 20–40% of its original constrained length. Because it is self-expandable, the stent progressively reaches its maximum diameter within 1–2 days following placement without need for dilation. Thus, the advantages of Wallstents include their pliability, self-expansion, and flexibility in the longitudinal axis. The first clinical trial using the biliary Wallstent was conducted by Huibregtse et al. in 1889 and was placed endoscopically in 33 patients [96]. Lammer et al. demonstrated the technical feasibility of primary percutaneous Wallstent placement without need for previous catheter drainage using stents mounted on a small diameter delivery catheter (7 French) in 61 patients [97]. The Wallstent was the most commonly used self-expandable biliary stent in the 1990s, and the duration of stent patency was found to be superior to that of rigid, large bore (10 Fr) plastic stents [98].

## Second Generation: Wire-Based Nitinol Stents

The successful application of the first-generation biliary stents brought rapid progress in SEMS development. The most substantial development was the use of nitinol rather than stainless steel as the metal of choice. Nitinol is an alloy of nickel and titanium and has the unique properties of super-elasticity and shape memory that make it particularly well suited for self-expandable stents. Several types of new, expandable stents have since been developed and tested in animals and most of them have eventually made their way into clinical practice.

The evolution of nitinol stents is linked to the evolution of nitinol, itself [99]. Initially, nitinol was only available in wire form, and the early nitinol stents were merely wire coils. The EndoCoil (InStent, Eden Prairie, MN, USA), first introduced in 1993, was a coil spring stent made of a flat nitinol wire. Advantages of the EndoCoil included increased radial force with rapid expansion, inhibition of tumor ingrowth caused by the stent's coil framework with close approximation of the loops, and the potential for endoscopic removal by unwinding the stent [100]. The ZA biliary stent (Cook) is a modified, knitted nitinol stent designed for use in the biliary tree. This stent is extremely flexible and does not shorten during deployment [101]. The Niti-S stent (Taewoong, Seoul, Korea) is made of a nitinol monofilament intertwined in a tight, net-shaped cylinder with platinum radiopaque markers at both ends. Various modifications, including the D-type, T-type, and Y-type, have also been developed in order to facilitate the insertion of a second stent in patients with hilar tumors [102, 103] (Fig. 3.7).

## Third Generation: Tube-Based Nitinol Stents

In the mid-1990s, nitinol seamless tubing appeared on the market. With subsequent advances in laser cutting technology, most biliary nitinol stents are now produced by laser cutting of nitinol tubing. An early example is the Memotherm stent (Angiomed, Karlsruhe, Germany). This stent has a rigid, closed-cell design with a diamond-shaped pattern and which became the first of the following stent designs. Most laser-cut nitinol stents use variations and/or combinations of these basic design features. This stent can be placed with great accuracy for its minimal foreshortening [104]. The biliary Zilver stent (Cook Endoscopy) is one of the most recently developed nitinol stents. The entire stent is configured as one wire by laser cutting a nitinol tube in a zigzag shape. This stent is mounted on a six French delivery system, which allows side-by-side insertion of predeployed stents through the working channel of a therapeutic duodenoscope for bilateral stent placement for hilar obstruction [105].

## Fourth Generation: Membrane-Coated Stents

With their mesh structure, uncovered stents occlude mainly by tumor or tissue ingrowth. Their nonremovability requires additional stent placement to manage stent occlusion. To overcome this disadvantage, covered stents have been developed. Two types of covered, biliary stents are currently available – partially and fully covered. The Wallstent (Boston Scientific, Natick, MA, USA) is available as partially covered while the Wallflex is available in partially and fully covered forms. The Wallflex is a silicone-covered, nitinol stent with a structure similar to that of the original uncovered Wallstent. The ComVi stent (Taewoong) is a combination stent that incorporates a layer of PTFE between two layers of nitinol stents and is considered fully covered and designed to simultaneously minimize tumor ingrowth as well as the risk of stent migration. The Viabil biliary stent (W. L. Gore & Associates, Flagstaff, AZ, USA) consists of a nitinol exoskeleton with PTFE and a fluorinated ethylene propylene tubular lining throughout its length (fully covered) and had anti-migration fins. It has not been convincingly shown whether covered stents provide longer patency than uncovered stents, though a recent meta-analysis of randomized trials suggests that they do [106].

The most important characteristic of covered SEMS is removability, thus allowing its use in patients with resectable malignancies and benign strictures. Recently, a number of authors have showed that covered stents can be successfully removed without complications, regardless of the patient's underlying disease [107, 108]. In addition, covered stents provide the possibility for the development of drug-eluting stents [109]. This concept heralds a new paradigm for the management of biliary malignancies in which the stent is not merely a palliative device but is used for treatment.

## References

1. Symonds CJ. A case of malignant stricture of the oesophagus illustrating the use of the new form of oesophageal catheter. Trans Chir Soc Lond. 1885;18:155–8.
2. Ogilvie AL, Dronfield MW, Percuson R, Atkinson M. Palliative intubation of oesophagogastric neoplasms at fiberoptic endoscopy. Gut. 1982;23:1060–7.
3. Liakakos TK, Ohri SK, Townsend ER, Fountain SW. Palliative intubation for dysphagia in patients with carcinoma of the esophagus. Ann Thorac Surg. 1992;53:460–3.
4. Domschke W, Foerster EC, Matek W, Rodl W. Self-expanding mesh stent for esophageal cancer stenosis. Endoscopy. 1990;22:134–6.
5. Bethge N, Knyrim K, Wagner HJ, et al. Self-expanding metal stents for palliation of malignant esophageal obstruction. A pilot study of eight patients. Endoscopy. 1992;24:411–5.
6. Knyrim K, Wagner HJ, Bethge N, et al. A controlled trial of an expansile metal stent for palliation of esophageal obstruction due to inoperable cancer. N Engl J Med. 1993;329:1302–7.
7. Acunas B, Rozanes I, Akpinar S, Tunaci A, et al. Palliation of malignant esophageal strictures with self-expanding nitinol stents: drawbacks and complications. Radiology. 1996;199:648–52.
8. Adam A, Ellul J, Watkinson AF, et al. Palliation of inoperable esophageal carcinoma: a prospective randomized trial of laser therapy and stent placement. Radiology. 1997;202:344–8.
9. Cwikiel W, Tranberg KG, Cwikiel M, et al. Malignant dysphagia: palliation with esophageal stents – long-term results in 100 patients. Radiology. 1998;207:513–8.
10. Song HY, Choi KC, Cho BH, et al. Esophagogastric neoplasms: palliation with a modified Gianturco stent. Radiology. 1991;180:349–54.
11. Song HY, Do YS, Han YM, et al. Covered, expandable esophageal metallic stent tubes: experiences in 119 patients. Radiology. 1994;193:689–95.
12. Saxon RR, Barton RE, Katon RM, et al. Treatment of malignant esophagorespiratory fistulas with silicone-covered metallic Z stents. J Vasc Interv Radiol. 1995;6:237–42.
13. Morgan RA, Ellul JP, Denton ER, et al. Malignant esophageal fistulas and perforations: management

with plastic-covered metallic endoprostheses. Radiology. 1997;204:527–32.

14. Shin JH, Song HY, Ko GY, et al. Esophagorespiratory fistulae: long-term results of palliative treatment with covered expandable metallic stents in 61 patients. Radiology. 2004;232:252–9.

15. Wu WC, Katon RM, Saxon RR, et al. Silicone-covered self-expanding metallic stents for the palliation of malignant esophageal obstruction and esophagorespiratory fistulas: experience in 32 patients and a review of the literature. Gastrointest Endosc. 1994;40:22–33.

16. Kozarek RA, Raltz S, Brugge WR, et al. Prospective multicenter trial of esophageal Z-stent placement for malignant dysphagia and tracheoesophageal fistula. Gastrointest Endosc. 1996;44:562–7.

17. Bartelsman JEW, Bruno MJ, Jensema AI, et al. Palliation of patients with esophagogastric neoplasm by insertion of a covered expandable modified Gianturco-Z endoprosthesis: experiences in 153 patients. Gastrointest Endosc. 2000;51:134–8.

18. Siersema PD, Hop WCJ, van Blankenstein M, et al. A comparison of 3 types of covered metal stents for the palliation of patients with dysphagia caused by esophagogastric carcinoma: a prospective, randomized study. Gastrointest Endosc. 2001;54:145–53.

19. Song HY, Park SI, Jung HY, et al. Benign and malignant esophageal strictures: treatment with a polyurethane-covered retrievable expandable metallic stent. Radiology. 1997;203:747–52.

20. Yoon CJ, Shin JH, Song HY, et al. Removal of retrievable esophageal and gastrointestinal stents: experience in 113 patients. AJR Am J Roentgenol. 2004;183:1437–44.

21. Song HY, Jung HY, Park SI, et al. Covered retrievable expandable nitinol stents in patients with benign esophageal strictures: initial experience. Radiology. 2000;217:551–7.

22. Kim JH, Song HY, Choi EK, et al. Temporary metallic stent placement in the treatment of refractory benign esophageal strictures: results and factors associated with outcome in 55 patients. Eur Radiol. 2009;19:348–90.

23. Dormann AJ, Eisendrath P, Wigginghaus B, et al. Palliation of esophageal carcinoma with self-expanding plastic stent. Endoscopy. 2003;35:207–11.

24. Conigliaro R, Battaglia G, Repici A, et al. Polyflex stents for malignant oesophageal and oesophagogastric stricture: a prospective, multicentric study. Eur J Gastroenterol Hepatol. 2007;19:195–203.

25. Fernández A, Vila JJ, Vázquez S, et al. Self-expanding plastic stents for the treatment of post-operative esophago-jejuno anastomosis leak. A case series study. Rev Esp Enferm Dig. 2010;102: 704–10.

26. Szegedi L, Gál I, Kósa I, Kiss GG. Palliative treatment of esophageal carcinoma with self-expanding plastic stents: a report on 69 cases. Eur J Gastroenterol Hepatol. 2006;18:1197–201.

27. Conio M, Repici A, Battaglia G, et al. A randomized prospective comparison of self-expandable plastic stents and partially covered self-expandable metal stents in the palliation of malignant esophageal dysphagia. Am J Gastroenterol. 2007;102:2667–77.

28. Do YS, Choo SW, Suh SW, et al. Malignant esophagogastric junction obstruction: palliative treatment with an antireflux valve stent. J Vasc Interv Radiol. 2001;12:647–51.

29. Dua KS, Kozarek R, Kim J, et al. Self-expanding metal esophageal stent with anti-reflux mechanism. Gastrointest Endosc. 2001;53:603–13.

30. Laasch HU, Marriott A, Wilbraham L, et al. Effectiveness of open versus antireflux stents for palliation of distal esophageal carcinoma and prevention of symptomatic gastroesophageal reflux. Radiology. 2002;225:359–65.

31. Guo JH, Teng GJ, Zhu GY, et al. Self-expandable esophageal stent loaded with [125] I seeds: initial experience in patients with advanced esophageal cancer. Radiology. 2008;247:574–81.

32. Won JH, Lee JD, Wang HJ, et al. Self-expandable covered metallic esophageal stent impregnated with beta-emitting radionuclide: an experimental study in canine esophagus. Int J Radiat Oncol Biol Phys. 2002;53:1005–13.

33. Repici A, Vleggaar FP, Hassan C, et al. Efficacy and safety of biodegradable stents for refractory benign esophageal strictures: the BEST (Biodegradable Esophageal Stent) study. Gastrointest Endosc. 2010;72:927–34.

34. Lei L, Liu X, Guo S, et al. 5-Fluorouracil-loaded multilayered films for drug controlled releasing stent application: drug release, microstructure, and ex vivo permeation behaviors. J Control Release. 2010;146:45–53.

35. Kim EY, Shin JH, Jung YY, et al. A rat esophageal model to investigate stent-induced tissue hyperplasia. J Vasc Interv Radiol. 2010;21:1287–91.

36. Fujino Y, Suzuki Y, Kamigaki T, et al. Evaluation of gastroenteric bypass for unresectable pancreatic cancer. Hepatogastroenterology. 2001;48:563–8.

37. Song HY, Yang DH, Kuhn JH, Choi KC. Obstructing cancer of the gastric antrum: palliative treatment with covered metallic stents. Radiology. 1993;187: 357–8.

38. Kozarek RA, Ball TJ, Patterson DJ. Metallic self-expanding stent application in the upper gastrointestinal tract: caveats and concerns. Gastrointest Endosc. 1992;38:1–6.

39. Strecker EP, Boos I, Husfeldt KJ. Malignant duodenal stenosis: palliation with peroral implantation of a self-expanding nitinol stent. Radiology. 1995;196: 349–51.

40. de Baere T, Harry G, Ducreaux M, et al. Self-expanding metallic stents as palliative treatment of malignant gastroduodenal stenosis. AJR Am J Roentgenol. 1997;169:1079–83.

41. Adler DG, Baron TH. Endoscopic palliation of malignant gastric outlet obstruction using self-expanding metal stents: experience in 36 patients. Am J Gastroenterol. 2002;97:72–8.

42. Yates MR, Morgan DE, Baron TH. Palliation of malignant gastric and small intestinal strictures with

self-expandable metal stents. Endoscopy. 1998;30: 266–72.

43. Nassif T, Prat F, Meduri B, et al. Endoscopic palliation of malignant gastric outlet obstruction using self-expandable metallic stents: results of a multicenter study. Endoscopy. 2003;35:483–9.

44. Jung GS, Song HY, Kang SG, et al. Malignant gastroduodenal obstructions: treatment by means of a covered expandable metallic stent-initial experience. Radiology. 2000;216:758–63.

45. Lopera JE, Alvarez O, Castano R, Castaneda-Zuniga W. Initial experience with Song's covered duodenal stent in the treatment of malignant gastroduodenal obstruction. J Vasc Interv Radiol. 2001;12: 1297–303.

46. Park KB, Do YS, Kang WK, et al. Malignant obstruction of gastric outlet and duodenum: palliation with flexible covered metallic stents. Radiology. 2001;219:679–83.

47. Jung GS, Song HY, Seo TS, et al. Malignant gastric outlet obstructions: treatment by means of coaxial placement of uncovered and covered expandable nitinol stents. J Vasc Interv Radiol. 2002;13: 275–83.

48. Kim JH, Song HY, Shin JH, et al. Membrane degradation of covered stents in the upper gastrointestinal tract: frequency and clinical significance. J Vasc Interv Radiol. 2008;19:220–4.

49. Song HY, Shin JH, Yoon CJ, et al. A dual expandable nitinol stent: experience in 102 patients with malignant gastroduodenal strictures. J Vasc Interv Radiol. 2004;15:1443–9.

50. Kim JH, Song HY, Shin JH, et al. Metallic stent placement in the palliative treatment of malignant gastroduodenal obstructions: prospective evaluation of results and factors influencing outcome in 213 patients. Gastrointest Endosc. 2007;66:256–64.

51. Katsanos K, Sabharwal T, Adam A. Stenting of the lower gastrointestinal tract: current status. Cardiovasc Intervent Radiol. 2011;34:462–73.

52. Jung MK, Park SY, Jeon SW, et al. Factors associated with the long-term outcome of a self-expandable colon stent used for palliation of malignant colorectal obstruction. Surg Endosc. 2010;24:525–30.

53. Dionigi G, Villa F, Rovera F, et al. Colonic stenting for malignant disease: review of literature. Surg Oncol. 2007;16(Suppl 1):S153–5.

54. Baron TH. Expandable metal stents for the treatment of cancerous obstruction of the gastrointestinal tract. N Engl J Med. 2001;344(22):1681–7.

55. Dohmoto M, Rupp KD, Hohlbach G. Endoscopically-implanted prosthesis in rectal carcinoma [German]. Dtsch Med Wochenschr. 1990;115:915.

56. Keen RR, Orsay CP. Rectosigmoid stent for obstructing colonic neoplasm. Dis Colon Rectum. 1992;35: 912–3.

57. Tejero E, Mainar A, Fernandez L, et al. New procedure for the treatment of colorectal neoplastic obstructions. Dis Colon Rectum. 1994;37:1158–9.

58. de Gregorio MA, Laborda A, Tejero E, et al. Ten-year retrospective study of treatment of malignant colonic obstructions with self-expandable stents. J Vasc Interv Radiol. 2011;22:870–8.

59. Fregonese D, Naspetti R, Ferrer S, et al. Ultraflex precision colonic stent placement as a bridge to surgery in patients with malignant colon obstruction. Gastrointest Endosc. 2008;67:68–73.

60. Camúñez F, Echenagusia A, Simó G, et al. Malignant colorectal obstruction treated by means of self-expanding metallic stents: effectiveness before surgery and in palliation. Radiology. 2000;216: 492–7.

61. Song HY, Kim JH, Shin JH, et al. A dual-design expandable colorectal stent for malignant colorectal obstruction: results of a multicenter study. Endoscopy. 2007;39:448–54.

62. Mauro MA, Koehler RE, Baron TH. Advances in gastrointestinal intervention: the treatment of gastroduodenal and colorectal obstructions with metallic stents. Radiology. 2000;215:659–69.

63. Kim JH, Song HY, Li YD, et al. Dual-design expandable colorectal stent for malignant colorectal obstruction: comparison of flared ends and bent ends. AJR Am J Roentgenol. 2009;193:248–54.

64. Keswani RN, Azar RR, Edmundowicz SA, et al. Stenting for malignant colonic obstruction: a comparison of efficacy and complications in colonic versus extracolonic malignancy. Gastrointest Endosc. 2009;69:675–80.

65. Saida Y, Sumiyama Y, Nagao J, Takase M. Stent endoprosthesis for obstructing colorectal cancers. Dis Colon Rectum. 1996;39:552–5.

66. Itabashi M, Hamano K, Kameoka S, Asahina K. Self-expanding stainless steel stent application in rectosigmoid stricture. Dis Colon Rectum. 1993;36: 508–11.

67. Spinelli P, Dal Fante M, Mancini A. Self-expanding mesh stent for endoscopic palliation of rectal obstructing tumors: a preliminary report. Surg Endosc. 1992;6:72–4.

68. Spinelli P, Dal Fante M, Mancini A. Rectal metal stents for palliation of colorectal malignant stenosis. Bildgebung. 1993;60(Suppl):48–50.

69. Tejero E, Fernandez-Lobato R, Mainar A, et al. Initial results of a new procedure for treatment of malignant obstruction of the left colon. Dis Colon Rectum. 1997;40:432–6.

70. Wallis F, Campbell KL, Eremin O, Hussey JK. Self-expanding metal stents in the management of colorectal carcinoma – a preliminary report. Clin Radiol. 1998;53:251–4.

71. Tack J, Gevers AM, Rutgeerts P. Self-expandable metallic stents in the palliation of rectosigmoidal carcinoma: a follow-up study. Gastrointest Endosc. 1998;48:267–71.

72. Canon CL, Baron TH, Morgan DE, et al. Treatment of colonic obstruction with expandable metal stents: radiologic features. AJR Am J Roentgenol. 1997;168:199–205.

73. Rey JF, Romanczyk T, Greff M. Metal stents for palliation of rectal carcinoma: a preliminary report on 12 patients. Endoscopy. 1995;27:501–4.

74. Choo IW, Do YS, Suh SW, et al. Malignant colorectal obstruction: treatment with a flexible covered stent. Radiology. 1998;206:415–21.

75. Kang SG, Jung GS, Cho SG, et al. The efficacy of metallic stent placement in the treatment of colorectal obstruction. Korean J Radiol. 2002;3:79–86.

76. Repici A, Reggio D, De Angelis C, et al. Covered metal stents for management of inoperable malignant colorectal strictures. Gastrointest Endosc. 2000;52:735–40.

77. Repici A, Fregonese D, Costamagna G, et al. Ultraflex precision colonic stent placement for palliation of malignant colonic obstruction: a prospective multicenter study. Gastrointest Endosc. 2007;66: 920–7.

78. Repici A, De Caro G, Luigiano C, et al. WallFlex colonic stent placement for management of malignant colonic obstruction: a prospective study at two centers. Gastrointest Endosc. 2008;67:77–84.

79. Park S, Cheon JH, Park JJ, et al. Comparison of efficacies between stents for malignant colorectal obstruction: a randomized, prospective study. Gastrointest Endosc. 2010;72:304–10.

80. Burcharth F. A new endoprosthesis for nonoperative intubation of the biliary tract in malignant obstructive jaundice. Surg Gynecol Obstet. 1978;146:76–8.

81. Pereiras Jr RV, Rheingold OJ, Huston D, et al. Relief of malignant obstructive jaundice by percutaneous insertion of a permanent prosthesis in the biliary tree. Ann Intern Med. 1978;89:589–3.

82. Lammer J, Stoffler G, Petek WW, Hofler H. In vitro long-term perfusion of different materials for biliary endoprostheses. Invest Radiol. 1986;21:329–31.

83. Sung JY, Leung JW, Shaffer EA, et al. Bacterial biofilm, brown pigment stone and blockage of biliary stents. J Gastroenterol Hepatol. 1993;8:28–34.

84. Wright KC, Wallace S, Charnsangavej C, Carrasco CH, Gianturco C. Percutaneous endovascular stents: an experimental evaluation. Radiology. 1985;156: 69–72.

85. Rosch J, Uchida BT, Hall LD, et al. Gianturco-Rosch expandable Z-stents in the treatment of superior vena cava syndrome. Cardiovasc Intervent Radiol. 1992;15:319–27.

86. Uchida BT, Putnam JS, Rosch J. Modifications of Gianturco expandable wire stents. AJR Am J Roentgenol. 1988;150:1185–7.

87. Carrasco CH, Wallace S, Charnsangavej C, et al. Expandable biliary endoprosthesis: an experimental study. AJR Am J Roentgenol. 1985;145:1279–81.

88. Coons HG. Self-expanding stainless steel biliary stents. Radiology. 1989;170:979–83.

89. Irving JD, Adam A, Dick R, et al. Gianturco expandable metallic biliary stents: results of a European clinical trial. Radiology. 1989;172:321–6.

90. Rossi P, Bezzi M, Rossi M, et al. Metallic stents in malignant biliary obstruction: results of a multicenter European study of 240 patients. J Vasc Interv Radiol. 1994;5:279–85.

91. LaBerge JM, Doherty M, Gordon RL, Ring EJ. Hilar malignancy: treatment with an expandable metallic transhepatic biliary stent. Radiology. 1990;177:793–7.

92. Yoshioka T, Sakaguchi H, Yoshimura H, et al. Expandable metallic biliary endoprostheses: preliminary clinical evaluation. Radiology. 1990;177: 253–7.

93. Kubota Y, Nakatani S, Nakahashi Y, et al. Bilateral internal biliary drainage of hilar cholangiocarcinoma with modified Gianturco Z stents inserted via a single percutaneous tract. J Vasc Interv Radiol. 1993;4:605–10.

94. Rossi P, Bezzi M, Salvatori FM, et al. Recurrent benign biliary strictures: management with self-expanding metallic stents. Radiology. 1990;175: 661–5.

95. Zollikofer CL, Antonucci F, Stuckmann G, et al. Historical overview on the development and characteristics of stents and future outlooks. Cardiovasc Intervent Radiol. 1992;15:272–8.

96. Huibregtse K, Cheng J, Coene PP, et al. Endoscopic placement of expandable metal stents for biliary strictures – a preliminary report on experience with 33 patients. Endoscopy. 1989;21:280–2.

97. Lammer J, Klein GE, Kleinert R, et al. Obstructive jaundice: use of expandable metal endoprosthesis for biliary drainage. Work in progress. Radiology. 1990;177:789–92.

98. Davids PH, Groen AK, Rauws EA, et al. Randomised trial of self-expanding metal stents versus polyethylene stents for distal malignant biliary obstruction. Lancet. 1992;340:1488–92.

99. Stoeckel D, Pelton A, Duerig T. Self-expanding nitinol stents: material and design considerations. Eur Radiol. 2004;14:292–301.

100. Goldin E, Beyar M, Safra T, et al. A new self-expandable and removable metal stent for biliary obstruction–a preliminary report. Endoscopy. 1993;25:597–9.

101. Varadarajulu S, Tutuian R, Gostout C, et al. Efficacy of the Za self-expandable metal stent for palliation of malignant biliary obstruction. J Clin Gastroenterol. 2004;38:77–80.

102. Kim CW, Park AW, Won JW, et al. T-configured dual stent placement in malignant biliary hilar duct obstructions with a newly designed stent. J Vasc Interv Radiol. 2004;15:713–7.

103. Lee JH, Kang DH, Kim JY, et al. Endoscopic bilateral metal stent placement for advanced hilar cholangiocarcinoma: a pilot study of a newly designed Y stent. Gastrointest Endosc. 2007;66:364–9.

104. Friedrich JM, Vogel J, Gorich J, et al. First clinical experience with a new nitinol stent in the biliary system. Rofo. 1995;162:429–35.

105. Chennat J, Waxman I. Initial performance profile of a new 6F self-expanding metal stent for palliation of malignant hilar biliary obstruction. Gastrointest Endosc. 2010;72:632–6.

106. Saleem A, Leggett CL, Murad MH, Baron TH. Meta-analysis of randomized trials comparing the patency of covered and uncovered self-expandable metal stents for palliation of distal malignant bile duct obstruction. Gastrointest Endosc. 2011;74(2):321–7.

107. Kuo MD, Lopresti DC, Gover DD, et al. Intentional retrieval of viabil stent-grafts from the biliary system. J Vasc Interv Radiol. 2006;17:389–97.

108. Baron TH. Covered self-expandable metal stents for benign biliary tract diseases. Curr Opin Gastroenterol. 2011;27:262–7.

109. Suk KT, Kim JW, Kim HS, et al. Human application of a metallic stent covered with a paclitaxel-incorporated membrane for malignant biliary obstruction: multicenter pilot study. Gastrointest Endosc. 2007;66: 798–803.

# Current Designs of Self-Expanding Stents

**4**

Hans-Ulrich Laasch

## General Considerations

The ideal stent for placement in the gastrointestinal tract would have the following properties: good visibility on fluoroscopy, predictable stent behavior on deployment, reliable expansion without causing pain, secure fixation yet the ability to be removed, resistance to obstruction, and high conformability around the flexures of the gut tube and the angled junctions of biliary tributaries. The latter is particularly important for the following reasons: If stents are too stiff to align around an anatomical curve, the ends may embed in the wall of the bowel or bile duct, resulting in impaired drainage or functional obstruction. Continuous pressure of the stent edges onto the mucosa can lead to ulceration, necrosis, and perforation (Fig. 4.1). This may also occur with stents that have either large throats or particularly sharp edges (Fig. 4.2). The stent must align within lumen and may not lie at angle to it; otherwise, reintervention becomes much more difficult (Fig. 4.3): Coaxial cannulation into the stent may not be possible, and further procedures may have to be performed through the gaps in the interstices, limiting positioning and expansion of secondary stents and increasing the risk of entanglement. Stents are also submitted to repetitive flexion forces, which lead

H.-U. Laasch, M.D. (✉)
Department of Radiology, The Christie NHS Foundation Trust, Wilmslow Road, Manchester, M20 4BX, UK
e-mail: hul@christie.nhs.uk

to material fatigue if there is insufficient elasticity within the stent skeleton [1–3]. Stent development has mainly been driven by commercial considerations on a trial-and-error basis, and a vast number of stent constructions have been developed and discarded. In 2011, 16 colonic, 23 biliary, and 32 different esophageal stent models were registered as commercially available with the stent registries of the British Society of Interventional Radiology and the Association of Coloproctology of the UK and Ireland. Stents differ considerably in their properties, as defined by the material used, the construction of their skeleton, their shape, and optional covering membranes.

## Stent Material

Most stents are constructed from metal. Stainless steel and other alloys are being superseded by a superelastic alloy developed by the US Navy (NiTiNOL – Nickel Titanium Naval Ordnance Laboratory). Since its first successful application for coupling hydraulic pipes in F-14 fighter jets in 1969, nitinol is now widely used in medicine as well as in products of daily life such as spectacle frames, underwired bras and pop-up tents. Nitinol exhibits two unusual properties, described in more detail by Kauffman and Mayo [4]:

1. Shape memory: A particular shape can be imprinted on a nitinol structure by heating it to around 500°C. This creates an ordered (austenite) atomic structure within the crystalline matrix of the metal. After cooling, it

R. Kozarek et al. (eds.), *Self-Expandable Stents in the Gastrointestinal Tract*, 
DOI 10.1007/978-1-4614-3746-8_4, © Springer Science+Business Media New York 2013

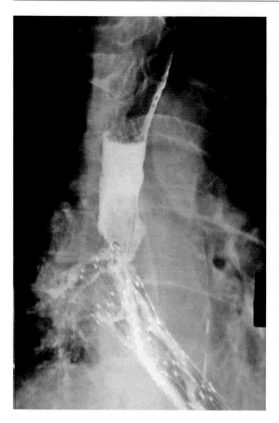

**Fig. 4.1** Necrosis of the esophageal wall caused by pressure from poor alignment (Dua stent)

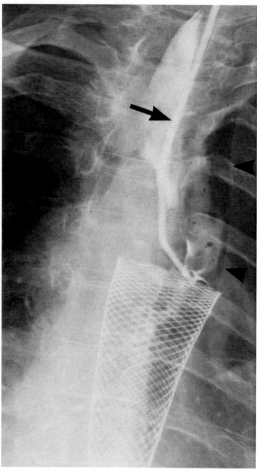

**Fig. 4.2** Esophageal perforation at the sharp edges of a large inlet funnel (Flamingo Wallstent): Injection of contrast through a catheter (arrow) fills the trachea (arrowheads)

can be easily deformed, which *subluxes* the atomic structure to a more complex (martenite) arrangement. On rewarming, the atoms attempt to regain the imprinted (austenite) configuration, and the structure recovers the original shape. The temperature range inducing the spontaneous recurrence to the austenite structure depends on the ratio of nickel to titanium within the alloy. For medical devices, this is essentially body temperature.

2. Super (pseudo-) elasticity: Nitinol can be deformed 20–30 times more than most other metals before a permanent (plastic) change is achieved. Applied mechanical force causes a reversible martenite transformation by displacing the atoms within the lattice against each other. This results in additional elasticity from within the material, whereas conventional alloys have to rely on the elasticity provided from within

the stent skeleton. These characteristics have also found application in kink-resistant nitinol guide wires.

Other materials used for stents include plastic (e.g., polyester) and biodegradable polymers (e.g., polydioxanone). Used as a monofilament, these are woven in a similar fashion to nitinol wire. Plastic stents are cheap; biodegradable stents allow temporary stenting without the need for stent removal. Both have the disadvantage of the stents needing to be loaded by the operator at the time of use, as they lack the elasticity of metal designs. There are a number of different ways in which stents can be constructed.

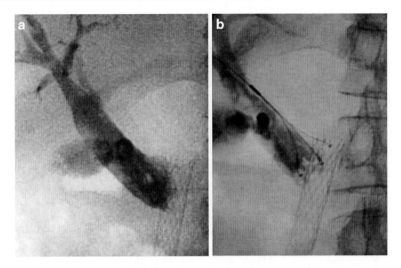

**Fig. 4.3**  (**a**) Poorly aligned and impacted laser-cut biliary stent (Memotherm). (**b**) Attempts at dislodging the top of the stent resulted in entanglement of the forceps

## Metal Stents

### Segmented Stents

Individual cylindrical metal baskets are connected to each other, resulting in a semirigid tube (Fig. 4.4). One of the earliest designs (Gianturco-Rösch Z-stent, Wilson Cook, Bloomington, USA) consists of multiple stainless steel segments, connected by sutures and covered by dipping into polyurethane. This stent has a low elasticity and needs to be loaded into the delivery sheath prior to use. The high straightening force prevents alignment around the gastroesophageal junction, at times leading to pressure necrosis and perforation of the esophageal wall [5].

The second-generation Ella esophageal stents (Boubella, Ella-CS, Hradec Kralove, Czech Republic) achieved greater flexibility with stainless steel segments; the first stent based on nitinol baskets was developed by a Korean manufacturer (Choo/Do stent, MI-Tech, Seoul, South Korea). Both were supplied preloaded into their delivery system. Due to the rigidity of the individual segments, this type of stent tends to buckle rather than bend. Repetitive strain occasionally leads to rupture at the junction of the segments (Fig. 4.5). Later, models were reinforced

by sutures (Boubella) or additional threads of nitinol (Choo/Hanaro stent).

### Laser-Cut Stents

A completely different approach to stent design is achieved by the construction of a solid nitinol tube, which is extensively perforated and sections cut out of it through the use of a laser (Fig. 4.6). Originally developed for the stenting of peripheral vascular stenoses, several manufacturers have adapted these for use in the biliary tree. These are not covered by a membrane, and their advantage is of a high initial radial force and the ability to fit into a small delivery system (6 French; *French* = circumference in mm). One covered esophageal version is available; the only enteral version was withdrawn due to complications. These stents excel by their minimal shortening (<10%) on release, which allows for more accurate stent placement. However, there are several trade-offs for this: Due to their angular struts, laser-cut stents cannot be repositioned or resheathed when partly deployed. The expanding cells of the stent skeleton act as barbs fixing the stent into the mucosa and engaging on the edge of the delivery sheath. The major limitation of

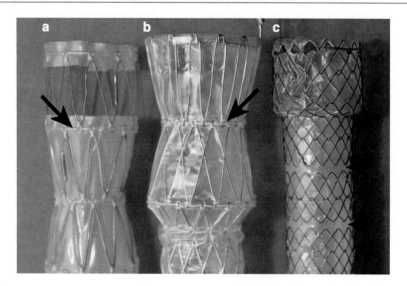

**Fig. 4.4** Segmented stents. (**a**) Gianturco-Z stent, Cook, Bloomington, USA; (**b**) Boubella stent, Ella-CS, Hradec Kralove, Czech Republic; (**c**) Hanaro stent, MI-Tech, Seoul, Korea. The two stainless steel stents consist of individual baskets sutured together (*arrows*), while the nitinol segments in the third stent are only connected by the covering membrane (*arrowheads*)

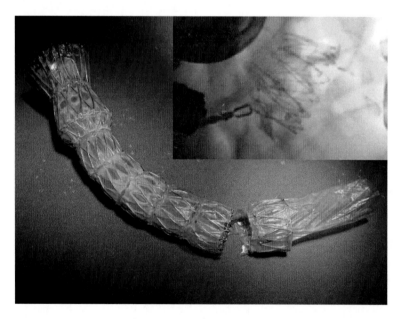

**Fig. 4.5** Ruptured membrane: After removal of a migrated stent (Boubella) from the stomach, the *lower* segment with the antireflux valve was found missing. It impacted in the sigmoid colon and was removed endoscopically (insert)

laser-cut stents however, is the reluctance to align smoothly around flexures (Fig. 4.7). This is due to the high straightening force caused by the memory effect of the tubular design. This type of stent is more likely to stretch the stented segment rather than conform to the natural anatomy. As a result, reintervention can be challenging (Fig. 4.8). Manufacturers have tried to address this by reducing the size of the metal struts. The memory effect of the metal tube also poses consistent resistance to natural flexion. If flexion is frequent and repetitive, it leads to metal fatigue

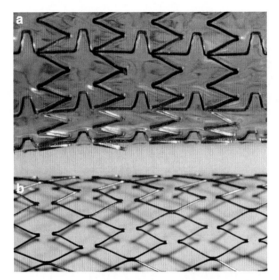

**Fig. 4.6** Close-up of laser-cut stents. (**a**) Covered Alimaxx-E esophageal stent; (**b**) Uncovered Luminexx biliary stent

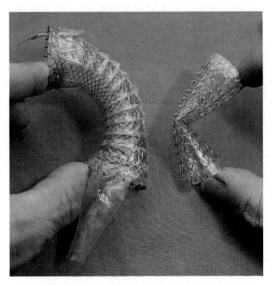

**Fig. 4.7** Better conformability of a braided esophageal stent (Ella-HV) compared to a laser-cut stent (Alimaxx-E, Merit Medical, South Jordan, Utah, USA)

and fracture (Fig. 4.9), reported as high as 6% in vivo [6] and as high as 100% in a vascular simulation model [3]. In the gut, this occurs from peristalsis, in the bile duct by excursion of the liver from breathing, coughing, laughing, and hiccups. The only laser-cut enteral stent (Memotherm, Bard) was discontinued due to a

high occurrence of stent fracture and colonic perforation [7–9].

## Woven Stents

There are two different ways of weaving a wire or monofilament into a tube and for the purpose of clarity will be called *braided* and *knitted* (Figs. 4.10 and 4.11). Braided stents consist of crisscrossing wires which are movable against each other. In contrast, with knitted stents, some of the wire junctions are looped around each other like a wire fence. This almost completely abolishes longitudinal straightening forces, resulting in great conformability as well as reduced stent lengthening on compression.

## Stent Manufacture

The wire is looped by hand around pins inserted into a metal mandrel. In case of nitinol, the completed stent skeleton undergoes heat treatment, imprinting the three-dimensional shape (Fig. 4.12). Following this, the metal is polished to reduce surface debris and microcracks. For covered versions, the stent may be dipped in liquid plastic, such as polyurethane or silicone, or covered with a polyethylene or PTFE membrane. Of all covering materials, PTFE is the most inert and resistant to degradation from gastric acid and bile, but it is also the most expensive and needs to be sutured by hand onto the stent skeleton. The finished stent is loaded manually into the delivery system, packed, and gas-sterilized.

## Braided Stents

A landmark stent design was achieved with the development of the biliary and enteral Wallstent (Boston Scientific, Natick, MA, USA). A continuous tube braided from cobalt alloy wires was cut into short sections, representing the individual stents. These stents were the first to be available for *through-the-scope* (TTS) placement for biliary and enteral use and are still a

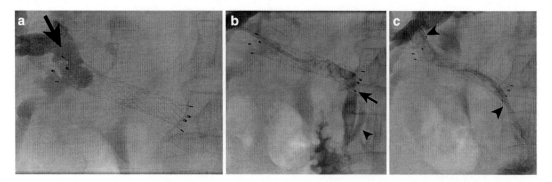

**Fig. 4.8** Poor alignment. (**a**) Blocked Luminexx stent. The *upper end* is impacted in the bile duct wall (*arrow*) making cannulation difficult. (**b**) Note the sharp angulation of the distorted bile duct at the *lower* stent end (*arrow*). The pancreatic duct is also demonstrated (*arrowhead*). (**c**) Insertion of a knitted biliary stent (Egis double bare) shows smoother alignment along the bile duct

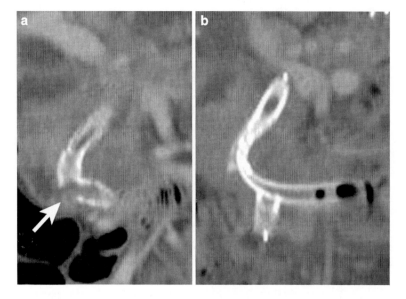

**Fig. 4.9** Fracture from metal fatigue. (**a**) CT reconstruction of a fractured laser-cut stent (Zilver); (**b**) After restenting with a braided stent (Ella-SX)

preferred stents for many endoscopists due to the high visibility on fluoroscopy. The drawback of this construction is the *crown* of sharp wire points, which forms the stent ends. If placed within a flexure, these may perforate the bowel wall. The wire ends are also at risk of intertwining when the delivery system is fed through the working channel of the endoscope. Once entangled, the stent may fail to open properly (Fig. 4.13). The follow-on Wallflex stent [10] now represents the commonest construction used in the GI tract. A single nitinol wire is

woven continuously around a metal mandrel, and the edges of the stent consist of loops of wire rather than sharp points.

Braided stents are very flexible but retain a significant straightening force. Esophageal stents tend to have greater radial force than enteral stents due to thicker wire gauge being used. This is possible, as the esophageal anatomy is essentially straight except for the gastroesophageal junction, and larger delivery systems (18–28 Fr) can be used. Softer stents for enteral use can be mounted in 10–10.5 Fr delivery systems, which

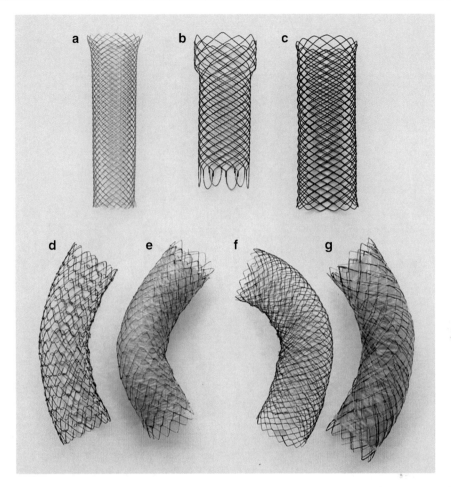

**Fig. 4.10** Woven enteral stents; *upper row* braided, *lower row* knitted stents (**a**) Wallstent; (**b**) Wallflex; (**c**) Ella-SX enteral; (**d**) Niti-S D-stent; (**e**) ComVi; (**f**) Egis single bare; (**g**) Egis double covered. Note the ability of the knitted stents to align in a *curve*

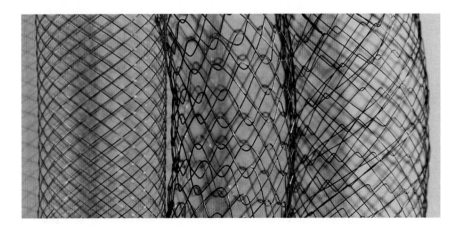

**Fig. 4.11** Close-up image showing the simple crossover of a braided construction Wallstent (*left*), and the interlocking wires of a single Niti-S D-stent (*center*), and a double knitted Egis stent (*right*)

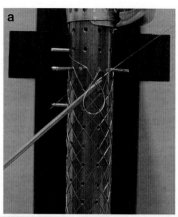

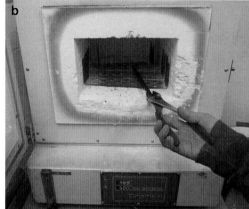
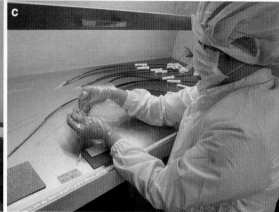

**Fig. 4.12** Manufacture of a nitinol colonic stent (Egis). (**a**) Weaving of the stent skeleton on a mandrel; (**b**) Heat treatment for imprinting shape memory; (**c**) Manual loading prior to sterilization (Courtesy of S&G Biotech, Seoul, Korea)

allows placement through large working channels (≥3.7 mm) of therapeutic endoscopes (*through-the-scope*, TTS). All stents lengthen when compressed into the delivery system and shorten again on deployment. This is most marked with braided stents (Fig. 4.14). Stent shortening can be as much as 50% in large-caliber stents. Note that this implies an initial doubling in length by compression (e.g., 10 cm ⇔ 20 cm); a shortening by one-third implies an original increase by 50% (e.g., 10 cm ⇔ 15 cm). A braided stent has a relatively smooth outer skeleton, which allows resheathing of a partially deployed stent. Equally stents may be gently repositioned by traction when already partly deployed. Indeed, this allows for a simple strategy to correct for stent shortening; the delivery system is intentionally inserted several centimeters too far and the stent partially deployed. Once the distal end has expanded and

shortened, the whole system is withdrawn carefully into the final position and deployment completed. This cannot be performed with laser-cut stents, as the barbs fix the stent into the mucosa.

## Knitted Stents

This construction results in very low straightening forces and excellent conformability to the host tube as well as reduced stent shortening (25–30%) on deployment compared to braided stents. Knitted esophageal stents have been in use for over 20 years; the commercially most successful version was the Ultraflex stent (Boston Scientific). Unfortunately, it was never possible to produce this within a pullback delivery system due to the high radial force. Instead, this stent

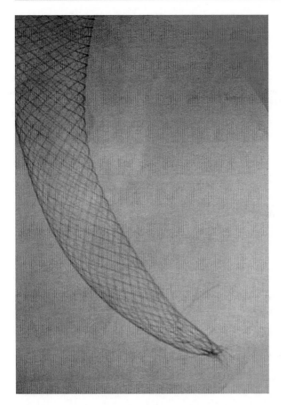

**Fig. 4.13** Enteral Wallstent placed endoscopically into a gastrojejunostomy immediately after deployment. The wires at the *lower* stent end have become entangled as the system was advanced through the working channel. This could be rectified by forceful passage of the endoscope

was tied down to the outside of the delivery catheter by silk thread. This made the system bulky and very rough, resulting in the highest need of all stents for predilatation to allow passage of the system through the stricture [11]. Being only partially covered, the Ultraflex was also not designed to be removable. The first removable knitted nitinol esophageal stent was introduced in 2011 (Egis, S&G Biotech, Seoul, Korea) (Fig. 4.15), available with optional antireflux valve.

Several enteral versions of a knitted stent were developed in South Korea. One system consists of two separate stents, one covered one uncovered [12, 13], but commercially more successful designs consist of a covering membrane sandwiched between two layers of nitinol (ComVi stent, Taewoong and Egis double covered stent, S&G Biotech). Intuitively, these constructions should combine the advantages of reduced migration due

to the outer layer of metal with the reduction of ingrowth from the covering membrane, but clinical results are ambiguous [14–16]. The drawback of this construction is the smaller wire gauge used, reducing radial force and visibility of the metal skeleton, although this is compensated for by the use of gold markers. These stents may be repositioned by traction if part-deployed but cannot be resheathed.

Knitted stents excel through their effortless conformability to flexures while retaining the ability to remodel and expand into the original configuration. This may however, take several days, and the urge to perform balloon dilatation immediately after insertion should be resisted.

## Biodegradable Stents

Early applications of biodegradable stents in the GI tract go back as far as 1997 [17, 18], but only one is commercially available at present (Ella-BD, Ella-CS, Hradec Kralove, Czech Republic). The stent is braided from a filament of a complex polymer (polydioxanone, PDX), which disintegrates through hydrolysis, over 3–4 months (Fig. 4.16). This is accelerated within an acidic environment [19]. The PDX skeleton is radiolucent, and only the gold markers are visible on fluoroscopy. Combined with the significant stent shortening, these stents require a conscientious and measured approach when used for the first time.

Due to the reduced elasticity biodegradable stents are currently supplied outside the delivery system and need to be loaded through a funnel prior to use. At present only licensed for the treatment of benign esophageal strictures [20], custom-made devices have been successfully used for fibrotic strictures of the bile duct and anastomotic strictures after gastrectomy and colectomy [21, 22].

They may have a role as an adjuvant for radical chemoradiotherapy for esophageal tumors (Fig. 4.17), but there are perceived difficulties with accurate radiotherapy planning and delivery of the target dose. Furthermore, successful stenting does not guarantee adequate oral intake [23].

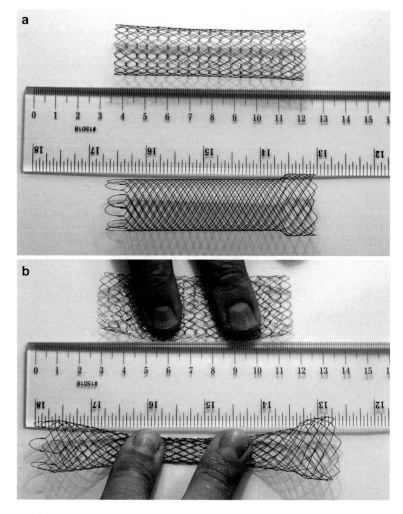

**Fig. 4.14** (**a**) and (**b**) Stent lengthening of a knitted (*Upper*: Niti-S D-stent) and a braided enteral stent (*Lower*: Wallflex)

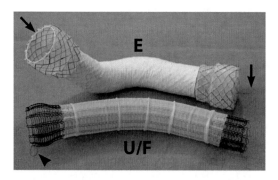

**Fig. 4.15** Knitted esophageal stents. Note the three-dimensional conformability. E: Fully covered removable Egis stent; U/F: partially covered Ultraflex stent. Purse strings for extraction (*arrows*) or repositioning (*arrowhead*) with forceps.

An expansion of the licensing for Ella-BD stents is expected over the next 2 years, and there are first case reports of alternate polymers being applied in the GI tract [24].

## Self-Expanding Plastic Stents

One self-expanding plastic stent (Polyflex, Boston Scientific) is currently available. It has similar characteristics to a metal stent but is cheaper. Not to be confused with the rigid plastic Atkinson tubes used in the beginnings of esophageal stenting, this stent has a braided polyester

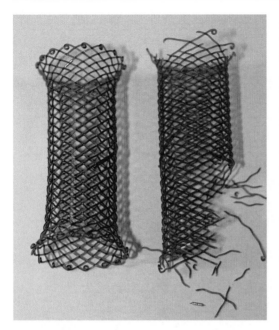

**Fig. 4.16** Biodegradable esophageal stent (Ella-BD) and spontaneous disintegration after 18-month exposure to room air

skeleton covered with silicone on the inside. It requires loading prior to delivery by withdrawing it into the delivery sheath with a flexible basket (Fig. 4.18). The disadvantage is the size of the delivery system, measuring 42 French for the biggest stents. The Polyflex is also radiolucent except for three bands of radiopaque markers. It has a rough outer texture and high radial force and has been used in a wide variety of benign and malignant indications [25–27]. A relatively high complication rate has been reported [28, 29] with migration as high as 63% [30] but can be removed endoscopically by extraction with forceps. Care must be taken that these do not cut through the stent wall.

Although the requirements for a stent within the esophagus and the bowel are very similar, designs for esophageal and enteral stents have pursued different directions.

## Migration of Esophageal Stents

Covered stents are used routinely in the esophagus, thus preventing stent occlusion by tumor ingrowth through the interstices of the stent. This does, however, result in an increased migration rate which is approximately 5% in the esophagus proper, but even with dedicated antimigration designs, at least 15% for stents placed across the gastroesophageal junction [11]. Most esophageal stents are of a *dog-bone* or a double-flared design with the stent ends being of a wider diameter than the stent trunk. In addition, some manufacturers have tried to specifically address the problem of migration. The Ella-HV stent (Ella-CS) has forward facing wings around the circumference of the proximal stent end, resulting in a collar, which anchors it against the stenosis (Fig. 4.19). The Niti-S double stent (Taewoong) is a dog-bone-shaped stent, which has an uncovered stent segment on the outside, designed to be gripped by the mucosa (Fig. 4.20). However, both stents migrate. The outer sleeve of the Niti-S double also stiffens the stent resulting in increased resistance to peristalsis and possibly a higher risk of migration. Whether softer knitted esophageal stents have a lower migration rate due to their better conformability remains to be seen.

Several stents are available with one or both of the ends uncovered. This allows better grip by the mucosa but makes future removal difficult, as there is invariably a degree of mucosal ingrowth into the uncovered mesh. This may be addressed by inserting a second covered stent resulting in pressure necrosis of the hyperplastic mucosa and subsequent removal of both stents together.

Older designs aimed at reducing migration included a conical shape (Flamingo Wallstent, Boston Scientific), but the large inlet funnel occasionally resulted in pressure necrosis of the esophageal wall.

The Gianturco-Z stent (Cook) had small barbs that protruded from the side of the stent to embed in the mucosa. However, this was associated with a high incidence of chest pain and prevented stent removal.

The majority of stents that migrate into the stomach do not cause significant problems. Stents that pass into the duodenum usually proceed to pass through the whole intestine and are often evacuated per ano without the patient noticing. However, impaction within the small bowel can

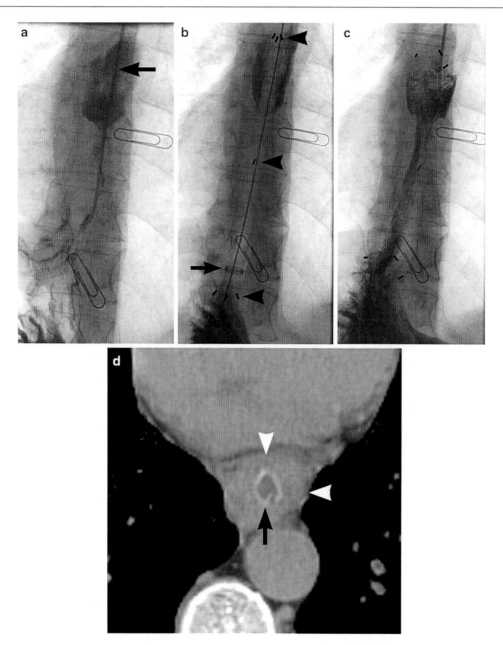

**Fig. 4.17** Biodegradable stent supporting radio-therapy. (**a**) Esophageal stent insertion. Injection of contrast through a biliary manipulation catheter (*arrow*) outlines a long distal stricture demarcated by paper clips on the patient's skin. (**b**) Stent deployment: Except for the gold markers (*arrowheads*), the stent is radiolucent. The three *lower* stent markers have begun to flare out as the delivery sheath is pulled back (*arrow*=distal metal marker on delivery sheath). (**c**) Deployed stent: Injection of contrast shows good position but limited initial expansion. (**d**) Radiotherapy planning CT: The stent (*arrow*) is just visible within the circumferential esophageal tumor (*arrowheads*)

occur (Fig. 4.21), and this may necessitate a laparotomy. With a few exceptions, all modern esophageal stents are removable, usually by a plastic or wire purse string around the stent end; this allows capture with endoscopic forceps and fairly atraumatic extraction. This offers the option of temporary stenting, for example, for the treatment of benign esophageal strictures.

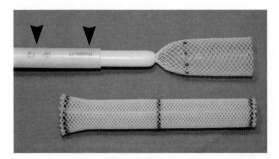

**Fig. 4.18** Self-expanding plastic stent (Polyflex) with capture basket for loading into the delivery system (*arrowheads*)

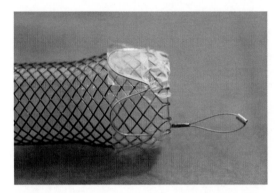

**Fig. 4.19** Esophageal stent with antimigration collar (Ella-HV+)

## Antireflux Stents

Stents placed with their lower end in the gastric fundus predispose the patient to reflux of gastric content. The fundus is the lowest part of the stomach in the supine position, and hydrostatic pressure will force gastric content through a stent into the mid and upper esophagus. This is readily demonstrated on CT scanning. Most esophageal stents are available with an antireflux valve (Fig. 4.22), but the clinical benefit of a valve is still controversial [31]. However, limited evidence suggests potential for a significant benefit, including reduced need for antireflux medication and prevention of aspiration pneumonia and fatal aspiration [5, 32–35] and increased quality of life [36]. A stand-alone retrofit valve (Vysera, Galway, Ireland) may be inserted into patients with an open stent who have troublesome regurgitation of gastric content (Fig. 4.23) [37].

## Bowel

Enteral stents are traditionally placed without covering membrane as the migration rate of covered stents is very high. The risk of displacement in the colon is increased by the passage of feces. It is important that constipation is avoided, but there is no consensus whether a low-residue diet or a diet high in soluble fiber is preferable. From a practical point of view, anything that keeps the patient regular must be a good thing, and stool-softening laxatives should be given routinely. Unfortunately, uncovered stents migrate less but occlude in almost 25%. Compound knitted stents, which sandwich a membrane between two layers of wire mesh, should be a good compromise, but initial outcome data are equivocal [15, 38]. The poor performance of laser-cut enteral stents however confirms that flexibility and conformability are a priority for enteral stents.

## Bile Duct

The greatest variety of different designs are seen in biliary stents, including membrane-based stents and numerous laser-cut stents as spin-offs from vascular designs (Fig. 4.24). Due to the nature of their tubular design, alignment of laser-cut stents is inferior to woven stents (Fig. 4.25), and fractures are not uncommon. Stent occlusion requiring reintervention is increasingly required due to extended patient survival from improved chemotherapy regimes. This becomes particularly challenging if the existing stent does not conform to the biliary anatomy, and reintervention is only possible through the side of the stent skeleton (Fig. 4.26). Care must be taken not to become entangled in the sharp edges of a laser-cut stent.

Covered stents are available for the biliary tree, but these should be considered with great caution. There is a high risk of irreversibly occluding biliary side branches: the cystic duct or the pancreatic duct. In case of a pancreatic head cancer, a covered stent may be a good choice if this can be placed below the origin of the cystic duct. However, obstruction of this can lead to

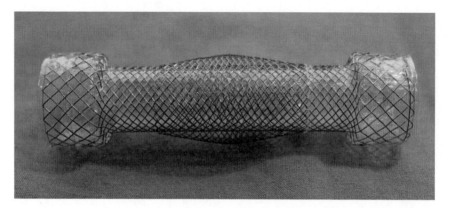

**Fig. 4.20** Esophageal stent with uncovered antimigration segment for mucosal ingrowth (Niti-S double)

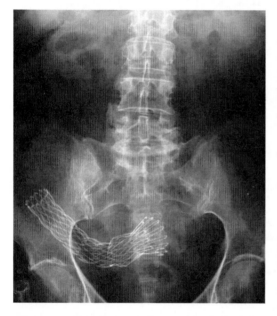

**Fig. 4.21** Migrated esophageal stent (Boubella) at ileo-cecal junction

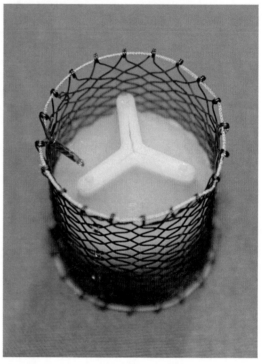

**Fig. 4.23** Antireflux valve for *retrofitting* into an open stent. The silicone valve is mounted in a segment of uncovered nitinol stent, which requires loading into a standard esophageal stent delivery system (viewed from below)

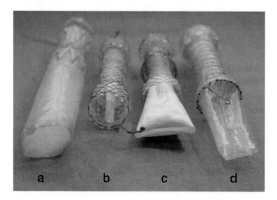

**Fig. 4.22** Stents with antireflux valves. (**a**) Dua (Cook); (**b**) Hanaro (MI-Tech); (**c**) Niti-S double (Taewoong); (**d**) Ella-HV (Ella-CS)

increasing dilatation of the gallbladder and chole-cystitis. The indiscriminate use of covered stents may result in unsalvageable occlusion of essential segmental ducts (Fig. 4.27).

Tumors of the biliary hilum represent a particular challenge. Skilled endoscopists will be able to place bilateral plastic stents in most cases, but these will occlude within 6–12 months. Larger-diameter

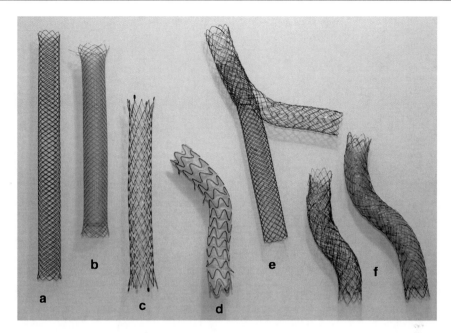

**Fig. 4.24** Biliary stents. (**a**) Ella-SX (braided); (**b**) Covered Wallstent (braided); (**c**) Luminexx (laser-cut); (**d**) PTFE membrane-based Viabil stent with nitinol struts (WL Gore, Flagstaff, AZ, USA); (**e**) T-stent for hilar strictures (Niti-S); (**f**) Bare and covered Egis (knitted)

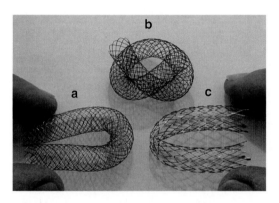

**Fig. 4.25** Luminal patency within a tight bend is well maintained in a knitted (**a**) and braided stent (**b**), whereas the laser-cut stent (**c**) kinks

metal stents tend to give a better long-term result, but bilateral placement is difficult endoscopically [39]. To allow stenting of both hepatic ducts through a single percutaneous approach, fenestrated stents are available, which allow initial placement from one hepatic duct to the other [40], with a further stent inserted downstream through the window, resulting in a coaxial T-configuration (Fig. 4.28). An uncovered stent must be used for this; otherwise, the contralateral side is excluded.

Biodegradable biliary stents are not routinely available, but custom-made devices have been used successfully for treatment of inflammatory biliary strictures [22]. They may play an important role in the future with the increasing numbers of liver transplantations and radical pancreaticoduodenectomies. At present, they are only available off-label with large delivery sheaths up to 13 French, which require very large transhepatic tracks and negate endoscopic insertion.

## Delivery Systems

Designs for delivery systems have converged onto pullback systems, where the stent is released by withdrawing the constraining sheath. The only remaining exception is the Ultraflex system (Boston Scientific) where the stent is tied down to the delivery system with loops of silk thread (Fig. 4.29). This unravels on traction like grandmother's jumper. The disadvantage is the large size and the very rough outer profile of the system, which frequently necessitates predilatation of the stricture in

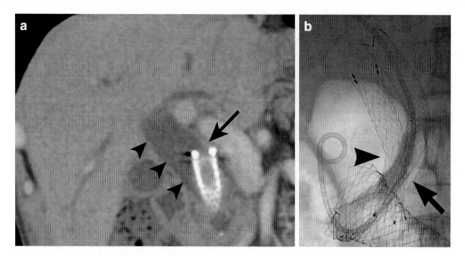

**Fig. 4.26** Reintervention for occluded laser-cut stent (pancreatic carcinoma) (**a**) Coronal CT reconstruction shows a poorly aligned, blocked stent (Luminexx) in a dilated bile duct (*arrowheads*). The *upper* end is partially embedded in the roof of the bile duct (*arrow*). An enteral Wallflex stent is present in the duodenum. (**b**) Attempts at cannulation of the stent failed, and the second stent (Niti-S) could only be placed through the side (*arrow*) of the first stent. The angulation of the laser-cut stent (*arrowhead*) indicates partial fracture. This became separated on follow-up CT (Courtesy of Dr. E. Bakir, North Manchester General Hospital, UK)

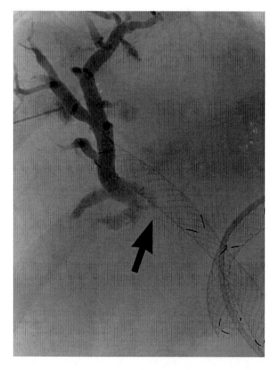

**Fig. 4.27** Occlusion of segmental ducts by placement of bilateral covered biliary stents. Percutaneous cholangiography shows holdup of contrast medium at the junction with the covered stent (*arrow*) (Courtesy of Dr. E. Bakir, North Manchester General Hospital, UK)

order to pass the stent. Pullback delivery systems for most metal esophageal stents measure 16–18 Fr (5–6 mm diameter) but can be considerably larger (e.g., Polyflex). A radiopaque ring at the end of the sheath reduces uncertainty about the degree of deployment. For resheathable stents, a marker indicating the *point of no return* is helpful. Increased control over the deployment process is offered by a pistol grip, where repeated pulling of the trigger slowly withdraws the sheath (Evolution, Cook); the process can be reversed to resheath the stent. It is available for esophageal, enteral, and biliary stents.

The tip of a large delivery system may impact in the deployed stent on withdrawal if the stent has not sufficiently expanded. A quirky delivery system for the early Ella-CS stents consisted of an angioplasty catheter, where the balloon formed the introducer tip. This was deflated prior to deployment, and impaction was completely avoided. It has now been replaced by a tip that sheds two parts of a plastic dilatation on release of the stent (Fig. 4.30). An interim design with a longer releasable tip was abandoned following a case of a perforated sigmoid diverticulum caused by impaction of the tip.

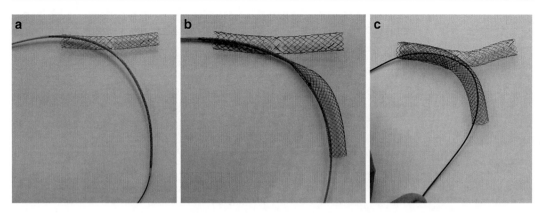

**Fig. 4.28** (**a–c**) Single puncture approach to hilar tumors affecting both hepatic ducts. A fenestrated knitted T-stent is placed from *right* to *left*, followed by a woven stent through the window into the common duct (Both Niti-S)

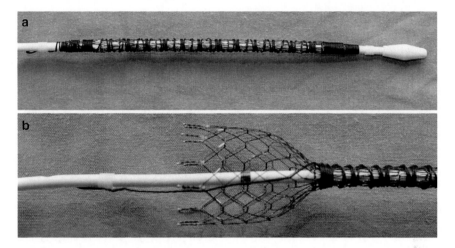

**Fig. 4.29** Thread-release delivery system (Ultraflex precision). (**a**) Undeployed; (**b**) Part-deployed colonic stent

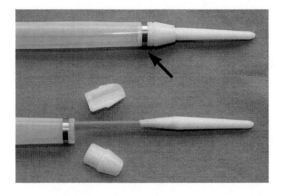

**Fig. 4.30** Compound tip of Ella delivery system. Two plastic dilator cones automatically detach from the flexible central tip on deployment. Note the metal marker ring on the distal end of the delivery sheath (*arrow*)

The DIY experience of loading the Polyflex system can be a challenge to the less playful operator. More importantly though, a balanced choice has to be made between the cost-savings of the stent against the large size and rigidity of the delivery system.

Some esophageal stents are available on a proximal release system for high strictures close to the upper esophageal sphincter (Fig. 4.31). Foreign body sensation increases above the upper margin of C7 vertebral body, and accurate positioning of the proximal end of the stent is essential in the cervical esophagus. The whole sheath is advanced distally and requires removal though the released stent. This requires sufficient

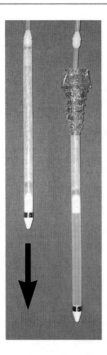

**Fig. 4.31** Proximal release system (Ella-HV). The delivery sheath pushes forward, releasing the stent from the *top*. It is removed through the deployed stent

length of guide wire below the stricture and adequate stent expansion for removal of the system through it.

Few differences between delivery systems for biliary and enteral stents exist; they are mainly limited to the presence of radiopaque markers and nitinol reinforcement of the constraining sheath.

## Summary

An understanding of the properties of different stent designs is helpful in choosing the most appropriate stent for each situation, but departments can only stock a limited supply. Better collaboration between scientists, industry, and clinicians is needed to change current trial-and-error development to purposeful optimization of designs. Ideally, this would involve mathematical modeling as well as a better understanding of stent behavior within the human body.

**Acknowledgments** The author would like to thank BVM Medical, COOK UK, Ella-CS, and UK Medical for their support with demonstration models and S&G Biotech for the provision of images from the manufacturing process.

## References

1. Robertson SW, Ritchie RO. In vitro fatigue-crack growth and fracture toughness behavior of thin-walled superelastic nitinol tube for endovascular stents: a basis for defining the effect of crack-like defects. Biomaterials. 2007;28:700–9.
2. Hajdinjak T, Patel M, Papatsoris A, Masood J, Buchholz N, Birch M. In vitro simulation of stent fracture mechanisms in ureteric nitinol wire stents. Urol Res. 2008;36:241–5.
3. Nikanorov A, Smouse HB, Osman K, Bialas M, Shrivastava S, Schwartz LB. Fracture of self-expanding nitinol stents stressed in vitro under simulated intravascular conditions. J Vasc Surg. 2008;48:435–40.
4. Kauffman GB, Mayo I. The story of nitinol: the serendipitous discovery of the memory metal and its applications. Chem Educ. 1996;2:1–21.
5. Laasch HU, Marriott A, Wilbraham L, Tunnah S, England RE, Martin DF. Effectiveness of open versus antireflux stents for palliation of distal esophageal carcinoma and prevention of symptomatic gastroesophageal reflux. Radiology. 2002;225:359–65.
6. Peck R, Wattam J. Fracture of Memotherm metallic stents in the biliary tract. Cardiovasc Intervent Radiol. 2000;23:55–6.
7. Odurny A. Colonic anastomotic stenoses and Memotherm stent fracture: a report of three cases. Cardiovasc Intervent Radiol. 2001;24:336–9.
8. Suzuki N, Saunders BP, Thomas-Gibson S, Marshall M, Halligan S, Northover JM. Complications of colonic stenting: a case of stent migration and fracture. Endoscopy. 2003;35:1085.
9. Stern N, Smart H. Repeated enteral stent fracture in patient with benign duodenal stricture. Gastrointest Endosc. 2010;72:655–7.
10. Piesman M, Kozarek RA, Brandabur JJ, et al. Improved oral intake after palliative duodenal stenting for malignant obstruction: a prospective multicenter clinical trial. Am J Gastroenterol. 2009;104:2404–11.
11. BSIR. British Society of Interventional Radiology. ROST – Registry of oesophageal stenting, first report 2004. Henley-on-Thames: Dendrite Clinical Systems; 2004. ISBN 1-903968-11-9.
12. Song HY, Shin JH, Yoon CJ, et al. A dual expandable nitinol stent: experience in 102 patients with malignant gastroduodenal strictures. J Vasc Interv Radiol. 2004;15:1443–9.
13. Song GA, Kang DH, Kim TO, et al. Endoscopic stenting in patients with recurrent malignant obstruction after gastric surgery: uncovered versus simultaneously deployed uncovered and covered (double) self-expandable metal stents. Gastrointest Endosc. 2007;65:782–7.

14. Isayama H, Kawabe T, Nakai Y, et al. Management of distal malignant biliary obstruction with the ComVi stent, a new covered metallic stent. Surg Endosc. 2010;24:131–7.

15. Moon CM, Kim TI, Lee MS, et al. Comparison of a newly designed double-layered combination covered stent and D-weave uncovered stent for decompression of obstructive colorectal cancer: a prospective multicenter study. Dis Colon Rectum. 2010;53:1190–6.

16. Kim YW, Choi CW, Kang DH, et al. A double-layered (comvi) self-expandable metal stent for malignant gastroduodenal obstruction: a prospective multicenter study. Dig Dis Sci. 2011;56:2030–6.

17. Tanaka T, Takahashi M, Nitta N, et al. Newly developed biodegradable stents for benign gastrointestinal tract stenoses: a preliminary clinical trial. Digestion. 2006;74:199–205.

18. Fry SW, Fleischer DE. Management of a refractory benign esophageal stricture with a new biodegradable stent. Gastrointest Endosc. 1997;45:179–82.

19. Zilberman M, Nelson KD, Eberhart RC. Mechanical properties and in vitro degradation of bioresorbable fibers and expandable fiber-based stents. J Biomed Mater Res B Appl Biomater. 2005;74:792–9.

20. Repici A, Vleggaar FP, Hassan C, et al. Efficacy and safety of biodegradable stents for refractory benign esophageal strictures: the BEST (Biodegradable Esophageal Stent) study. Gastrointest Endosc. 2010;72:927–34.

21. Janik V, Horak L, Hnanicek J, Malek J, Laasch HU. Biodegradable polydioxanone stents: a new option for therapy-resistant anastomotic strictures of the colon. Eur Radiol. 2011;21(9):1956–61.

22. Petrtyl J, Bruha R, Horak L, Zadorova Z, Dosedel J, Laasch HU. Management of benign intrahepatic bile duct strictures: initial experience with polydioxanone biodegradable stents. Endoscopy. 2010;42(Suppl 2): E89–90.

23. Stivaros SM, Williams LR, Senger C, Wilbraham L, Laasch HU. Woven polydioxanone biodegradable stents: a new treatment option for benign and malignant oesophageal strictures. Eur Radiol. 2010;20:1069–72.

24. Laukkarinen J, Sand J, Leppiniemi J, Kellomaki M, Nordback I. A novel technique for hepaticojejunostomy for nondilated bile ducts: a purse-string anastomosis with an intra-anastomotic biodegradable biliary stent. Am J Surg. 2010;200:124–30.

25. Szegedi L, Gal I, Kosa I, Kiss GG. Palliative treatment of esophageal carcinoma with self-expanding plastic stents: a report on 69 cases. Eur J Gastroenterol Hepatol. 2006;18:1197–201.

26. Fukumoto R, Orlina J, McGinty J, Teixeira J. Use of Polyflex stents in treatment of acute esophageal and gastric leaks after bariatric surgery. Surg Obes Relat Dis. 2007;3:68–71, discussion 71–62.

27. Karbowski M, Schembre D, Kozarek R, Ayub K, Low D. Polyflex self-expanding, removable plastic stents: assessment of treatment efficacy and safety in a variety of benign and malignant conditions of the esophagus. Surg Endosc. 2008;22:1326–33.

28. Ott C, Ratiu N, Endlicher E, et al. Self-expanding Polyflex plastic stents in esophageal disease: various indications, complications, and outcomes. Surg Endosc. 2007;21:889–96.

29. Dua KS, Vleggaar FP, Santharam R, Siersema PD. Removable self-expanding plastic esophageal stent as a continuous, non-permanent dilator in treating refractory benign esophageal strictures: a prospective two-center study. Am J Gastroenterol. 2008;103: 2988–94.

30. Pennathur A, Chang AC, McGrath KM, et al. Polyflex expandable stents in the treatment of esophageal disease: initial experience. Ann Thorac Surg. 2008;85:1968–72, discussion 1973.

31. Blomberg J, Wenger U, Lagergren J, et al. Antireflux stent versus conventional stent in the palliation of distal esophageal cancer. A randomized, multicenter clinical trial. Scand J Gastroenterol. 2009;45:208–16.

32. Nunes CC, Waechter FL, Sampaio JA, Pinto RD, Alvares-Da-Silva MR, Pereira-Lima L. Comparative post-operative study of prostheses, with and without an anti-reflux valve system, in the palliative treatment of esophageal carcinoma. Hepatogastroenterology. 1999;46:2859–64.

33. Osugi H, Lee S, Higashino M, et al. Usefulness of self-expandable metallic stent with an antireflux mechanism as a palliation for malignant strictures at the gastroesophageal junction. Surg Endosc. 2002;16: 1478–82.

34. Homs MY, Wahab PJ, Kuipers EJ, et al. Esophageal stents with antireflux valve for tumors of the distal esophagus and gastric cardia: a randomized trial. Gastrointest Endosc. 2004;60:695–702.

35. Wenger U, Johnsson E, Arnelo U, Lundell L, Lagergren J. An antireflux stent versus conventional stents for palliation of distal esophageal or cardia cancer: a randomized clinical study. Surg Endosc. 2006;20:1675–80.

36. Power C, Byrne PJ, Lim K, et al. Superiority of antireflux stent compared with conventional stents in the palliative management of patients with cancer of the lower esophagus and esophago-gastric junction: results of a randomized clinical trial. Dis Esophagus. 2007;20:466–70.

37. Hirdes MM, Vleggaar FP, Laasch HU, Siersema PD. Technical feasibility and safety of a new, implantable reflux control system to prevent gastroesophageal reflux in patients with stents placed through the lower esophageal sphincter (with video). Gastrointest Endosc. 2012;75(1):174–178.

38. Park S, Cheon JH, Park JJ, et al. Comparison of efficacies between stents for malignant colorectal obstruction: a randomized, prospective study. Gastrointest Endosc. 2010;72:304–10.

39. Saleem A, Baron TH, Gostout CJ. Large-diameter therapeutic channel duodenoscope to facilitate simultaneous deployment of side-by-side self-expandable metal stents in hilar cholangiocarcinoma. Gastrointest Endosc. 2010;72:628–31.

40. Chahal P, Baron TH. Expandable metal stents for endoscopic bilateral stent-within-stent placement for malignant hilar biliary obstruction. Gastrointest Endosc. 2010;71:195–9.

# Part 3

# Overview of Available Prostheses

# Esophageal Prostheses

## Massimo Conio and Antonella De Ceglie

Self-expandable metal stents (SEMS) represent a major breakthrough in the endotherapy field. Esophageal SEMS have acquired a pivotal role in palliation of malignant dysphagia due to esophageal-esophagogastric junction cancers (EC-EGJC) and mediastinal malignancy. Newly available SEMS have been proven safe and effective in relieving such distressing symptoms [1–3] to include dysphagia and chest pain. SEMS improve the quality of life (QoL) of these patients, allowing better nutrition intake which prevents dehydration and aspiration [4–6].

Recanalization of the esophageal lumen can be also achieved by other methods such as laser, argon plasma coagulation, and brachyradiotherapy with or without chemotherapy [7, 8]. However, chemoradiation therapy alone, as primary treatment, can improve dysphagia but requires several weeks. Randomized trials have shown similar efficacy for SEMS and brachytherapy with the consistent result that dysphagia improved more rapidly after stent placement, but the duration of relief was longer after brachytherapy [9–11].

While the role of stents in palliation of malignant strictures has been well established, their use in benign strictures has gained increasing acceptance in the last few years. Severe dysphagia can occur with benign esophageal strictures following radiotherapy, caustic ingestion, peptic injury, and surgery. Placement of a stent in benign strictures is challenging and sometimes risky [12, 13]. Endoscopic dilatation with bougies or through-the-scope (TTS) balloons is the standard treatment for such lesions, but in 10% of patients who develop refractory and recurrent strictures, the temporary placement of a stent should be considered [14–23]. In addition, stents have also been proven effective in management of esophagorespiratory fistula (ERF), anastomotic leaks, and ruptures. Their use has also been promulgated for patients with bleeding esophageal varices [24–26]. This chapter describes the esophageal stents currently used for malignant and benign conditions.

## Available Esophageal Stents

In the United States, the Food and Drug Administration (FDA) has approved esophageal metal stents for palliation of malignant dysphagia: Ultraflex stent (Boston Scientific, Natick, MA, USA); Niti-S stent (Taewoong Medical, Seoul, Korea); Evolution stent (Cook Medical, Winston Salem, NC, USA); Alimaxx-ES (Merit Medical System); Esophageal Z-stent (Cook Medical, Winston Salem, NC, USA); Dua antireflux (Cook Medical, Winston Salem, NC, USA); Wallflex®

M. Conio, M.D. (✉)
Department of Gastroenterology and Digestive Endoscopy, General Hospital Sanremo, C.so Garibaldi 187, 3, Sanremo (IM) 18038, Italy
e-mail: mxconio@libero.it

A. De Ceglie, M.D.
Department of Gastroenterology and Digestive Endoscopy, Cancer Institute Giovanni Paolo II, Bari, Italy

R. Kozarek et al. (eds.), *Self-Expandable Stents in the Gastrointestinal Tract*,
DOI 10.1007/978-1-4614-3746-8_5, © Springer Science+Business Media New York 2013

(Boston Scientific, Natick, MA, USA), and Bonastent® (Standard Sci Tech, Seoul, Korea). Additional stents are currently available in Europe, including Hanaro stent and Choo stent (MI Tech, Seoul, South Korea), the ENDO-FLEX (GmbH, Voerde, Germany), and the FerX-ELLA and SX-ELLA stent (ELLA-CS, Hradec Kralove, Czech Republic). A biodegradable version of ELLA is also available. Table 5.1 displays the variety of SEMS that are marketed. Figure 5.1 shows the most commonly used SEMS types.

Both in Europe and the United States, a removable, fully covered, self-expanding plastic stent (SEPS), the Polyflex (Boston Scientific, Natick, MA, USA), has been introduced as an alternative to SEMS. Because of its removability, the FDA has approved it for benign disease.

We have summarized the technical characteristics of the most commonly available self-expanding metal and plastic stents:

- Ultraflex stent (Boston Scientific, Natick, MA, USA) is a partially covered SEMS with a mesh knitted from a single elastic wire of nitinol. It is mounted with a long thread that holds the compressed stent. The end of the thread is pulled through the catheter lumen to the opposite end of the catheter and tied to a plastic ring. The stent is released by pulling the thread. There are four radiopaque markers. The inner 2 markers indicate the final position of the covered part of the deployed stent and the outer 2 the position of the uncovered portion.
- Wallflex® (Boston Scientific, Natick, MA, USA) is a partially or fully covered stent constructed of multiple braided wires with an internal silicone covering and uncoated flanges on both ends. The fully covered esophageal Wallflex presents the silicone covering extending over the full length of the stent. The presence of *progressive step flared ends* creates a wedge at either end to reduce the migration.
- Niti-S stent (Taewoong Medical, Seoul, Korea) is composed of a single thread of 0.2-mm nitinol wire and an inner polyurethane layer. The stent is delivered in a compressed form inside an introducer sheath of 4 mm in diameter. The company also produces esophageal

SEMS with a delivery system of 10 F that can be introduced through the operative channel of a therapeutic endoscope. To prevent migration, the stent has a *dog-bone* shape: the diameter of the body can be 16, 18, and 20 mm, while that of both ends can be 24, 26, and 28 mm. Another characteristic is the conformability, as the stent adapts to the morphology of the stricture after its release.

- For cancer involving the distal esophagus and the esophagogastric junction, there is a Niti-S *double* stent, with a double-layer configuration over the body, consisting of an inner polyurethane layer (covering the whole stent) and an outer uncovered nitinol wire. The ingrowth of the malignant tissue through the mesh of this outer wire is thought to prevent migration of the stent into the stomach. The Conio stent is a modified Niti-S prosthesis for hypopharyngeal strictures; it is characterized by small diameters (12, 14, and 16 mm in the body; 14, 16, and 18 mm for the flared upper end), and the available lengths are 8, 10, and 12 cm.
- Evolution® stent (Cook Endoscopy, Limerick, Ireland) is made of a single nitinol wire, and it is preloaded on a gun-like delivery system. The stent can be recaptured before it has been completely deployed. In November 2010, the Evolution® Controlled Release Esophageal Fully Covered Stent was approved by the FDA. This stent is characterized by an inner and outer silicone layer that resists tumor ingrowth. Another type of fully covered Esophageal Z-Stent with a DUA antireflux valve (Cook Endoscopy, Winston Salem, NC, USA) is also available.
- Alimaxx-E (Alveolus, Charlotte, NC, USA) is a laser-cut stent from a nitinol tube and fully covered with polyurethane. Small metal struts project from the outer part of the stent to avoid migration. It can be placed over a guide wire in the esophagus. In March 2009, Merit Medical Systems, Inc. (South Jordan, Utah, USA) acquired the products formerly manufactured and distributed by Alveolus, and the Alimaxx-ES™ is the stent now produced.
- SX-ELLA stent (ELLA-CS, Hradec Kralove, Czech Republic) is a SEMS composed of

**Table 5.1** Self-expanding stents marketed

| Stent | Manufacturer | Material | Covered | Length (cm) | Diameter shaft/flare (mm) | Type | Antireflux valve | Retrievable | FDA-approved |
|---|---|---|---|---|---|---|---|---|---|
| Alimaxx–ES | Merit Endotek | Nitinol | Polyurethane | 7/10/12 | 12/14/16/18/22 | FC | No | Yes | Yes not for retrieval |
| Bonastent | Standard Sci Tech | Nitinol | Silicone | 6/8/10/12/15 | 18/23 20/25 22/27 | PC/FC | Yes/no | No | Yes |
| Choo stent | MI Tech | Nitinol | Polyurethane | 8–17 | 18/24 20/26 | PC/FC | Yes (Dostent) | No | No |
| Esophageal Z | Cook | Stainless steel | Polyurethane | 8/10/12/14 | 18/25 | FC/uncoated flanges | Yes (Dua variant) | No | Yes |
| Evolution | Cook | Nitinol | Silicone | 8/10/12.5/15 8/10/12 | 20/25 18/23; 20/25 | PC FC | No | No | Yes |
| SX-ELLA | ELLA-CS | Nitinol | Polyethylene | 8.5/11/13.5/15 | 20/25 | FC | Yes/no | No | No |
| FerX-ELLA | | Stainless steel | | 9/10.5/1213.5/ 15/16.5/19.5/21 | 20/36 | PC/FC | Yes/no | No | |
| SX-ELLA BD | | Polydioxane | | 6/8/10/13.5 | 18/23 20/25 23/28 25/31 | BD | No | Yes | |
| Hanaro | MI Tech | Nitinol | Silicone | 8–17 | 18/24 | FC | Yes/no | No | No |
| Hanaro benign BS | | | | 8–12 | 20/26 22/28 | FC | No | Yes | |
| Niti-S | Taewoong Medical | Nitinol | Polyurethane | 8/10/12/15 | 16/24 18/26 20/28 | PC FC | Yes/no | No Yes | Yes |

(continued)

**Table 5.1** (continued)

| Stent | Manufacturer | Material | Covered | Length (cm) | Diameter shaft/flare (mm) | Type | Antireflux valve | Retrievable | FDA-approved |
|---|---|---|---|---|---|---|---|---|---|
| Polyflex | Boston Scientific | Polyester | Silicone | 9/12/15 | 16/20 18/23 21/28 | FC | No | Yes | Yes |
| Song | Stentech | Nitinol | Polyurethane | 5–18 | 16 18 | NC/PC/FC Double stent | | No | No |
| Ultraflex | Boston Scientific | Nitinol | Polyurethane | 10/12/15 | 18/23 23/28 | NC PC | No | No | Yes |
| Wallflex | Boston Scientific | Nitinol | Silicone | 10/12/15 | 18/23 18/25 23/28 | FC PC | No | Yes No | Yes |

*FDA* Food and Drug Administration, *FC* fully covered, *PC* partially covered, *NC* not covered, *BD* biodegradable

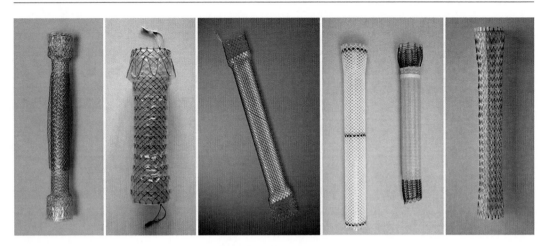

**Fig. 5.1** A variety of partially and fully covered self-expanding stents. From *left* to *right*: Niti-S *double stent*, SX-ELLA stent, Evolution stent, Polyflex, Ultraflex stent, Alimaxx-E stent

nitinol. The metal stents are coated with a polyethylene layer and are also available with an antireflux flap. At the proximal end, there is an antimigration ring designed to invert with antegrade traction, opposing peristalsis and preventing migration. A biodegradable version of the SX-ELLA made of polydioxanone is now available.

- Polyflex® stent (Boston Scientific, Natick, MA, USA) is a self-expanding plastic stent made of a polyester monofilament netting embedded in silicone. The diameter of the delivery system ranges between 12 and 14 mm contingent upon stent diameter. The stent needs to be loaded into the delivery device using a back loader, which is provided in the kit.

- Another type of stent (the ENDO-FLEX, GmbH, Voerde, Germany), both covered and partially covered, with nylon threads on both ends for easy repositioning or removal, has also been marketed, but no published data are available.

## Comparison Among Stents

Since the early 1990s, SEMS have become the most used device for palliation of malignant dysphagia, replacing plastic prosthesis, which are still widely used in many developing countries because of their low cost [1, 27]. However, the extra cost of SEMS is offset by the cost of man-

aging the complications occurring more frequently after plastic stents deployment [28, 29].

Esophageal SEMS can be (1) uncovered, (2) partially covered, or (3) fully covered.

In a meta-analysis, Yakoub et al. evaluated the outcome from 12 studies comparing SEMS and plastic stents (6 randomized controlled trials; 6 nonrandomized/retrospective studies) and 8 studies comparing covered SEMS versus uncovered SEMS (1 randomized controlled trial; 7 retrospective studies) for a total of 911 patients. Data suggested that the use of SEMS, in comparison with plastic stents, was associated with less stent insertion-related mortality (1.7% vs. 11.1%), less incidence of esophageal perforation (1,4% vs. 9.4%), and less stent migration (2.1% vs. 13.1%), whereas no significant difference was noticed in terms of other stent-related morbidity and 30-day mortality.

Uncovered SEMS had a higher rate of tumor ingrowth (63% vs. 37%) despite a decreased migration rate (3.09% vs. 12.59%) [30]. The use of uncovered SEMS has been largely abandoned due to the high rate of restenosis causing recurrent dysphagia because of tumor or granulation tissue ingrowth, requiring repeated endoscopic intervention [31–33]. Furthermore, uncovered stents should not be used for patients with malignant extrinsic compression because the pressure of the mesh can cause necrosis of the wall and fistula formation.

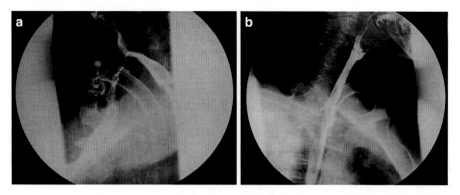

**Fig. 5.2** (a) Esophagocutaneous fistula postlaryngectomy. (b) A "dog-bone" $16 \times 24 \times 80$-mm Taewoong SEMS has been placed, sealing the fistula

Currently, several types of SEMS exist and vary by type of alloy, configuration, degree of shortening after release, length and diameter, type and extent of covering, delivery system, expandable force, presence or absence of antireflux valve, and removability. Almost all SEMS are made of nitinol, an alloy of nickel and titanium, whose peculiarity is superelasticity and shape memory. The covering is either polyurethane or silicone or polytetrafluoroethylene (PTFE). Their flexibility, the small diameter of the delivery system, and the large availability of models allow the treatment of any type of malignant esophageal obstruction and esophagorespiratory fistula (ERF) [34–36] (Fig. 5.2).

In patients treated with SEMS, dysphagia is relieved in approximately 90%, and these patients undergo significantly fewer procedures, spending fewer days in the hospital [36, 37].

Randomized studies have been carried out to identify the ideal prosthesis having favorable outcome in terms of clinical results and complications. There are no data to date demonstrating significant differences in outcomes or complications among SEMS types. Therefore, the choice of specific SEMS is often based on availability or endoscopist's preference and experience, although the initial stent selection has a significant impact on the clinical outcome in patients with inoperable malignancy [27, 38]. In some countries, such as Italy, cost has become an important factor in stent acquisition and availability, although the difference in the cost among SEMS is potentially small [26, 39].

Table 5.2 lists all prospective randomized trials comparing two or more types of esophageal stents published since 2001. The technical success rate for SEMS release was 100% in the majority of studies, and dysphagia score was improved in 83–100% of patients [32, 35, 40].

Placement of a Polyflex can improve malignant dysphagia in 86–100% of patients [35, 41–43]. It should be stressed that the major drawback of Polyflex stent is the excessively large delivery system, requiring dilatation before placement, increasing the risk of severe complications.

The degree of immediate dysphagia improvement did not differ among studies comparing different types of covered SEMS [32, 35, 44], covered versus uncovered SEMS, or SEMS versus SEPS, although significantly more interventions were needed for uncovered SEMS to treat recurrent dysphagia [32, 35, 44, 45].

Comparing three different types of partially covered expandable metal stents (Gianturco Z-stent, Ultraflex, and Flamingo Wallstent) for the palliation of dysphagia due to esophageal cancer (EC) or esophagogastric junction cancer (EGJC), Siersema et al. reported no statistically significant differences among stent types in the improvement of dysphagia score, recurrent dysphagia, migration, or survival. Placement of Gianturco Z-stents was associated with a trend toward more complications when compared with Ultraflex stents and Flamingo Wallstents (36% vs. 24% and 18%) [44]. Retrospective data reported more stent-related complications in

**Table 5.2** Prospective randomized studies on esophageal stents

| Author/year | n pts | Site tumor | Stent type (n pts) | Technical success n (%) | Dysphagia pre | Dysphagia post | CT/RT pre (n pts) | CT/RT post (n pts) | Predilation type mm (mean) | Complications early | Complications late | Survival (median) |
|---|---|---|---|---|---|---|---|---|---|---|---|---|
| Blomberg et al. (2010) [52] | 65 | Esophagus EGJ | Esophageal Z Dua stent (Cook) [28] | 28/28 (100%) | Scores 62 | Scores 56 | ND | ND | Balloon up to 15 | ND | Migration: 7% Obstruction: 18% Hemorrhage: 7% Severe pain: 4% Others: 14% | 63 days (4–393) |
| | | | Esophageal Z-stent (Cook) | 37/37 (100%) | Scores 45 | Scores 45 | ND | ND | Balloon up to 15 | ND | Perforation: 3% | 70 days (4–511) |
| | | | Ultraflex (Boston) | | | | | | | | Migration: 11% | |
| | | | Wallstent (Boston) [37] | | | | | | | | Obstruction: 11% Hemorrhage: 3% Severe pain: 14% Other: 11% | |
| Kim et al. (2009) [64] | 37 | Esophagus EGJ | Niti-S covered (Taewoong) [19] | 19/19 (100%) | Mean 2.95±0.52 | Mean 1.00±0.64 | 9 CT/RT | 2 CT/RT | None | Pneumonia: 5% | Migration: 5% Hemorrhage: 11% Overgrowth: 26% Reflux: 11% | 62 days |
| | | | Niti-S double-layered (Taewoong) [18] | 17/18 (94%) | Mean 2.94±0.41 | Mean 1.08±0.49 | 7 CT/RT | 3 CT/RT | | | Fistula: 6% Bolus impaction: 6% | 74 days |
| Sabharwal et al. (2008) [51] | 48 | Lower third of esophagus EGJ | Ultraflex (Boston) [26] | 26/26 (100%) | Median 3 | Median 0 | 6 CTRT 13 CT 1 RT | ND | Balloon 14 | Migration: 8% Reflux: 8% Severe pain: 35% | Migration: 15% Hemorrhage: 8% Fistula: 4% Obstruction: 27% | Mean follow-up 101 days |
| | | | FerX-ELLA valve (ELLA CS) [22] | 22/22 (100%) | Median 3 | Median 0 | 5 CTRT 6 CT 2 RT | ND | | Reflux: 9% Severe pain: 9% | Migration: 32% Hemorrhage: 5% Reflux: 4% Obstruction: 9% | Mean follow-up 78 days |

(continued)

**Table 5.2** (continued)

| Author/year n pts | Site tumor | Stent type (n pts) | Technical success n (%) | Dysphagia pre | Dysphagia post | CT/RT pre (n pts) | CT/RT post (n pts) | Predilation type mm (mean) | Complications early | Complications late | Survival (median) |
|---|---|---|---|---|---|---|---|---|---|---|---|
| Verschuur et al. 125 (2008) [45] | Esophagus | Polyflex (Boston) [41] | 34/41 (83%) | Median 3 | Median 1 | 7 CT | 2 CT | Savary up to 12 | Perforation: 5% | Hemorrhage: 12% | 102 days |
| | EGJ | | | | | 5 CTRT | | | Pneumoniae: 2% | Mild pain: 2% | |
| | | | | | | | | | | Reflux: 5% | |
| | | | | | | | | | | Migration: 29% | |
| | | | | | | | | | | Tissue growth: 10% | |
| | | | | | | | | | | Bolus impaction: 5% | |
| | | Ultraflex (Boston) [42] | 42/42 (100%) | Median 3 | Median 0 | 8 CT | 7 CT | | Severe pain: 2% | Hemorrhage: 12% | 132 days |
| | | | | | | 3 RT | | | Fever: 2% | Fistula: 5% | |
| | | | | | | 3 CTRT | | | | Mild pain: 5% | |
| | | | | | | | | | | Reflux: 2% | |
| | | | | | | | | | | Migration: 17% | |
| | | | | | | | | | | Tissue growth: 31% | |
| | | | | | | | | | | Bolus impaction: 24% | |
| | | Niti-S (Taewoong) [42] | 40/42 (95%) | Median 3 | Median 0 | 7 CT | 15 CT | | Hemorrhage: 2% | Hemorrhage: 2% | 159 days |
| | | | | | | 1 RT | | | Severe pain: 5% | Fistula: 2% | |
| | | | | | | 3 CTRT | | | | Mild pain: 5% | |
| | | | | | | | | | | Reflux: 7% | |
| | | | | | | | | | | Migration: 12% | |
| | | | | | | | | | | Tissue growth: 24% | |
| | | | | | | | | | | Bolus impaction: 2% | |

Gianturco Z-stent with a large diameter compared with a large-diameter Ultraflex or Flamingo Wallstent [46]. In a prospective study, recurrent dysphagia due to tumor overgrowth was noticed less frequently with Ultraflex stents ($P=0.05$) in comparison with Flamingo Wallstents and Z-stents, while migration occurred more frequently ($P=0.05$) [47].

Tissue ingrowth was more frequent in partially, than fully, covered stents, although the difference was not statistically significant (31% in Ultraflex vs. 24% in Niti-S stents and 10% in Polyflex stents) [45]. Conio et al. reported recurrent dysphagia caused by tumor overgrowth in the same percentage of patients treated with Polyflex and Ultraflex stents (20% vs. 19%), but the median time for the occurrence of tumor overgrowth was longer in Polyflex group (107 vs. 97 days). Significantly more complications, in particular late stent migration, were observed in the Polyflex group [35]. Because of the high rate of stent migration, great radial pressure, and the excessively large delivery system, SEPS should not be used in patients with malignancy [35, 45].

## Antireflux Stents

Stents placed across the gastroesophageal junction provide inferior palliation and an increased number of complications to include migration and severe gastroesophageal reflux, risk of pulmonary aspiration, and pneumonia [36]. Conflicting data have been reported on the efficacy of antireflux stents in relieving symptoms (Table 5.2).

Antireflux stents (ARSs) of different designs have been introduced [48–52]. Studies comparing ARSs with conventional stents have shown better reflux control in the former [48, 53, 54]. However, a recent meta-analysis did not corroborate these data [55].

Considering the health-related quality of life (HRQL) in patients with EC or EGJC, treated with Esophageal Z-stent, with a Dua antireflux valve, or without it (Esophageal Z-stent, Ultraflex, and Wallstent), no statistically significant difference was observed. Unexpectedly, more reflux symptoms were reported in patients treated with antireflux stent compared to the conventional ones [52].

These results are similar to those reported by Homs et al. who compared, in patients with EGJC, FerX-ELLA stents with a windsock-type antireflux valve and open stents of similar design but without the antireflux system. No significant improvement of dysphagia, occurrence of complications, survival, gastroesophageal reflux symptoms, or difference in 24-h pH monitoring existed between the two groups [50].

## Fully Covered/Retrievable SEMS

Fully covered self-expanding metal stents (FCSEMS) have been introduced recently to counter the shortcomings of SEPS. They have been developed for malignant esophageal disease, and only occasionally have they been used in benign disorders.

Because of the low incidence of benign refractory strictures, only small case series, case reports, and retrospective studies considering removable FCSEMS (plastic and metal) have been published.

A meta-analysis, including eight studies (two receiving nitinol stents and six, Polyflex), showed that the efficacy of these stents in benign refractory strictures was 46%. However, they were associated with a migration rate of 26%. Polyflex stents have been purported to have a significantly better primary result than nitinol stents (55.3% vs. 21.8%), but a higher migration rate (30% vs. 21.8%, $p>0.05$). Analysis suggests that the migration rate may be related to the number of pre-stent dilatations, while on meta-regression analysis, confounding variables (sex, age, race, etiology, stricture location and length, time to removal, duration of follow-up) had no significant influence on the outcome [16].

A removable stent might also be used in malignant strictures as a *bridge to surgery* in patients undergoing neoadjuvant chemoradiation in order to improve the nutritional intake [11, 56–60]. FDA-approved FCSEMS include the Niti-S, the covered Wallflex, and the Alimaxx-ES, all approved only for malignant strictures.

FCSEMS, as well as Polyflex prostheses, should be easily removable because of their limited tissue reaction, although migration occurs more frequently [59]. However, the removal of these stents is more traumatic and risky than covered nitinol SEMS, which are more flexible. Recently, Uidehaag et al. found a 16% incidence of recurrent dysphagia due to tissue overgrowth in patients with EC/EGJC treated with the Alimaxx-E stent; this value was in line with the rates reported in literature with Polyflex stents, but lower than those reported with fully covered and partially covered metal stents. A high migration rate has also been reported (36%) [61]. Removability of Alimaxx has been demonstrated also by Bakken et al., but the authors highlighted the relative moderate clinical efficacy because of stent migration [62].

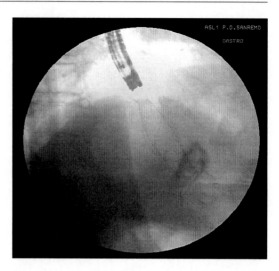

**Fig. 5.3** *Double-layer* SEMS in patient with esophagogastric junction cancer

The treatment of benign esophageal disease by FCSEMS (Alimaxx) placement was successful in 31% of patients in a study by Eloubedi et al. and was particularly useful in patients with esophageal leaks/perforations. Migration occurred in 34% of cases. All stents were retrieved successfully, except one which was fractured [21]. Stent fragmentation during removal has been reported in a few case reports because of disintegration of the polyurethane coating; this problem has been partly solved by coating the inner lining of the stent with silicone (Alimaxx-ES) [63]. To prevent migration, a double-layered Niti-S stent was introduced (Fig. 5.3). A reduction in the rate of recurrent malignant dysphagia has been reported when comparing the double-layer Niti-S stent with Ultraflex and Polyflex (31% vs. 52% and 37%), due, in part, to reduced migration (12% vs. 17% and 29%) [45]. The absence of tissue overgrowth has been reported in double-layered Niti-S stents when compared to the covered Niti-S (0% vs. 26%) in malignant strictures. The overall complication rate was higher with the covered Niti-S than in the double-layer group (58% vs. 12%) [64].

The treatment of benign esophageal strictures by temporary placement of Niti-S stents has been safe and effective during the period of the stent placement, in spite of the high rates of tissue hyperproliferation and migration, particularly

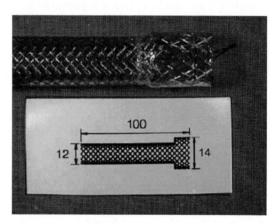

**Fig. 5.4** The modified Niti-S stent for hypopharyngeal strictures (*Conio stent*)

when stents were placed in the proximal and distal esophagus. Dysphagia caused by stricture recurrence following stent removal occurred in 69% of subjects, and a long length of stricture (>7 cm) was the only significant factor associated with decreased long-term patency [65].

In refractory hypopharyngeal strictures after laryngectomy and radiotherapy, Conio et al. used a Niti-S stent designed by the authors (Niti-S Conio Cervical Stent) (Figs. 5.4 and 5.5). These stents were characterized by small diameters that avoided a foreign body sensation. The cover prevented ingrowth of granulation tissue and allowed a safe removal of the stent [18].

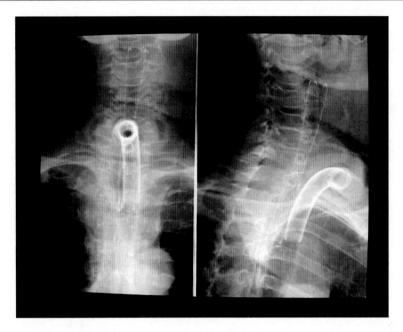

**Fig. 5.5** A *Conio stent* in a patient with refractory hypopharyngeal stricture following laryngectomy and radiotherapy

The ELLA stents (the FerX-ELLA made of stainless steel and the SX-ELLA made of nitinol) fully coated with a polyethylene wrap have been recently introduced in Europe. In a prospective study, the SX-ELLA has provided good symptomatic relief of malignant dysphagia, with a low rate of tissue overgrowth compared to previously reported, other, fully covered stents, possibly due to the large size of the midportion of the SX-ELLA (20 mm). Despite the stent design, the frequency of stent migration does not differ from that of other SEMS [66]. Case reports also have evaluated the safety and efficacy of SX-ELLA stent in the management of refractory variceal bleeding [67–69].

## Newly Available Stents

In 2008, a biodegradable (BD) SX-ELLA stent was introduced. The stent is manufactured from woven polydioxanone monofilament, which degrades by random hydrolysis accelerated by a low ambient pH. Stent integrity and radial force are maintained for 6–8 weeks following deployment, and its disintegration usually occurs by 11–12 weeks postdeployment. The degradation products are harmful; the stent material is partly

absorbed and partly travels through the gastrointestinal tract. The diameter of the stent is 25 mm with both ends flaring to 31 mm; different lengths are available, ranging from 60 to 135 mm. Recently, smaller sized [18, 20, 23] stents have been made available in Europe. The stent design is similar to an uncovered enteral stent, and it needs to be loaded into a 28-F applicator. After release, the stent expands gradually achieving its preformed diameter after 24–48 h. Generally, predilatation of the stenosis is recommended, as BD stents have a radial force lower than nitinol stents. This stent does not require removal, even after migration. Currently, it is only approved for use in benign strictures, although it has been applied in malignant disease.

The utility of BD stents was evaluated in small series from Japan and Europe. In benign strictures, Saito et al., using an Ultraflex stent made of poly-L-lactic monofilaments (PLLA), reported stent migration in 77% of the cases within 10–21 days of placement, without development of a primary stricture or restenosis during 2 years of follow-up [70]. The same investigators reported encouraging results in two patients with benign stenosis from endoscopic submucosal dissection for early esophageal cancer [71]. A low migration

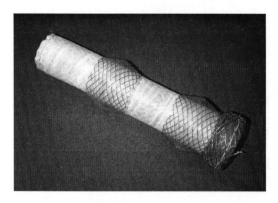

**Fig. 5.6** A new prototype stent with antimigration rings (Taewoong) for benign esophageal strictures

rate and complete relief of dysphagia in nearly 50% of patients with benign, refractory strictures have also been reported obtained by Repici et al., using the BD SX-ELLA [19].

Severe granulomatous in- and overgrowth leading to stent obstruction can occur with these stents [19, 72]. The relief of dysphagia was 30% and 33%, respectively, in a prospective, nonrandomized study comparing the efficacy and safety of the Polyflex with ELLA BD stents in the treatment of benign refractory esophageal strictures. Patients with BD stents required fewer procedures than patients with SEPS (33% vs. 50%); however, more stent-related complications occurred after BD stent placement (44%) than after SEPS placement (25%) [73].

A new prototype of nitinol stent has been recently proposed in patients with benign refractory esophageal strictures. It is completely covered and has two covered rings in its outer part, which should mitigate migration. The stent is under evaluation by our group, and no preliminary data are available (Fig. 5.6).

Drug-eluting, partially covered stents have gained interest for esophageal stenting as they might inhibit granulation tissue overgrowth. However, no human trials have been reported. In animal study on dogs, SEMS coated with the antiproliferative chemotherapeutic agent paclitaxel caused little tissue hyperplastic reaction and were easily removed [74]. A study using a 5-fluorouracil-containing SEMS in a rabbit model demonstrated maximal drug levels in a sustained manner for 45 days in the tissue in direct contact with the stent, with low levels in the serum and liver [75].

## Conclusions

At present, the endoscopist can select a stent among a wide variety of models. However, there are no striking differences among the marketed stents. It is important to consider the flexibility of the stent before using it, as we believe that the incidence of complications can be reduced (pressure necrosis, ERF) with increased flexibility.

The ideal stent does not exist yet. Migration and benign or malignant tissue overgrowth are unsolved problems. The introduction of conformable stents represents an interesting evolution in this field, even if randomized studies are lacking. Technical improvements are essential in the treatment of benign strictures, where results are unsatisfactory due to recurrence of the stricture in almost 50% of patients. In this subgroup of patients, drug-eluting stents with antifibrosis agents could represent a useful approach.

## References

1. Schembre DB. Recent advances in the use of stents for esophageal disease. Gastrointest Endosc Clin N Am. 2010;20:103–21.
2. Mohan V, Kozarek RA. Placement of conventional and expandable stents for malignant esophageal stenoses. Tech Gastrointest Endosc. 2001;3: 166–75.
3. Xinopoulos D, Dimitroulopoulos D, Moschandrea I, et al. Natural course of inoperable esophageal cancer treated with metallic expandable stents: quality of life and cost-effectiveness analysis. J Gastroenterol Hepatol. 2004;19:1397–402.
4. Madhusudhan C, Saluja SS, Pal S, Ahuja V, et al. Palliative stenting for relief of dysphagia in patients with inoperable esophageal cancer: impact on quality of life. Dis Esophagus. 2009;22:331–6.
5. Maroju NK, Anbalagan P, Kate V, et al. Improvement in dysphagia and quality of life with self-expanding metallic stents in malignant esophageal strictures. Indian J Gastroenterol. 2006;25:62–5.
6. White RE, Parker RK, Fitzwater JW, et al. Stents as sole therapy for oesophageal cancer: a prospective analysis of outcomes after placement. Lancet Oncol. 2009;10:240–6.

7. Langer FB, Zacherl J. Palliative endoscopic interventions in esophageal cancer. Eur Surg. 2007;39: 288–94.

8. Siersema PD. New developments in palliative therapy. Best Pract Res Clin Gastroenterol. 2006;20:959–78.

9. Hayter CR, Huff-Winters C, Paszat L, et al. A prospective trial of short-course radiotherapy plus chemotherapy for palliation of dysphagia from advanced esophageal cancer. Radiother Oncol. 2000;56: 329–33.

10. Homs MY, Steyerberg EW, Eijkenboom WM, et al. Single-dose brachytherapy versus metal stent placement for the palliation of dysphagia from oesophageal cancer: multicentre randomised trial. Lancet. 2004;364:1497–504.

11. Bower M, Jones W, Vessels B, et al. Nutritional support with endoluminal stenting during neoadjuvant therapy for esophageal malignancy. Ann Surg Oncol. 2009;16:3161–8.

12. Spechler SJ. American Gastroenterological Association medical position statement on treatment of patients with dysphagia caused by benign disorders of the distal esophagus. Gastroenterology. 1999;117:229–33.

13. Ferguson DD. Evaluation and management of benign esophageal strictures. Dis Esophagus. 2005;18:359–64.

14. Lew RJ, Kochman ML. A review of endoscopic methods of esophageal dilation. J Clin Gastroenterol. 2002;35:117–26.

15. Kochman ML, McClave SA, Boyce HW. The refractory and the recurrent esophageal stricture: a definition. Gastrointest Endosc. 2005;62:474–5.

16. Thomas T, Abrams KR, Subramanian V, et al. Esophageal stents for benign refractory strictures: a meta-analysis. Endoscopy. 2011;43:386–93.

17. Repici A, Hassan C, Sharma P, et al. Systematic review: the role of self-expanding plastic stents for benign oesophageal strictures. Aliment Pharmacol Ther. 2010;31:1268–75.

18. Conio M, Blanchi S, Filiberti R, et al. A modified self-expanding Niti-S stent for the management of benign hypopharyngeal strictures. Gastrointest Endosc. 2007;65:714–20.

19. Repici A, Vleggaar FP, Hassan C, et al. Efficacy and safety of biodegradable stents for refractory benign esophageal strictures: the BEST (Biodegradable Esophageal Stent) study. Gastrointest Endosc. 2010;72: 927–34.

20. Repici A, Conio M, De Angelis C, et al. Temporary placement of an expandable polyester silicone-covered stent for treatment of refractory benign esophageal strictures. Gastrointest Endosc. 2004;60:513–9.

21. Eloubeidi MA, Talreja JP, Lopes TL, et al. Success and complications associated with placement of fully covered removable self-expandable metal stents for benign esophageal diseases (with videos). Gastrointest Endosc. 2011;73:673–81.

22. Baron TH. Role of endoscopy in the management of esophageal diseases. Minerva Gastroenterol Dietol. 2008;54:415–27.

23. Schembre D. Advances in esophageal stenting: the evolution of fully covered stents for malignant and benign disease. Adv Ther. 2010;27:413–25.

24. Ross WA, Alkassab F, Lynch PM, et al. Evolving role of self-expanding metal stents in the treatment of malignant dysphagia and fistulas. Gastrointest Endosc. 2007;65:70–7.

25. Dai Y, Chopra SS, Kneif S, Hünerbein M. Management of esophageal anastomotic leaks, perforations, and fistulae with self-expanding plastic stents. J Thorac Cardiovasc Surg. 2011;141:1213–7.

26. Sharma P, Kozarek R. Role of esophageal stents in benign and malignant diseases. Practice parameters committee of American College of gastroenterology. Am J Gastroenterol. 2010;105:258–73.

27. Ramirez FC, Dennert B, Zierer ST, Sanowski RA. Esophageal self-expandable metallic stents–indications, practice, techniques, and complications: results of a national survey. Gastrointest Endosc. 1997;45: 360–4.

28. O'Donnell CA, Fullarton GM, Watt E, et al. Randomized clinical trial comparing self-expanding metallic stents with plastic endoprostheses in the palliation of oesophageal cancer. Br J Surg. 2002;89: 985–92.

29. Siersema PD, Hop WC, Dees J, et al. Coated self-expanding metal stents versus latex prostheses for esophagogastric cancer with special reference to prior radiation and chemotherapy a controlled, prospective study. Gastrointest Endosc. 1998;47:113–20.

30. Yakoub D, Fahmy R, Athanasiou T, et al. Evidence-based choice of esophageal stent for the palliative management of malignant dysphagia. World J Surg. 2008;32:1996–2009.

31. Conio M, Blanchi S, Filiberti R, De Ceglie A. Self-expanding plastic stent to palliate symptomatic tissue in/overgrowth after self-expanding metal stent placement for esophageal cancer. Dis Esophagus. 2010;23:590–6.

32. Vakil N, Morris AI, Marcon N, et al. A prospective, randomized, controlled trial of covered expandable metal stents in the palliation of malignant esophageal obstruction at the gastroesophageal junction. Am J Gastroenterol. 2001;96:1791–6.

33. Saranovic DJ, Djuric-Stefanovic A, Ivanovic A, et al. Fluoroscopically guided insertion of self-expandable metal esophageal stents for palliative treatment of patients with malignant stenosis of esophagus and cardia: comparison of uncovered and covered stent types. Dis Esophagus. 2005;18:230–8.

34. Baron TH. A practical guide for choosing an expandable metal stent for GI malignancies: is a stent by any other name still a stent? Gastrointest Endosc. 2001;54:269–72.

35. Conio M, Repici A, Battaglia G, et al. A randomized prospective comparison of self-expandable plastic stents and partially covered self-expandable metal stents in the palliation of malignant esophageal dysphagia. Am J Gastroenterol. 2007;102:2667–77.

36. Baron TH. Expandable metal stents for the treatment of cancerous obstruction of the gastrointestinal tract. N Engl J Med. 2001;344:1681–7.

37. Nicholson DA, Haycox A, Kay CL, et al. The cost effectiveness of metal oesophageal stenting in malignant disease compared with conventional therapy. Clin Radiol. 1999;54:212–5.

38. Rao C, Haycock A, Zacharakis E, et al. Economic analysis of esophageal stenting for management of malignant dysphagia. Dis Esophagus. 2009;22:337–47.

39. Conio M, De Ceglie A, Blanchi S, Fisher DA. Esophageal strictures, tumors, and fistulae: stents for primary esophageal cancer. Tech Gastrointest Endosc. 2010;12:191–202.

40. Sabharwal T, Hamady MS, Chui S, et al. A randomised prospective comparison of the Flamingo Wallstent and Ultraflex stent for palliation of dysphagia associated with lower third oesophageal carcinoma. Gut. 2003;52:922–6.

41. Karbowski M, Schembre D, Kozarek R, et al. Polyflex self-expanding, removable plastic stents: assessment of treatment efficacy and safety in a variety of benign and malignant conditions of the esophagus. Surg Endosc. 2008;22:1326–33.

42. Siersema PD, Dees J, van Blankenstein M. Palliation of malignant dysphagia from oesophageal cancer. Rotterdam oesophageal tumor study group. Scand J Gastroenterol. 1998;225(Suppl):75–84.

43. Costamagna G, Shah SK, Tringali A, et al. Prospective evaluation of a new self-expanding plastic stent for inoperable esophageal strictures. Surg Endosc. 2003;17:891–5.

44. Siersema PD, Hop WC, van Blankenstein M, et al. A comparison of 3 types of covered metal stents for the palliation of patients with dysphagia caused by esophagogastric carcinoma: a prospective, randomized study. Gastrointest Endosc. 2001;54:145–53.

45. Verschuur EM, Repici A, Kuipers EJ, et al. New design esophageal stents for the palliation of dysphagia from esophageal or gastric cardia cancer: a randomized trial. Am J Gastroenterol. 2008;103:304–12.

46. Verschuur EM, Steyerberg EW, Kuipers EJ, Siersema PD. Effect of stent size on complications and recurrent dysphagia in patients with esophageal or gastric cardia cancer. Gastrointest Endosc. 2007;65:592–601.

47. Homs MY, Steyerberg EW, Kuipers EJ, et al. Causes and treatment of recurrent dysphagia after self-expanding metal stent placement for palliation of esophageal carcinoma. Endoscopy. 2004;36:880–6.

48. Dua KS, Kozarek R, Kim J, et al. Self-expanding metal esophageal stent with anti-reflux mechanism. Gastrointest Endosc. 2001;53:603–13.

49. Do YS, Choo SW, Suh SW, et al. Malignant esophagogastric junction obstruction: palliative treatment with an antireflux valve stent. J Vasc Interv Radiol. 2001;12:647–51.

50. Homs MY, Wahab PJ, Kuipers EJ, Steyerberg EW, et al. Esophageal stents with antireflux valve for tumors of the distal esophagus and gastric cardia: a randomized trial. Gastrointest Endosc. 2004;60:695–702.

51. Sabharwal T, Gulati MS, Fotiadis N, et al. Randomised comparison of the FerX Ella antireflux stent and the Ultraflex stent: proton pump inhibitor combination for prevention of post-stent reflux in patients with esophageal carcinoma involving the esophago-gastric junction. J Gastroenterol Hepatol. 2008;23:723–8.

52. Blomberg J, Wenger U, Lagergren J, et al. Antireflux stent versus conventional stent in the palliation of distal esophageal cancer. A randomized, multicenter clinical trial. Scand J Gastroenterol. 2010;45:208–16.

53. Laasch HU, Marriott A, Wilbraham L, et al. Effectiveness of open versus antireflux stents for palliation of distal esophageal carcinoma and prevention of symptomatic gastroesophageal reflux. Radiology. 2002;225:359–65.

54. Shim CS, Jung IS, Cheon YK, et al. Management of malignant stricture of the esophagogastric junction with a newly designed self-expanding metal stent with an antireflux mechanism. Endoscopy. 2005;37:335–9.

55. Sgourakis G, Gockel I, Radtke A, et al. The use of self-expanding stents in esophageal and gastroesophageal junction cancer palliation: a meta-analysis and meta-regression analysis of outcomes. Dig Dis Sci. 2010;55:3018–30.

56. Adler DG, Fang J, Wong R, et al. Placement of Polyflex stents in patients with locally advanced esophageal cancer is safe and improves dysphagia during neoadjuvant therapy. Gastrointest Endosc. 2009;70:614–9.

57. Siddiqui AA, Glynn C, Loren D, et al. Self-expanding plastic esophageal stents versus jejunostomy tubes for the maintenance of nutrition during neoadjuvant chemoradiation therapy in patients with esophageal cancer: a retrospective study. Dis Esophagus. 2009;22:216–22.

58. Langer FB, Schoppmann SF, Prager G, et al. Temporary placement of self-expanding oesophageal stents as bridging for neo-adjuvant therapy. Ann Surg Oncol. 2010;17:470–5.

59. Lopes TL, Eloubeidi MA. A pilot study of fully covered self-expandable metal stents prior to neoadjuvant therapy for locally advanced esophageal cancer. Dis Esophagus. 2010;23:309–15.

60. Vleggaar FP. Stent placement in esophageal cancer as a bridge to surgery. Gastrointest Endosc. 2009;70:620–2.

61. Uitdehaag MJ, van Hooft JE. A fully-covered stent (Alimaxx-E) for the palliation of malignant dysphagia: a prospective follow-up study. Gastrointest Endosc. 2009;6:1082–9.

62. Bakken JC, Wong Kee Song LM, de Groen PC, Baron TH. Use of a fully covered self-expandable metal stent for the treatment of benign esophageal diseases. Gastrointest Endosc. 2010;72:712–20.

63. Irani S, Kozarek R. Esophageal stents: past, present, and future. Tech Gastrointest Endosc. 2010;12:178–90.

64. Kim ES, Jeon SW, Park SY, et al. Comparison of double-layered and covered Niti-S stents for palliation of malignant dysphagia. J Gastroenterol Hepatol. 2009;24:114–9.

65. Kim JH, Song HY, Choi EK, et al. Temporary metallic stent placement in the treatment of refractory benign esophageal strictures: results and factors associated with outcome in 55 patients. Eur Radiol. 2009;19:384–90.

66. Uitdehaag MJ, Siersema PD, Spaander MC, et al. A new fully covered stent with antimigration properties for the palliation of malignant dysphagia: a prospective cohort study. Gastrointest Endosc. 2010;71:600–5.

67. Mishin I, Ghidirim G, Dolghii A, et al. Implantation of self-expanding metal stent in the treatment of severe bleeding from esophageal ulcer after endoscopic band ligation. Dis Esophagus. 2010;23: E35–8.

68. Wright G, Lewis H, Hogan B, et al. A self-expanding metal stent for complicated variceal hemorrhage: experience at a single center. Gastrointest Endosc. 2010;71:71–8.

69. Zehetner J, Shamiyeh A, Wayand W, Hubmann R. Results of a new method to stop acute bleeding from esophageal varices: implantation of a self-expanding stent. Surg Endosc. 2008;22:2149–52.

70. Saito Y, Tanaka T, Andoh A, et al. Usefulness of biodegradable stents constructed of poly-l-lactic acid monofilaments in patients with benign esophageal stenosis. World J Gastroenterol. 2007;13:3977–80.

71. Tanaka T, Takahashi M, Nitta N, et al. Newly developed biodegradable stents for benign gastrointestinal tract stenoses: a preliminary clinical trial. Digestion. 2006;74:199–205.

72. Hair CS, Devonshire DA. Severe hyperplastic tissue stenosis of a novel biodegradable esophageal stent and subsequent successful management with high-pressure balloon dilation. Endoscopy. 2010;42(Suppl 2): E132–3.

73. van Boeckel PG, Vleggaar FP, Siersema PD. A comparison of temporary self-expanding plastic and biodegradable stents for refractory benign esophageal strictures. Clin Gastroenterol Hepatol. 2011;9: 653–9.

74. Jeon SR, Eun SH, Shim CS, et al. Effect of drug-eluting metal stents in benign esophageal stricture: an in vivo animal study. Endoscopy. 2009;41: 449–56.

75. Guo SR, Wang ZM, Zhang YQ, et al. In vivo evaluation of 5-fluorouracil-containing self-expandable nitinol stent in rabbits: efficiency in long-term local drug delivery. J Pharmacol Sci. 2010;99: 3009–18.

## Further Reading

1. Power C, Byrne K, Lim K, et al. Superiority of anti-reflux stent compared with conventional stents in the palliative management of patients with cancer of the lower esophagus and esophago-gastric junction: results of a randomized clinical trial. Dis Esophagus. 2007;20:466–70.

2. Wenger U, Johnsson E, Arnelo U, et al. An antireflux stent versus conventional stents for palliation of distal esophageal or cardia cancer: a randomized clinical study. Surg Endosc. 2006;20: 1675–80.

## Mohan Ramchandani and D. Nageshwar Reddy

It has been three decades since endoscopic biliary drainage was first introduced. In 1979, Cotton et al. first described transnasal endoscopic biliary drainage [1]; in 1980, biliary stents were introduced by Soehendra and Reynders-Frederix [2]. Small-caliber endoprosthesis (6–7 Fr) was used, but the size of endoprosthesis has increased with developments in design of accessory devices and endoscopes. However, clogging leading to stent blockage has turned out to be a major problem. Self-expandable metal stents (SEMS) were developed to overcome this issue. Endoscopic placement of SEMS was first described in 1989 [3, 4]. SEMS prolong the duration of patency by increasing the stent diameter overcoming the limitation of the diameter of the endoscope. SEMS are delivered into the bile duct while constrained by a sheath, allowing insertion as a small-circumference delivery system. When the sheath is retracted, the wire mesh stent expands to a diameter up to 10 mm when fully deployed. The large diameter of the lumen in fully deployed SEMS is associated with significantly prolonged stent patency when compared to plastic biliary stents [5–11]. Over time, the open mesh is subsequently covered by biliary epithelial cells. In contrast to plastic stents, repositioning or removal of uncovered

SEMS is difficult or impossible once they have been deployed. Covered SEMS were introduced in the 1990s to improve the patency of SEMS by preventing tissue ingrowth. Unlike uncovered SEMS, which are integrated into the tumor or duct wall, covered SEMS do not embed and therefore can be removed easily. However, there is increased risk of stent migration. Recently, fully covered metal stents have been increasingly used in benign biliary diseases including biliary strictures and biliary leaks.

## Types of Biliary Self-Expanding Metal Stents

There are a variety of commercially available SEMS (Tables 6.1 and 6.2) which vary moderately in price, mechanical properties, size of the open cells of the mesh, anchoring mechanisms, design of the ends, etc. [12–14]. Since there are few studies comparing the different stents, the effect of these parameters on clinical outcome is difficult to determine.

## Mechanical Properties

Many types of SEMS with varying mechanical properties are available. The mechanical properties of SEMS include radial force (RF), chronic outward force (radial resistance force), axial force, flexibility, shortening ratio, radiopacity, and trackability [15]. A high radial expansion force might

M. Ramchandani, M.D., D.M. • D.N. Reddy, M.D., D.M., D.Sc., F.A.M.S, F.R.C.P(✉)
Gastroenterology Department, Asian Institute of Gastroenterology, 6-3-661, Somajiguda, Hyderabad, AP 500 082, India
e-mail: aigindia@yahoo.com.in

R. Kozarek et al. (eds.), *Self-Expandable Stents in the Gastrointestinal Tract*,
DOI 10.1007/978-1-4614-3746-8_6, © Springer Science+Business Media New York 2013

**Table 6.1** Uncovered self-expandable metal stents

| | Zilver | WallFlex | Niti-S S-type | Niti-S D-type | Nitinella Plus | Bonastent | X-Suit NIR® |
|---|---|---|---|---|---|---|---|
| Material | Nitinol | Platinol | Nitinol | Nitinol | Nitinol | Nitinol | Nitinol |
| Construction | Laser cut | Braided multiple wire | Braided single wire | Braided multiple wire | Braided single wire | Braided single wire | Laser cut |
| Diameter delivery catheter | 6 F/7 Fr | 8 Fr | 7 Fr | 8 Fr | 7 Fr | 7 Fr | 7.5 Fr |
| Diameter deployed stent | 6, 8, or 10 mm | 8 or 10 mm | 6, 8, or 10 mm | 6, 8, or 10 mm | 8 or 10 mm | 10 | 8 or 10 mm |
| Length of stent | 4, 6, or 8 cm | 4, 6, 8, or 10 cm | 4, 5, 6, 7, 8, 10, or 12 cm | 4, 5, 6, 7, 8, 10, or 12 cm | 4, 6, 8, or 10 cm | 4, 5, 6, 8, 10 or 12 cm | 4, 6, 8, or 10 cm |
| Shortening ratio | 0 | 45% | 37% | 26% | 27% | 30% | 0 |
| Stent recapture | No | Yes, to 80% of full deployment | No | No | Yes, to 50% of full deployment | Yes, to 76% of full deployment | No |
| Manufacturer | Cook Endoscopy, North Carolina, USA | Boston Scientific, Natick, Massachusetts, USA | Taewoong, Seoul, Korea | Taewoong, Seoul, Korea | ELLA-CS, Hradec Kralove, Czech Republic | Sewoon Medical, Seoul, Korea | Olympus Med |

**Table 6.2** Commonly used covered self-expandable metal stents

| | Wallstent | WallFlex | ComVi | Niti-S | Nitinella Plus | Bonastent |
|---|---|---|---|---|---|---|
| Material | Elgiloy | Platinol | Nitinol | Nitinol | Nitinol | Nitinol |
| Construction | Braided multiple wired | Braided multiple wire | Braided multiple wire | Braided single wire | Braided single wire | Braided single wire |
| | Permalume | Permalume | PTFE | Silicone | Silicone | Silicone |
| | Partly covered | Partly for fully covered | Fully covered | Fully covered | partially covered | Fully covered |
| Diameter delivery catheter | 8 Fr | 8.5 Fr | 8 Fr | 8 Fr | 9 Fr | 8.5 Fr |
| Diameter deployed stent | 6 or 10 mm | 8 or 10 mm | 6, 8, or 10 mm | 6, 8, or 10 mm | 8 or 10 mm | 10 mm |
| Length of stent | 4, 6, or 8 cm | 4, 6, 8, or 10 cm | 4, 5, 6, 7, 8, 10, or 12 cm | 4, 5, 6, 7, 8, 10, or 12 cm | 4, 6, 8, or 10 cm | 4, 6, 8, or 10 cm |
| Shortening ratio (%) | 45 | 45 | 25 | 35 | 27 | 30 |
| Stent recapture | Yes, to 80% of full deployment | Yes, to 80% of full deployment | No | No | Yes, to 50% of full deployment | Yes, to 76% of full deployment |
| Manufacturer | Boston Scientific, Natick, Massachusetts, USA | Boston Scientific, Natick, Massachusetts, USA | Taewoong, Seoul, Korea | Taewoong, Seoul, Korea | ELLA-CS, Hradec Kralove, Czech Republic | Sewoon Medical, Seoul, Korea |

**Table 6.3** Classification of stents based on radial and axial forces

| Low AF | Moderate AF | High AF |
| --- | --- | --- |
| Moderate RF | Moderate to high RF | Low RF |
| Zilver stent | Sinus superflex | Wallstent |
| Viabil | Flexxus stent | |
| ComVi | SMART | |
| Zeo | | |
| SelfX | | |
| Diamond stent | | |
| ZA stent | | |
| Niti-S stent | | |

From Isayama et al. [15], with permission

**Table 6.4** Stent structure

| Braided | Specially braided | Laser cut |
| --- | --- | --- |
| Wallstent | Viabil stent | SMART stent |
| Diamond stent | ComVi stent | Sinus-Endoscopic stent |
| Za stent | | Flexxus stent |
| | | JOSTENT SelfX stent |
| | | Zilver stent |
| | | ZEO stent |

be preferable as long-term patency has been reported to be higher if expansion of the SEMS approximates 70% at 24 h. A high flexibility is particularly important in some locations such as the left intrahepatic ducts. RF is important because in SEMS radial force maintains and expands the luminal patency at the stricture once the SEMS is deployed. The axial force (AF) is defined as a recovery force to keep the stent straight after it was bent. Axial force is related to conformability. If AF is too high, the stent may exert forces to change its shape, which could result in adverse clinical events in a bile duct. There are four clinical events to which AF values are related; these are kinking, biliary wall damage, sludge formation, and migration. Tendencies to kinking have been reported in Wallstents, which exhibit the highest AF values among SEMS. In contrast, no kinking is reported in ComVi, Viabil, Diamond, SelfX, and Zilver stents, all of which have very low AF values (Table 6.3) [15]. During self-expansion, SEMS shorten by 0–50%; SEMS with a low shortening ratio are preferable in some circumstances (e.g., long SEMS in long tight strictures), but they may be associated with jerky deployment [12]. Large open cells in the mesh may allow tissue to protrude into the SEMS lumen, making it ineffective for biliary drainage either immediately after insertion or during follow-up. Most SEMS have identical mesh cell sizes along their whole length, but some models, designed for hilar strictures, have a section with larger cells in order to facilitate the passage of instruments through the mesh at this point.

## Structure

There are three types of structures, namely, braided, specially braided, and laser-cut types (Table 6.4). Among them, the specially braided SEMS (i.e., ComVi and Viabil stents) have unique structures and may need further explanation. ComVi stents consist of two uncovered SEMS overlapping each other with an expanded polytetrafluoroethylene (e-PTFE) membrane sandwiched between them. As a result of this structure, the two wires are not attached to each other, and there is no bonding between the wire and the membrane. Viabil stents, on the other hand, consist of one spiral Z-shaped wire with an e-PTFE membrane attached to it.

## Material

There are two types of materials: nitinol and stainless steel. Most SEMS for ERCP applications are made of nitinol, a superelastic nickel-titanium alloy with thermal shape memory, a property of reassuming a predetermined shape through heating. Elgiloy, a cobalt-based alloy, is employed in some stents.

## Membrane

Some stents are covered in order to prevent stent occlusion by tissue ingrowth and to facilitate SEMS removal. The covering may be made of various materials, including silicone, polyurethane, and expanded polytetrafluoroethylene; it may extend over the entire length of the stent (fully covered SEMS), or small areas at the ends may be left uncovered (partly covered SEMS) [15].

## Uncovered Self-Expandable Stent

### Wallstent

The Wallstent is a self-expanding stent made from a biomedical stainless-steel alloy with a radiopaque core, filaments woven in a tubular fashion, and flexible construction [16, 17]. The Wallstent is available in 40-, 60-, 80-, and 100-mm lengths. The available diameters of the fully expanded Wallstent are 8 and 10 mm. The delivery device has an outside diameter of 7.5 Fr and consists of a 0.035-in. guidewire compatible introducer catheter, on which the compressed SEMS is constrained by a hydrophilic-coated outer sheath. The delivery device has a tapered tip to allow ease of passage. The stent is deployed by withdrawing the outer sheath releasing the SEMS in the desired location. The Wallstent is radiopaque (Fig. 6.1), and there are four radiopaque markers on the delivery device to guide precision deployment. The stent can be recaptured, if need be, and repositioned to 90% of full stent release. Wallstents can be deployed entirely within the bile duct or in transpapillary position. There is 33% foreshortening of the Wallstent postdeployment. Transpapillary positioned, uncovered Wallstents may be reliably removed within 12–24 h after insertion. Subsequently, the stent becomes embedded into the bile duct wall, and it is more difficult, if not impossible, to remove.

### WallFlex Biliary RX Stent

This new SEMS features an improved metal material to form the wire of the stent. Platinol (platinum-cored nitinol) wire achieves a 30–40% reduction in axial force while conferring sufficient expandability comparable to that of the Wallstent. This may preclude complications immediately after stent placement, including stent kinking and migration. Furthermore, the stent is designed

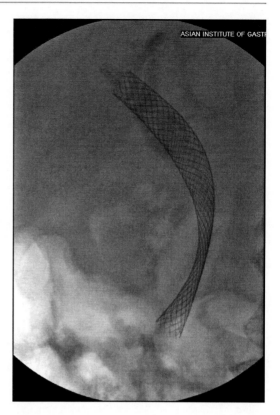

**Fig. 6.1** Wallstent (Courtesy of Asian Institute of Gastroenterology, Somajiguda, India)

with flared and looped wire ends, which may reduce the risk of migration and tissue trauma. It gives the stent flexibility to aid placement in tortuous anatomies and maintain luminal patency. The stents are uncovered, partially covered, and fully covered and are available in multiple sizes. The stent has braided construction with close cell design, and the covered stents have Permalume covering. There is enhanced full-length radiopacity to aid visibility during stent placement. There is an integrated retrieval loop to aid in removal of this stent. Due to the integrated braided design of the fully and partially covered stents, when the retrieval loop is pulled using forceps, the entire length and diameter of the stent are designed to narrow to help facilitate repositioning and removal of the stent during the initial placement procedure. The delivery system is RX Biliary System compatible, designed for physician control and locking of the guidewire. The stent is reconstrainable for up to 80% of deployment, to aid in repositioning. There is a yellow transition zone on the catheter, four fluoroscopy markers, and a reconstrainment limit marker on the handle to aid in placement.

## Zilver Stent

The Zilver biliary stent [18–21] was the first stent of its kind made of flexible laser-cut nitinol tubing, which makes it an open-cell-design stent. The cells of an open-cell-design stent are simply connected, without the tight weaving or interlocking of closed-cell-design stents. Laser cut and polished from solid tubing, this SEMS produces more metal coverage with smaller interstices than previous designs, theoretically impeding tissue ingrowth. Zilver "Z" configuration applies uniform radial strength evenly to the biliary duct. Nitinol, which is inherently kink resistant, allows the stent to conform to the ductal wall while providing reliable patency. Stent ends are atraumatic, potentially reducing the risk of ulceration or perforation. The four gold markers on each end and 0% foreshortening of the stent assist in precise positioning of the stent. The Zilver stent is, in fact, a modification of the original Gianturco-Rosch "Z" stent. The "Z" stent was a stainless steel wire bent into a continuous Z-shaped pattern forming a cylinder. This was modified by stringing together individual cages by adding small eyelets making the stent more flexible and compressible. This is known as the spiral Z stent. The spiral Z stent is available in 5.7- and 7.5-cm lengths and 10 mm in diameter. There are silver radiopaque markers along the length of the stent. Another modification of the design, the Za stent, incorporates nitinol in place of stainless steel making the stent more flexible. The available lengths of the Za stent are 4, 6, and 8 cm with a diameter of 10 mm. There are gold radiopaque markers in the middle and at the end of the Za stent for fluoroscopic visualization. A novel, self-expanding nonforeshortening metal stent has been developed with a 6-Fr delivery system (Zilver 635; Cook Medical, Winston-Salem, NC) to potentially enable simultaneous side-by-side bilateral hilar deployment [21]. The current commercially available iteration of the 6-Fr Zilver 635 system is 200 cm long and available in diameters of 6, 8, and 10 mm and stent lengths of 4, 6, and 8 cm.

Recently, a randomized, prospective, controlled study was conducted to compare the nitinol 6- and 10-mm Zilver stents with the 10-mm stainless steel Wallstent and determine the mechanism of obstruction [18]. At interim, analysis noted a significant increase in occlusions in the 6-mm Zilver group resulting in arm closure. Final study arms were 64, 88, and 89 patients receiving a 6-mm Zilver, 10-mm Zilver, and 10-mm Wallstent, respectively. Stent occlusions occurred in 25 (39.1%) of the patients in the 6-mm Zilver arm, 21 (23.9%) of the patients in the 10-mm Zilver arm, and 19 (21.4%) of the patients in the 10-mm Wallstent arm. The mean number of days of stent patency was 142.9, 185.8, and 186.7, respectively.

## Niti-S Stent

The stent is made of nitinol wire. It is a flexible, fine mesh tubular prosthesis, and it has radiopaque markers to enhance fluoroscopic visibility (Fig. 6.2). It has a diameter of 8 or 10 mm, and the length ranges from 40 to 120 mm. Various types of Niti-S biliary stents are available.

## Niti-D Biliary Uncovered Stent

The Niti-D biliary uncovered stent (NDS) (Taewoong Medical, Gimpo City, Korea) was introduced to improve the efficacy of the SEMS. It is manufactured from nitinol, a nickel-titanium alloy, and has both a "hook-and-cross"-type wire structure to make a D-shaped cavity between wires at deployment and a wide stent mesh. It has an unfixed cell with woven construction. These characteristics are designed to maximize the flexibility and conformability of the stent and to minimize shortening of the stent without loss of radial forces. In addition, radiopaque markers located at the ends and middle of the stent increase its fluoroscopic visibility during stent insertion. Yang et al. examined the efficacy and complication

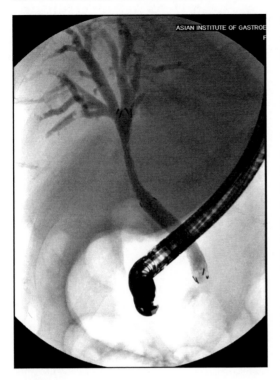

**Fig. 6.2** Niti-S biliary stent (Courtesy of Asian Institute of Gastroenterology, Somajiguda, India)

which helps to improve conformability. Three radiopaque markers are fixed to both ends as well as two at the middle.

## Niti-S Biliary Y Stent

This is a transverse stent with the Y configuration, called a Y stent (Niti-S biliary Y stent; Taewoong, Seoul, Korea), and was developed as a hybrid of spiral and Z stents. The mesh of the central part of the Y stent becomes bigger by omitting the Z component (forming a central area of relatively wide-open mesh), resulting in an open-weave portion that is 10 mm long in the middle of the stent [23, 24]. The Y stent has a 6–7-cm length and a diameter of 10 mm, with gold markers indicating the central mesh. The second stent, a spiral or Z stent (Niti-S or Niti-D stent, respectively; Taewoong), introduced via the central mesh of the Y stent, had a 6–8-cm length and a diameter of 10 mm.

## Niti-S Large Cell D-Type Biliary Stent

The newly designed nitinol metallic stent (Niti-S large cell D-type [LCD] biliary stent; Taewoong Corporation, Seoul, Korea) with an 8.5-Fr delivery system has a larger cell size (7 mm) than the conventional D-type stent (4 mm) facilitating passage of a second stent through the mesh for hilar biliary obstruction. Unlike the recently developed new stents, the cell size of the Niti-S stent is uniform with the LCD, allowing both unilateral and bilateral biliary drainage. Despite the large cell size, the radial force of the LCD is maintained by using thicker nitinol wire (0.178 mm) than the conventional D-type (0.127 mm). The unique chain-like connection of each stent cell allows low axial force. Kogure et al. evaluated the feasibility and efficacy of the Niti-S large cell D-type biliary stent with a uniform large cell for both unilateral and bilateral drainage of malignant hilar biliary obstruction [25]. All 12 patients successfully underwent stenting. Five of the patients underwent bilateral LCD placement. The median stent patency period was 202 days.

rates of the Niti-D biliary uncovered metal stent (NDS), which is more conformable than the uncovered Wallstent [22]. One hundred and one patients received an NDS (41 cases) or a Wallstent (60 cases) for malignant biliary obstruction. Stent occlusion occurred in 11 patients (26.8%) with the NDS and 17 patients (28.3%) with the Wallstent. The results of this study showed no significant differences between the NDS and the Wallstent for the palliative endoscopic management of malignant biliary obstruction. There were no significant differences in patency, complication rates, and patient survival between the more conformable NDS and the conventional Wallstent. However, the NDS, because of its conformability, may be preferred for hilar obstruction.

## Niti-S Biliary Uncovered Stent, S-Type

The stent is a fixed cell type with braided construction. It has atraumatic ends that help to reduce tissue hyperplasia and has low axial force

## Bonastent M-Hilar

The stent (Bonastent M-Hilar, Standard Sci Tech Inc., Seoul, South Korea) has a nitinol wire with a high degree of flexibility and elasticity, a narrower stent mesh, a thin delivery shaft (7 Fr), and good pushability. To facilitate placement of a contralateral stent, the first stent has two spiral radiopaque markings (X mark) in the midsection and four spot markings on both ends. This nitinol stent has the hook and cross wire on the proximal and distal portion. In the 25-mm-long central portion, only the cross-wired structure is present with two spiral markings to facilitate placement of a contralateral stent.

## Flexxus Biliary Stent

The Flexxus stent (ConMed, USA), which was formerly known as Memotherm and Luminexx stent, is fabricated from a single tube of nitinol. This stent is laser cut to minimize foreshortening and provide appropriate flexibility and radial force. Four tantalum spoons have been added to each end of the stent to provide enhanced visibility under fluoroscopy. This nitinol stent design conforms even to torturous anatomy [24]. It has flared ends which provide stent anchoring within the duct, reducing the potential for migration. The interstices of the latticework are large enough to permit cannulation of the interstices and dilation for placement of another stent to create a "Y" configuration for palliation of hilar strictures. The proprietary S.A.F.E.™ pistol grip delivery system provides a controlled incremental release to maximize placement accuracy. It is available in 8- and 10-mm diameter and 4-, 6-, 8-, and 10-cm length.

## JOSTENT SelfX Stent

The JOSTENT SelfX stent (Abbott Vascular Devices, Redwood City, CA) is an uncovered SEMS made from the nitinol. The unique character of this stent depends on its special configuration. This stent has 15 wave-shaped struts that do not cross the circumference. Because every fifth zigzag element is connected, only three are connected in one circumference. Therefore, this stent has high flexibility. When bent, the gap of the stent mesh widens. As such, a Y configuration deployment is easy to achieve. The JOSTENT SelfX stent exhibits a high degree of flexibility and elasticity. It is also designed to exhibit minimal shortening. These characteristics are suitable for precise stent placement in hilar biliary strictures. Furthermore, this stent has a wide stent mesh, a thin delivery shaft (7 Fr), and good pushability. The stent is available in a 10-mm diameter and lengths of 48, 68, or 92 mm. Endoscopic partial stent-in-stent deployment with multiple JOSTENT SelfX prostheses has been reported in treatment of malignant hilar biliary strictures [26, 27].

## Nitinella Plus

SX-ELLA Stent Biliary (Nitinella Plus) Stent system (ELLA-CS, Hradec Králové, Czech Republic) is available for endoscopic or percutaneous transhepatic insertion. It is a self-expandable, braided, nitinol stent preloaded in a pullback delivery system. Both covered and uncovered stents are marketed. Both stent ends of covered stents are uncovered for 5 mm in order to prevent stent migration. It has atraumatic edges and is flexible which is helpful for smooth and kink-free alignment with torturous bile ducts. Radiopaque markers are at both stent ends. Covered stents have a silicone covering and are delivered through a 9-Fr delivery system.

## X-Suit NIR® Biliary Metallic Stents

X-Suit NIR stent (Olympus Med) is made of nitinol with a NIRflex TM Cell Design. In this design, there are alternating narrow strut rings and wide strut rings. The alternating strut width optimizes stability and flexibility while maintaining a relatively uniform cell area, even in curved lumens. The wide struts contribute to stability, radial strength, and resistance to recoil. The conformability is attributed to its fine-strutted, closed-cell design. It thus maintains full wall coverage and consistent stent uniformity while conforming to the bile duct anatomy. The closed-cell design also accounts for the minimal fore-shortening of the X-Suit NIR upon deployment.

## Sinus-Endoscopic Stent

Sinus-Endoscopic stent (OptiMed, Ettlingen, Germany) is made of nitinol. It has a braided structure and an open-cell design. The insertion device is 7 Fr in diameter with braided outer sheath and coiled distal end. The stent diameter is available from 7 to 10 mm. The length of stent varies from 4 to 10 cm.

## Covered Stents

Covered stents (CSEMS) have been developed in an attempt to prolong SEMS patency [28–37]. The covering membrane on the stent prevents stent occlusion due to tumor ingrowth and reactive tissue hyperplasia through the mesh. This also prevents the metal wires from imbedding into the tissue and thus allows for removability, particularly when the distal end is positioned across the papilla into the duodenum. However, this type of stent tends to migrate. The initially designed CSEMS were coated in the midportion, and the ends were uncovered (partially CSEMS); fully CSEMS are now available: Clinically, stent patency and complications differ according to the type of stent. However, very few studies have compared various stents and analyzed the factors influencing the clinical results.

## Covered Wallstent

The covered Wallstent [37, 38] biliary endoprosthesis is a stainless steel stent with a silicone polymer membrane (Permalume [Boston Scientific]) covering the inner lumen. At both the distal and proximal ends, 5-mm lengths are uncovered so that the stent can be anchored at the site of placement within the bile duct. A fully expanded covered biliary Wallstent has a 30-Fr lumen. The fully braided flexible delivery catheter

is designed to resist kinking in tortuous anatomy. Four radiopaque markers on the sheath and catheter enhance deployment control. This stent has a high axial force and low radial force. The stent is designed to exert gentle outward radial pressure, thus establishing and maintaining luminal patency. The outer surface of the stent is relatively rough due to its coating, which is thought to work as an antimigration system.

## ComVi Stent

The ComVi stent [39] (Niti-S stent, ComVi type; Taewoong Medical) is made with an e-PTFE membrane sandwiched between two uncovered nitinol self-expanding metallic stent layers. Thus, this stent is constructed in three layers: a covered membrane sandwiched (not attached) between two uncovered metal stents (Niti-S D-type) (Fig. 6.3). This unique construction results in no additional AF and RF by attaching the cover with wires. The Niti-S D-type stent has a very low AF, and the ComVi stent has almost no AF. The outer uncovered layer may work as an antimigration system, while the inner surface (uncovered layer) may result in the impaction of food scraps. Wire is exposed on both the inner and outer surfaces.

## Niti-S Biliary Covered Stent S-Type

Niti-S biliary covered stent S-type (Niti-S stent; Taewoong Medical) has double-coated silicone-covered membrane. A smooth inner surface helps in hydrodynamic flow of bile and may reduce sludge formation. The outer layer prevents direct contact of metal with tissue, but metal mesh may still embed into the bile duct. A nylon drawstring at the end of the stent helps in easy capture and collapse of the stent for uncomplicated extraction (Fig. 6.4).

## Viabil Biliary Stent

The Viabil [40] is a self-expanding covered stent (GORE® VIABIL® Biliary Endoprosthesis)

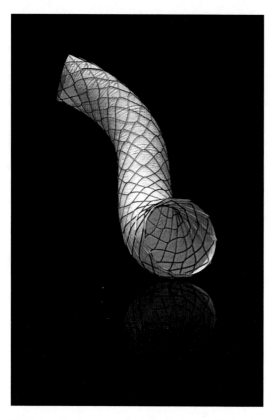

**Fig. 6.3** ComVi stent (Taewoong Medical, Gveonggi-Do, Korea)

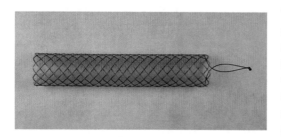

**Fig. 6.4** Niti-S biliary covered stent (Taewoong Medical, Gveonggi-Do, Korea)

made of an ePTFE/FEP tubular lining externally supported by a helical nitinol stent with radiopaque markers at both ends. The inner lining is made of low-porosity, ultrathin, 0.010-mm-thick ePTFE/FEP. Multiple sections of the wires near each end of the nitinol stent project outward from the external surface of the tubular lining and act as anchoring fins. The presence of these lateral anchoring fins reduces the risk of stent

migration, and the delivery system consists of an 8–10-Fr outer sheath. There is no foreshortening. The basement wire construction is a spiraled, wavy wire. No migration has been reported for this stent. The AF is low and the RF moderate. Two versions are available on the market, one with transmural drainage side holes which are present in the lining for 2 cm along the proximal end and a fully covered one. The purpose of these holes is to avoid obstruction of the intrahepatic side ducts or the cystic duct. If an endoprosthesis with transmural drainage holes is selected, the middle and hepatic end radiopaque rings demarcate the boundaries of the holed region. The endoprosthesis is available in a diameter of 8 or 10 mm and a length of 4, 6, 8, or 10 cm in both the fenestrated and the fully covered version. According to the manufacturer, the Viabil should extend at least 2 cm proximal and distal to the margins of the stricture. Due to the nitinol lining, total expansion is reached approximately 24 h after placement, but the endoprosthesis length is not subject to variation.

## Covered Zeostent

There are several characteristics unique to covered Zeostent (Zeon Medical Inc., Tokyo, Japan) other than its fully covered structure. One is the shape of the stent after full expansion. It has a wavy contour with an uneven outer surface, which expectedly contributes to prevention of stent migration. A very low shortening ratio (about 3%) is another characteristic, which facilitates accurate deployment of the stent. Furthermore, the axial force is lower compared with that of other covered SEMS, which presumably avoids kinking of the bile duct.

## Niti-S Stent

This removable covered self-expandable metal stent (RCSEMS) is a Niti-S (Kaffes) [41] biliary stent, which consists of an implantable metal stent and a flexible introducer system (Taewoong Medical Co Ltd., South Korea). The stent is a semirigid, flexible, and expandable tubular device made of nitinol (nickel-titanium alloy) wire. Upon deployment, the RCSEMS imparts an outward radial force on the luminal surface of the biliary duct to establish patency. The RCSEMS is available in one diameter (8-mm midportion and 10 mm at either end) and one length (40 mm). This stent is designed especially for posttransplant strictures where the stricture length is usually short (0.5–1.0 cm) and the rest of the bile duct is usually of normal caliber. There are two characteristic features of this stent to address these characteristics of posttransplant biliary strictures. First, a 10-cm radiopaque nylon string is incorporated into the distal end of the stent to facilitate endoscopic retrieval. Second, it has a waist that is 2 mm narrower than each end which helps to prevent stent migration. The removal of RCSEMS can be performed using a standard endoscopy biopsy forceps by grasping the string attached at the distal end of the RCSEMS and then pulling it via the working channel of the scope.

### Hanarostent

Three types of stents are available: Hanarostent noncovered biliary, covered biliary, and covered biliary with lasso (MI Tech Co., Ltd., Seoul, South Korea). It is self-expanding nitinol tubular prosthesis with a silicone membrane. There are flared ends which minimize the migration. A total of 12 radiopaque markers, 4 on each end and 4 at the center, give a clear flouroscopic view of the stent. Recapture of the stent is possible using the delivery device. It has a flexible structure for natural fitting to the lumen with minimum shortening.

### Comparison Between Covered and Uncovered Stents

CSEMS were developed to provide prolongation in patency over USEMS. Advantages of using CSEMS over USEMS for palliation of distal malignant biliary obstruction are controversial.

Two recent prospective, randomized trials did not show a difference in stent patency between CSEMS and USEMS [42, 43]. These findings, combined with the substantial increase in cost of CSEMS, the higher migration rate, and the potential for an increase in cholecystitis, have limited the adoption of CSEMS over USEMS. However, a recently published meta-analysis based on five randomized, controlled studies comparing CSEMS and USEMS for palliative decompression of distal malignant biliary obstruction suggests that covered biliary SEMS have a significantly longer duration of patency compared with USEMS in patients with malignant distal bile duct obstruction [44]. Stent dysfunction occurs at a similar rate, although there is a trend toward later obstruction with CSEMS. CSEMS dysfunction is more likely to result from tumor overgrowth, sludge formation, and stent migration. USEMS more commonly occlude from tumor ingrowth or tissue hyperplasia.

### Comparison Between Various SEMS

Several trials have compared different metal stents. One study found the spiral Z stent (Wilson-Cook, Winston-Salem, North Carolina) to be comparable to the Wallstent in terms of technical and therapeutic efficacy and rate of stent occlusion [20]. Recently, Weston and colleagues reported a comparison of the clinical outcomes of nitinol and stainless steel uncovered metal stents for malignant distal biliary stricture [45]. In this study, a total of 81 nitinol and 96 stainless steel stents were placed to relieve malignant biliary strictures. The most common cancer diagnosis was pancreatic (80.2% of nitinol stents and 62.5% of stainless steel stents), and the most frequent site of stricture was the common bile duct (85.2% nitinol and 86.5% stainless steel). Biliary decompression was achieved in 93.8% of the nitinol group and 86.4% of the stainless steel group. The overall duration of stent patency in the nitinol and stainless steel groups was similar (median, 129 and 137 days, respectively; $P = 0.61$). At the present time, it seems there is no clear clinical advantage in one type of SEMS over the other.

## Conclusion

Biliary stenting is the treatment of choice for inoperable malignant strictures of the common bile duct. Effective palliation can be achieved using conventional plastic stents. The major drawback of plastic stents is the high rate of clogging, requiring frequent stent exchange. Self-expanding metal stents have been shown to be associated with fewer episodes of stent occlusion compared with plastic stents. All available biliary metal stents are effective for treating malignant obstructive jaundice, but definitive data favoring one stent over another are currently lacking. More recently introduced covered SEMS have been associated with significantly prolonged stent patency and longer stent survival; however, stent migration, tumor overgrowth, and sludge formation are significantly higher with covered SEMS.

## References

1. Cotton PB, Burney PG, Mason RR. Transnasal bile duct catheterization after endoscopic sphincterotomy: method for biliary drainage, perfusion, and sequential cholangiography. Gut. 1979;20:285–7.
2. Soehendra N, Reynders-Frederix V. Palliative bile duct drainage – a new endoscopic method of introducing a transpapillary drain. Endoscopy. 1980;12:8–11.
3. Neuhaus H, Hagenmuller F, Classen M. Self-expanding biliary stents: preliminary clinical experience. Endoscopy. 1989;21:225–8.
4. Huibregtse K, Cheng J, Coene PP, et al. Endoscopic placement of expandable metal stents for biliary strictures: a preliminary report on experience with 33 patients. Endoscopy. 1989;21:280–2.
5. Davids PH, Groen AK, Rauws EA, et al. Randomized trial of self-expanding metal stents versus polyethylene stents for distal malignant biliary obstruction. Lancet. 1992;340:1488–92.
6. Knyrim K, Wagner HJ, Pausch J, et al. A prospective, randomized, controlled trial of metal stents for malignant obstruction of the common bile duct. Endoscopy. 1993;25:207–12.
7. Wagner HJ, Knyrim K, Vakil N, et al. Plastic endoprostheses versus metal stents in the palliative treatment of malignant hilar biliary obstruction: a prospective and randomized trial. Endoscopy. 1993;25:213–8.
8. Prat F, Chapat O, Ducot B, et al. A randomized trial of endoscopic drainage methods for inoperable malignant strictures of the common bile duct. Gastrointest Endosc. 1998;47:1–7.
9. Kaassis M, Boyer J, Dumas R, et al. Plastic or metal stents for malignant stricture of the common bile duct? Results of a randomized prospective study. Gastrointest Endosc. 2003;57:178–82.
10. Moses PL, Alan BN, Gordon SR, et al. A randomized multicenter trial comparing plastic to covered metal stents for the palliation of lower malignant biliary obstruction [abstract]. Gastrointest Endosc. 2006;63:AB289.
11. Soderlund C, Linder S. Covered metal versus plastic stents for malignant common bile duct stenosis: a prospective, randomized, controlled trial. Gastrointest Endosc. 2006;63:986–95.
12. Dumonceau JM, Heresbach D, Devière J, et al. Biliary stents: models and methods for endoscopic stenting. Endoscopy. 2011;43:617–26.
13. Lee JH. Self-expandable metal stents for malignant distal biliary strictures. Gastrointest Endosc Clin N Am. 2011;21:463–80. viii–ix.
14. Gerges C, Schumacher B, Terheggen G, et al. Expandable metal stents for malignant hilar biliary obstruction. Gastrointest Endosc Clin N Am. 2011;21:481–97.
15. Isayama H, Nakai Y, Toyokawa Y, et al. Measurement of radial and axial forces of biliary self-expandable metallic stents. Gastrointest Endosc. 2009;70:37–44.
16. Huibregtse K. The Wallstent for malignant biliary obstruction. Gastrointest Endosc Clin N Am. 1999;9:491–501.
17. Adam A, Chetty N, Roddie M, et al. Self-expandable stainless steel endoprostheses for treatment of malignant bile duct obstruction. AJR Am J Roentgenol. 1991;156:321–5.
18. Loew BJ, Howell DA, Sanders MK, et al. Comparative performance of uncoated, self-expanding metal biliary stents of different designs in 2 diameters: final results of an international multicenter, randomized, controlled trial. Gastrointest Endosc. 2009;70:445–53.
19. Varadarajulu S, Tutuian R, Gostout C, et al. Efficacy of the Za self-expandable metal stent for palliation of malignant biliary obstruction. J Clin Gastroenterol. 2004;38:77–80.
20. Shah RJ, Howell DA, Desilets DJ, et al. Multicenter randomized trial of the spiral Z-stent compared with the Wallstent for malignant biliary obstruction. Gastrointest Endosc. 2003;57:830–6.
21. Chennat J, Waxman I. Initial performance profile of a new 6F self-expanding metal stent for palliation of malignant hilar biliary obstruction. Gastrointest Endosc. 2010;72:632–6.
22. Yang KY, Ryu JK, Seo JK, et al. A comparison of the Niti-D biliary uncovered stent and the uncovered Wallstent in malignant biliary obstruction. Gastrointest Endosc. 2009;70:45–51.
23. Lee JH, Kang DH, Kim JY, et al. Endoscopic bilateral metal stent placement for advanced hilar cholangiocarcinoma: a pilot study of a newly designed Y stent. Gastrointest Endosc. 2007;66:364–9.
24. Ramchandani M, Lakhtakia S, Gupta R, et al. A new biliary "Y" stent for hilar tumors. Endoscopy. 2007;39(Suppl 1):E47–8.

25. Kogure H, Isayama H, Kawakubo K, et al. Endoscopic bilateral metallic stenting for malignant hilar obstruction using newly designed stents. J Hepatobiliary Pancreat Sci. 2011;18:653–7.

26. Kawamoto H, Tsutsumi K, Harada R, et al. Endoscopic deployment of multiple JOSTENT SelfX is effective and safe in treatment of malignant hilar biliary strictures. Clin Gastroenterol Hepatol. 2008;6:401–8.

27. Kawamoto H, Tsutsumi K, Fujii M, et al. Endoscopic 3-branched partial stent-in-stent deployment of metallic stents in high-grade malignant hilar biliary stricture (with videos). Gastrointest Endosc. 2007;66:1030–7.

28. Siddiqui AA, Mehendiratta V, Loren D, et al. Fully Covered self-expandable metal stents are effective and safe to treat distal malignant biliary strictures, irrespective of surgical resectability status. J Clin Gastroenterol. 2011;45:824–7.

29. Poley JW, van Tilburg AJ, Kuipers EJ, et al. Breaking the barrier: using extractable fully covered metal stents to treat benign biliary hilar strictures. Gastrointest Endosc. 2011;74:916–20.

30. Isayama H, Nakai Y, Kawakubo K, et al. Covered metallic stenting for malignant distal biliary obstruction: clinical results according to stent type. J Hepatobiliary Pancreat Sci. 2011;18:673–7.

31. Kasher JA, Corasanti JG, Tarnasky PR, et al. A multicenter analysis of safety and outcome of removal of a fully covered self-expandable metal stent during ERCP. Gastrointest Endosc. 2011;73:1292–7.

32. Hwang JC, Kim JH, Yoo BM, et al. Temporary placement of a newly designed, fully covered, self-expandable metal stent for refractory bile leaks. Gut Liver. 2011;5:96–9.

33. Costamagna G, Tringali A, Reddy DN, et al. A new partially covered nitinol stent for palliative treatment of malignant bile duct obstruction: a multicenter single-arm prospective study. Endoscopy. 2011;43:317–24.

34. Bakhru M, Ho HC, Gohil V, Wang AY, et al. Fully-covered, self-expandable metal stents (CSEMS) in malignant distal biliary strictures: mid-term evaluation. J Gastroenterol Hepatol. 2011;26:1022–7.

35. Tsuchiya T, Itoi T, Gotoda T, et al. A multicenter prospective study of the short-term outcome of a newly developed partially covered self-expandable metallic

36. Baron TH. Covered self-expandable metal stents for benign biliary tract diseases. Curr Opin Gastroenterol. 2011;27:262–7.

37. Nakai Y, Isayama H, et al. New method of covered Wallstents for distal malignant biliary obstruction to reduce early stent-related complications based on characteristics. Dig Endosc. 2011;23:49–55.

38. Yoon WJ, Lee JK, Lee KH, et al. A comparison of covered and uncovered Wallstents for the management of distal malignant biliary obstruction. Gastrointest Endosc. 2006;63:996–1000.

39. Isayama H, Kawabe T, Nakai Y, et al. Management of distal malignant biliary obstruction with the ComVi stent, a new covered metallic stent. Surg Endosc. 2010;24:131–7.

40. Van Steenbergen W. The first prospective endoscopic experience with the ePTFE-covered Viabil stent in patients with a distal malignant biliary stenosis. Acta Gastroenterol Belg. 2010;73:18–24.

41. Tee HP, James MW, Kaffes AJ. Placement of removable metal biliary stent in post-orthotopic liver transplantation anastomotic stricture. World J Gastroenterol. 2010;16:3597–600.

42. Kullman E, Frozanpor F, Söderlund C, et al. Covered versus uncovered self-expandable nitinol stents in the palliative treatment of malignant distal biliary obstruction: results from a randomized, multicenter study. Gastrointest Endosc. 2010;72:915–23.

43. Telford JJ, Carr-Locke DL, Baron TH, et al. A randomized trial comparing uncovered and partially covered self-expandable metal stents in the palliation of distal malignant biliary obstruction. Gastrointest Endosc. 2010;72:907–14.

44. Saleem A, Leggett CL, Murad MH, et al. Meta-analysis of randomized trials comparing the patency of covered and uncovered self-expandable metal stents for palliation of distal malignant bile duct obstruction. Gastrointest Endosc. 2011;74:321–7.

45. Weston BR, Ross WA, Liu J, et al. Clinical outcomes of nitinol and stainless steel uncovered metal stents for malignant biliary strictures: is there a difference. Gastrointest Endosc. 2010;72:1195–200.

biliary stent (WallFlex(®)). Dig Dis Sci. 2011;56:1889–95.

# Enteric Prostheses

**7**

## Chan Gyoo Kim and Il Ju Choi

Enteral stents are devices used to relieve gastroduodenal stenosis, resulting from advanced gastric, pancreatic, biliary, and duodenal cancers, or postsurgical anastomotic stenosis. The anatomy at the stenosis is usually angulated and thus requires more flexible stents and longer delivery systems than esophageal stenosis. A large stent diameter is mandatory for patients to tolerate a solid diet, particularly when the proximal end is within the stomach. Bending of the delivery system at sites such as the greater curvature of the stomach is frequent. These anatomic characteristics led to the development of a dedicated delivery system for enteral stents that is flexible, long, and of small predeployed diameters to pass through the working channel of therapeutic endoscopes. This chapter provides an overview of the available enteric self-expandable metallic stents (SEMS) including general characteristics and specific features.

## Early Stents

The first attempts to relieve enteral obstruction or stenosis with stents were made in the 1990s using modified or unmodified esophageal, biliary, or vascular stents [1, 2]. Examples include the Z

C.G. Kim, M.D., Ph.D. • I.J. Choi, M.D., Ph.D. (✉)
Center for Gastric Cancer, National Cancer Center,
323 Ilsan-ro, Ilsandong-gu, Goyang, Gyeonggi-do
410-769, Republic of Korea
e-mail: cij1224@ncc.re.kr

stent (Wilson-Cook Medical, Inc., Winston-Salem, NC, USA) [3]; Song esophageal stent (Doosung Medi-tech, Seoul, Korea) [4]; esophageal Wallstent (Schneider AG, Bulach, Switzerland) [5]; Ultraflex Esophageal Stent (Boston Scientific, Natick, MA, USA) [6]; and Alimaxx (Alveolus, Charlotte, NC, USA) [7]. Bard (Bard, Tempe, AZ, USA) [7], Memotherm (C.R. Bard, Inc., Murray Hill, NJ, USA) [8], Strecker stent (Boston Scientific) [8], Choo esophageal stent (Solco Intermed, Seoul, Korea) [9], and InStent (Eden Prairie, MN, USA) [10] were also used for the same purpose, and most are no longer used for enteral purposes. Biliary or vascular stents had diameters of 10–16 mm, which limited their use as enteral stents.

The first widely used enteral stent was the enteral Wallstent, initially made by Schneider and subsequently acquired by Boston Scientific/Microvasive, Natick, MA, USA (Fig. 7.1a) [11, 12], and was a modification of the biliary Wallstent (Schneider, Minneapolis, MN, USA, now Boston Scientific) which has a small-caliber lumen (10 mm diameter) [1]. The enteral Wallstent is of a similar design but with large luminal diameters (18–22 mm) which allowed patients with malignant gastroduodenal stenosis [13] the ability to eat solid diets and are available in lengths of 6 and 9 cm. The enteral Wallstent, still commercially available, has a small-diameter delivery system (10 F) that can be passed through the working channel of a therapeutic endocope and allows controlled release under both endoscopic

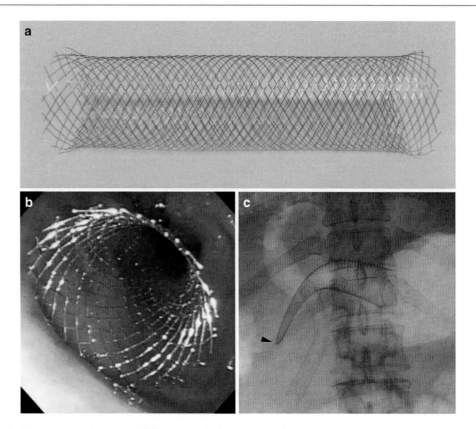

**Fig. 7.1** Wallstent enteral stent. (**a**) Wallstent enteral, the first widely used enteral stent, is still commercially available. (**b**) Endoscopic view of Wallstent showing sharp wire ends (**c**) The sharp ends of the individual wires at the distal side are twisting during deployment and prevent expansion (*arrowhead*)

and fluoroscopic views. In addition, the delivery system is long (230 cm) enough to access obstruction sites up to the distal duodenum and proximal jejunum. It is composed of multiple strands of Elgiloy [11], a corrosion-resistant alloy composed primarily of cobalt, nickel, and chromium with high radial strength. One disadvantage of the Wallstent is sharp ends of cut wire; with the tendency to straighten, the wires would erode into the bowel wall and were felt to increase the risk of perforation. Stent failure occurs from twisting of the individual wires during deployment, preventing expansion (Fig. 7.1b, c) [14].

## Stent Compositions

An alloy of nickel and titanium (nitinol) has replaced Elgiloy in most currently available enteral stents. Nitinol has increased flexibility but less radial strength than Elgiloy. Stents made from nitinol have smoother finished wire ends, which reduce the risk of trauma to the bowel wall and stent failure from entanglement of wire ends. In addition, nitinol enables manufacture of softer and more flexible stents and produces a predictable self-expanding shape due to shape memory of the original stent configuration after deployment at body temperature [15]. Although nitinol is a nonferromagnetic alloy which enables patients to safely undergo magnetic resonance imaging (MRI), the stent produces a mild local-field inhomogeneity on MRI which may make interpretation of images more difficult [16]. The stent also creates a beam-hardening artifact on computed tomography, which causes brighter appearance at the edges than the center. Some enteral stent models have several gold or platinum markers on the wire mesh to provide clear fluoroscopic view in addition to the radiopacity of the mesh structure.

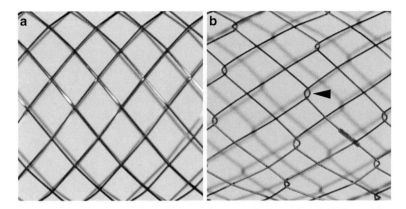

**Fig. 7.2**  A close-up of wire structure. (**a**) The basic cross-wire structure of currently available stents. (**b**) Hooked type (*arrowhead*) can be added to the cross-wire structure

Although diverse woven structures are available from several manufacturers, the basic structure of currently available stents is cross wire, and hooked type can be added to the cross structure (Fig. 7.2). Crossed wire type enables small-diameter delivery systems, but often with substantial stent shortening after deployment. The labeled stent length indicates the length at full expansion, and a variable degree of foreshortening is anticipated during stent deployment depending on the manufacturer.

## Delivery Systems

Enteral stents are packaged in compressed form and constrained on a delivery device (Fig. 7.3a) for endoscopic placement with or without fluoroscopic assistance, or by interventional radiologists using only fluoroscopic guidance. Experienced interventional radiologists can pass guidewires across obstructive lesions and deploy stents over the wire (OTW). Endoscopic placement through the scope (TTS) requires therapeutic endoscopes with a large working channel (>3.7 mm; Fig. 7.3b–d). Because of frequent excess bending of the delivery system at the greater curvature of the distended stomach when the fluoroscopic approach is used, the TTS method has the advantage of straightening the

access route and for direct visualization of the stricture site. Shortening of woven stents during deployment may result in stent misplacement. Thus, most delivery systems allow recapturing of a partially deployed stent so that the stent position can be precisely adjusted during deployment.

## Covered and Uncovered Stents

Uncovered enteral stents consist of nitinol mesh without a covering membrane and are susceptible to restenosis due to progressive tumor ingrowth and/or tissue hyperplasia through the openings between the stent wire filaments. Covered enteral stents with a membrane on the nitinol mesh reduce restenosis by preventing tumor ingrowth or tissue hyperplasia. However, migration is more frequent in covered than in uncovered stents leading to special stent designs with flared ends for better anchorage. The initial models of covered enteral stents could only be inserted under fluoroscopic guidance due to the large-diameter delivery systems [17], but current covered models have delivery systems of small enough diameter (10–10.5 F) to be inserted by the TTS method. Materials used for membrane covering of enteral stents are silicone or polytetrafluoroethylene (PTFE), which are more durable and resilient than older polyurethane fabrics [18].

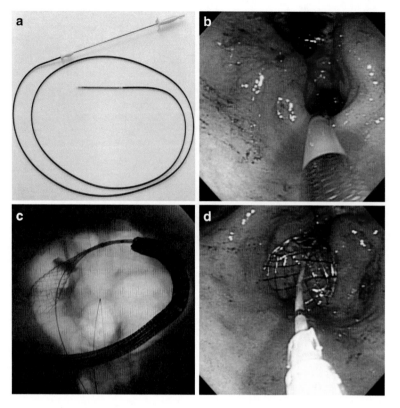

**Fig. 7.3** Delivery system for through the scope (TTS) deployment method. (**a**) The long-length and small-diameter delivery system can be passed through the working channel of an endoscope. (**b**) Delivery system is being inserted into the stenosis using the TTS method. (**c**) Fluoroscopic guidance enables precise stent deployment. (**d**) Endoscopic view immediately after stent deployment using TTS placement. The delivery system has not yet been withdrawn

## WallFlex Duodenal Stent

The WallFlex duodenal stent (Boston Scientific) is one of the most popular enteral stents currently available. This TTS, self-expandable metal uncovered stent is woven from braided nitinol wire (Fig. 7.4a). The use of nitinol has made this stent more flexible than the earlier Wallstent. The WallFlex has a flare (27 mm diameter and 15 mm long) at the proximal end to reduce the risk of stent migration and looped ends to minimize the possibility of mucosal injury and subsequent bowel perforation (Fig. 7.4a). The unconstrained body diameter is 22 mm, and unconstrained lengths are available in 6, 9, and 12 cm. Although this stent does not have radiopaque markers, the mesh itself is radiopaque well visualized fluoroscopically.

The WallFlex comes preloaded on a 10-F anchor lock delivery system, which is 230 cm long for insertion by the TTS or OTW method. It shortens up to 45% after complete deployment [19]. It is reconstrainable up to 70% stent deployment (the point of no return), allowing easy repositioning. Three radiopaque markers are on the delivery system (Fig. 7.4b), including an exterior tube marker on the distal tip of the delivery system. A deployment limit marker indicates the point of no return. The point of no return where the stent can no longer be reconstrained is identified when the exterior tube marker band (arrow) reaches the deployment limit marker band (closed arrowhead). The postdeployment marker identifies the approximate final position of the proximal end of the deployed stent (open arrowhead).

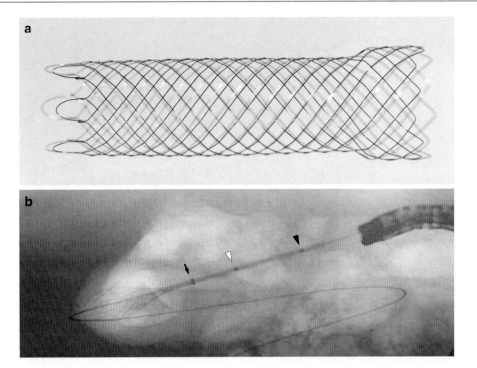

**Fig. 7.4** WallFlex enteral stent. (**a**) WallFlex enteral stent has a flare at the proximal end and roundly angled edges. (**b**) Three radiopaque markers on the delivery system enable precise stent deployment. The stent can be reconstrained at any time up to when the exterior tube marker band (*dark solid arrow*) reaches the deployment limit marker band (*closed arrowhead*). A postdeployment marker band (*open arrowhead*) identifies the approximate final position of the proximal end of the stent when fully expanded

## Evolution Duodenal Stent

The Evolution duodenal stent is manufactured by Cook Medical Inc. (Winston-Salem, NC, USA; Fig. 7.5). This is a TTS, self-expandable metal uncovered stent made of braided nitinol with a single-wire woven structure. This stent has proximal and distal flanges to prevent stent migration. The diameter of the flared ends is 27 mm with a length of 20 mm. The unconstrained body diameter is 22 mm and unconstrained lengths are 6, 9, and, 12 cm. The stent comes preloaded on a 10-F, 230-cm delivery system.

There are eight radiopaque markers on the stent (four on each end) in addition to the radiopaque mesh structure to provide fluoroscopic visualization. An endoscopic marker on the introducer system indicates the proximal end of the stent within the sheath. The Evolution duodenal stents are recapturable up to approximately 50% of stent deployment. The stents foreshorten by approximately 45–50%.

## Niti-S Pyloric/Duodenal Stent

Niti-S is the registered trademark of Taewoong Medical, Seoul, Korea. The Niti-S (ComVi type) is a unique triple-layered covered stent sandwiched designed to overcome tumor ingrowth and an uncovered outer stent to reduce migration.

### Niti-S Pyloric/Duodenal Uncovered Stent: D Type
The Niti-S pyloric/duodenal uncovered stent – D type – is a self-expandable metal uncovered stent made of braided nitinol, which is woven with knitted-interlock structure (D type, Fig. 7.6a). "D type" denotes "double wire type" in which two separate wires are woven into a stent mesh. Unlike the S type (single wire type), individual cells of D-type stent are not fixed and can overlap with each other at the curved areas where the stent is bent (Fig. 7.6b, c), designed to avoid abrupt luminal narrowing at the flexed area. The

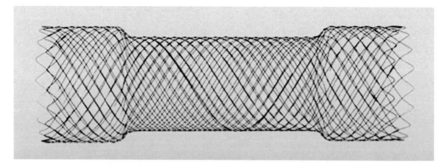

**Fig. 7.5** Evolution duodenal stent. This stent is a through the scope, uncovered enteral stent with flanges at both ends to prevent stent migration

structural characteristics provide high flexibility and conformability.

This stent is a straight type, with the same diameter on body and both ends with round edges to reduce the risk of tissue injury. The unconstrained body diameter is available in 18, 20, 22, and 24 mm, and unconstrained lengths are 6, 8, 10, and 12 cm. In addition to the radiopacity of the mesh structure, there are ten platinum radiopaque markers – four each at the distal/proximal end and two at middle portion to provide optimal fluoroscopic visualization. The stent can be inserted by TTS or OTW methods and comes preloaded on a 10-F delivery system. The length of the delivery system is 180 cm for TTS and 135 cm for OTW placement. After complete deployment, the shortening rate of this enteral stent is 17%. It is not reconstrainable at any point during deployment.

## Niti-S Pyloric/Duodenal Stent: ComVi Type

This is a newly designed covered enteral stent to overcome both stent migration and reocclusion. This stent has a unique design of a triple-layered sandwich structure. The stent is made of two nitinol-braided outer and inner D-type stents with a PTFE membrane between them (Fig. 7.6d, e). The outer exposed stent mesh is expected to reduce migration by embedding itself into the tumor and surrounding normal tissue and a central PTFE membrane that prevents tumor ingrowth [20]. There are 5 or 15-mm uncovered portions at each end and also looped edges to reduce the risk of mucosal injury.

Available unconstrained body diameters are 18 and 20 mm, and unconstrained lengths and radiopaque markers, and are same as the uncovered stent (D type). The stent comes preloaded on a 10.5 F for TTS or OTW delivery. Other characteristics of the delivery system and the shortening rate of stent are similar to the D-type stent.

## Niti-S Pyloric/Duodenal Stent: S Type

The Niti-S pyloric/duodenal stent – fully covered – is an older model but still currently available. It is a self-expandable metal stent woven into single-wired structure (Fig. 7.6c, f). The covering material is silicone. It has flanges (24 mm diameter and 15 mm long) at the ends to minimize the risk of migration and rounded edges to reduce the risk of tissue injury. A repositioning lasso on the proximal end is optional. Although the default model has coated flanges on both ends, the manufacturer provides uncoated flanges at the proximal and/or distal ends.

The unconstrained body diameter, lengths, radiopaque markers, and delivery system are the same as the ComVi-type stent. After complete deployment, the shortening rate of this enteral stent is 50–60%, and it is reconstrainable up to 70% stent deployment, allowing easy repositioning and improved control.

## HANAROSTENT® Duodenum/Pylorus

HANAROSTENT is the registered trademark of M.I. Tech Co. Ltd., Seoul, Korea. It is available either uncovered stent or covered, both of similar design other than the silicone-coated body.

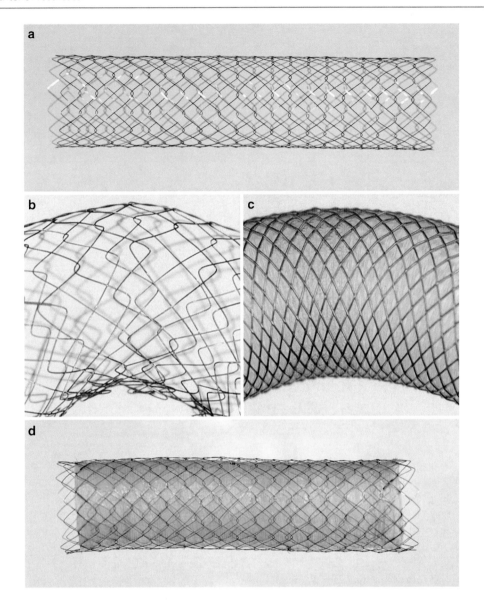

**Fig. 7.6** Niti-S pyloric/duodenal stents (**a**) Niti-S pyloric/ duodenal uncovered stent (D type) is an uncovered enteral stent. (**b**) A close-up of the bent D-type (double-wire knitted-interlock structure) stent shows overlapping cells because the individual cells are not fixed. (**c**) A close-up of the bent S-type stent shows that individual cells do not overlap. (**d**) Niti-S pyloric/duodenal stent (ComVi type) is a covered enteral stent. (**e**) ComVi type consists of three layers; an outer and inner nitinol meshes and a PTFE membrane between the meshes. (**f**) Niti-S pyloric/duodenal stent (S type) is the old model of covered enteral stent. A reposition lasso (arrowhead) is optional

## HANAROSTENT Duodenum/Pylorus, Noncovered (NNN)

This is an uncovered enteral stent. NNN denotes noncovered distal, center, and proximal parts of the stent, respectively. It is a self-expandable metal stent woven with the hook-type nitinol structure (Fig. 7.7a, b). A repositioning lasso can be attached at the proximal end if needed.

The unconstrained body diameter is 20 mm, and unconstrained lengths are 6, 8, 10, 12, 14, or 16 cm. This stent has flares (diameter 25 mm and length 13 mm) on both ends to reduce the risk of migration and rounded edges to reduce the risk of tissue injury. In addition to the radiopacity of the mesh structure, there are 12 gold radiopaque markers – four each located at the center and both

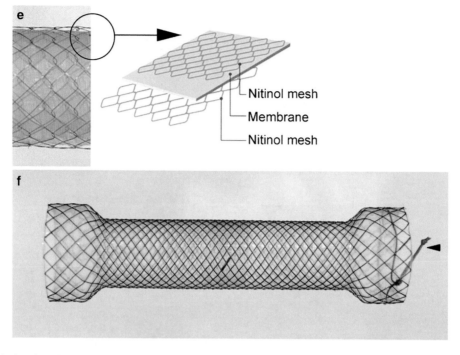

**Fig. 7.6** (continued)

ends for excellent fluoroscopic visualization, (Fig. 7.7b, c).

This stent can be inserted TTS or OTW. The stent comes preloaded on a 10.2-F, 230-cm-long (for TTS delivery) or 10.5-F, 120-cm-long (for OTW delivery) HANARO delivery device. The olive tip of the delivery device is radiopaque, and the distal end of outer sheath has radiopaque tungsten rings. After complete deployment, there is a 20% foreshortening. It is reconstrainable up to 80% of fully stent deployment, allowing easy repositioning and improved control. The point of no return is marked in red on the inner shaft of handle (Fig. 7.7f, open arrowhead).

### HANAROSTENT Duodenum/Pylorus (NCN and CCN)

HANAROSTENT® duodenum/pylorus (NCN) is a covered enteral stent. NCN means noncovered distal, covered center, and noncovered proximal portions. CCN means covered distal and center, and uncovered proximal portions. The body of this stent is coated by silicone. Flared uncovered portions are present on both ends

(NCN) or proximal end (CCN) to reduce the risk of migration (Fig. 7.7d, e).

The covered stent has a similar design to the uncovered HANAROSTENT, except the number and location of radiopaque markers. There are 16 gold radiopaque markers (four each distal and proximal to the uncovered end, and distal and proximal to the covered end) to provide improved fluoroscopic visualization.

### BONASTENT® Pyloric/Duodenal

The BONASTENT has a design similar to the HANAROSTENT, but another uniquely designed stent, BONASTENT M-Duodenal, is available and developed to enable biliary stent placement and adequate expansion through the lumen of the duodenal stent.

### BONASTENT Pyloric/Duodenal Uncovered

BONASTENT is the registered trademark of Standard Sci-Tech Inc., Seoul, Korea. This is a self-expandable metal uncovered stent made of

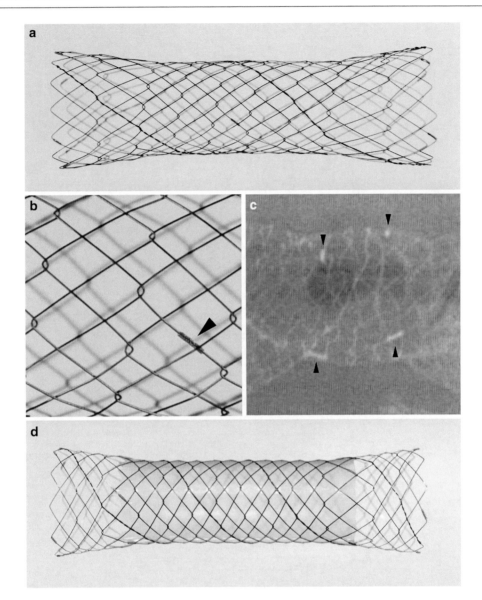

**Fig. 7.7** HANAROSTENT® duodenum/pylorus stents. (**a**) HANAROSTENT duodenum/pylorus uncovered stent. This enteral stent has flares on both ends. (**b**) A close-up view of HANAROSTENT duodenum/pylorus uncovered stent shows hook-type wire structure and gold radiopaque marker (*arrowhead*). (**c**) Fluoroscopic view of radiopaque markers (*arrowhead*). (**d**) HANAROSTENT duodenum/ pylorus covered stent (NCN). Flares on both ends remain uncovered. (**e**) HANAROSTENT duodenum/pylorus covered stent (CCN). Proximal end flare remains uncovered. (**f**) Recapturing *red* marker (*open arrowhead*) and deployment *black* markers. *Left* closed arrowhead denotes the starting point of stent deployment, and the *right* closed arrowhead indicates the finishing point of deployment

braided nitinol with a fixed hook and cross-wired structure (Fig. 7.8a). The cell size of the stent mesh is 4 mm. The diameter of the flared ends is 6 mm larger than that of the body, and the length of flare is 15 mm to minimize the risk of migra- tion, and it has smooth ends to reduce the risk of tissue injury. The unconstrained body diameter is available in 18 and 20 mm, and unconstrained lengths are 6, 8, 10, 12, 14, and 16 cm. There are 12 platinum wire spring radiopaque markers

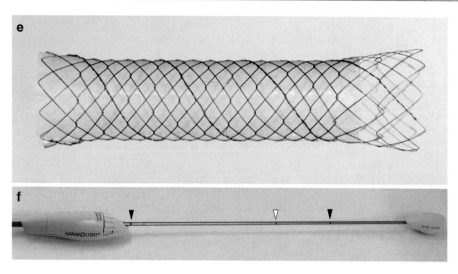

**Fig. 7.7** (continued)

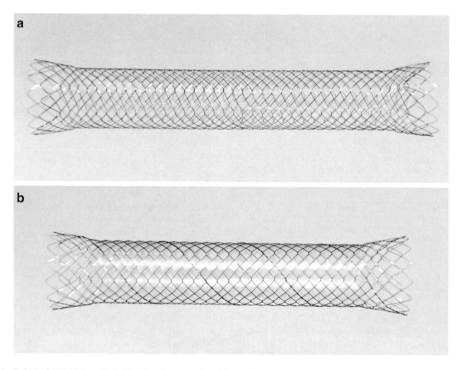

**Fig. 7.8** BONASTENT® pyloric/duodenal stents. (**a**) BONASTENT pyloric/duodenal uncovered stent. This enteral stent has flares on both ends. (**b**) BONASTENT pyloric/duodenal covered stent. Flares on both ends are uncovered

(four each at the distal, center, and proximal portions of the stent).

The stent comes preloaded on a 10-F delivery system for TTS or OTW placement. The lengths for TTS delivery are 180 and 230 cm, and 120 cm for OTW placement. Stainless steel radiopaque bands are on the proximal and distal parts of the delivery system inner shaft. After complete deployment, the stent shortens by up to 30%. It is reconstrainable up to 80% stent deployment. There is a red marker on the stainless steel outer shaft of the delivery system to denote the point of no return.

## BONASTENT Pyloric/Duodenal Covered

This partially covered enteral stent has same design as the BONASTENT pyloric/duodenal, except that the body is coated with silicone. Flares on both ends remain uncovered to reduce the risk of migration (Fig. 7.8b).

## BONASTENT M-Duodenal

Patients with malignant gastric outlet obstruction often have combined or impending biliary obstruction [21]. In these patients, a biliary stent is recommended prior to duodenal stent insertion through a percutaneous or an endoscopic approach. If a conventional enteral stent is placed, access to the papilla and biliary tree can be very difficult, and special maneuvers such as cutting the overlying wires or balloon dilating to widen the mesh structure of the duodenal stent are often required [21]. Moreover, biliary stents placed through the mesh of a conventional enteral stent rarely expand adequately because of the shape memory property of nitinol [14]. The BONASTENT M-Duodenal was developed to enable biliary stent placement and allow adequate expansion though the mesh structure of the duodenal stent.

The stent consists of two portions: a fixed portion with a woven fixed hook and cross-wired structure similar to the uncovered BONASTENT pyloric/duodenal and a 3-cm unfixed portion (M-portion) with an unfixed cross-wired structure. There are two stent types according to the location of the unfixed portion. The central type has the unfixed portion at the center of the stent, which is designed for type II bilioduodenal strictures that involve the second portion of duodenum with involvement of the papilla (Fig. 7.9a). The lateral type has the unfixed portion at either the distal or proximal part of the stent (Fig. 7.9b). The former is for type I bilioduodenal stenosis involving the duodenal bulb or the first portion without papillary involvement. The latter is for type III bilioduodenal stenosis involving the third portion of the duodenum with sparing of the papilla. These features contribute to easy insertion of a biliary stent through the mesh wall of the unfixed portion of the duodenal stent without resistance (Fig. 7.9c, d). There are 16 platinum wire spring radiopaque markers (four each at both ends of the unfixed portion, and proximal and distal ends) for improved fluoroscopic visualization of the entire stent and the unfixed portions.

Although the initial model had a smaller stent mesh cell size of 2.5–2.75 mm, the current model has 4-mm cells in both fixed and unfixed portions [22]. The available diameter of BONASTENT M-Duodenal is 22 mm. Other specifications of the flared ends and body are compatible with BONASTENT pyloric/duodenal uncovered.

## EGIS Pyloric Stent

The EGIS pyloric stent is the enteral stent from S&G Biotech (Seongnam, Korea), which provides various types of stents including EGIS pyloric stent-single bare, double bare, single-covered, double-covered, and Hercules SP pyloric stent, which consists of two stents. EGIS pyloric stent-double bare and Hercules SP pyloric stents have unique designs to minimize tumor ingrowth and stent migration.

### EGIS Pyloric Stent, Single Bare and Double Bare

These are self-expandable metal uncovered stents made of braided nitinol, which are woven into a cross and hooked structures. There are two types of stents that differ in the number of layers of mesh wire: single bare and double bare (Fig. 7.10a, b). Double bare is a unique double-layered structure created by crossing two stents resulting in a smaller diameter cell size (2–3 mm) with denser, numerous cells designed to reduce tumor ingrowth. EGIS pyloric stents lack flared ends and have round edges to reduce the risk of tissue damage and perforation. The unconstrained body diameters are 18, 20, 22, and 24 mm, and unconstrained lengths are 6, 8, 10, and 12 cm. There are ten gold radiopaque markers (four at each end and two in the midportion). The stent comes preloaded on a 10-F delivery system for either TTS (length, 180 cm) or OTW (length, 120 cm) deployment. There is radiopaque tungsten at the distal end of the outer sheath. After complete deployment, the stent foreshortens by 32% in

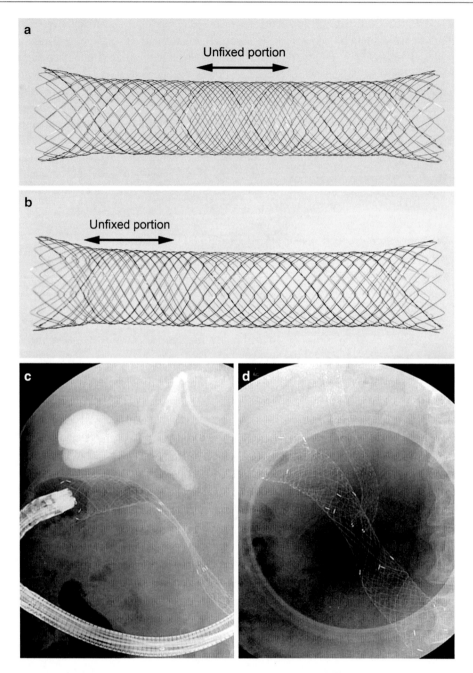

**Fig. 7.9** BONASTENT® M-duodenal. Unfixed portion of BONASTENT® M-duodenal enables biliary stents to be placed and allows expansion though the lumen of the duodenal stent. (**a**) Central type. Unfixed portion is located on the center of the stent body for the second portion of duodenal strictures. (**b**) Lateral type. Unfixed portion is located on the distal or proximal part. (**c**) Fluoroscopic view showed placement of a BONASTENT M-duodenal central type across the duodenal stricture. (**d**) Fluoroscopic view showed biliary stent successfully placed through the unfixed mesh of the duodenal stent (c and d, Courtesy of Prof. JH Moon, Soon Chun Hyang University School of Medicine, Bucheon/Seoul, Korea)

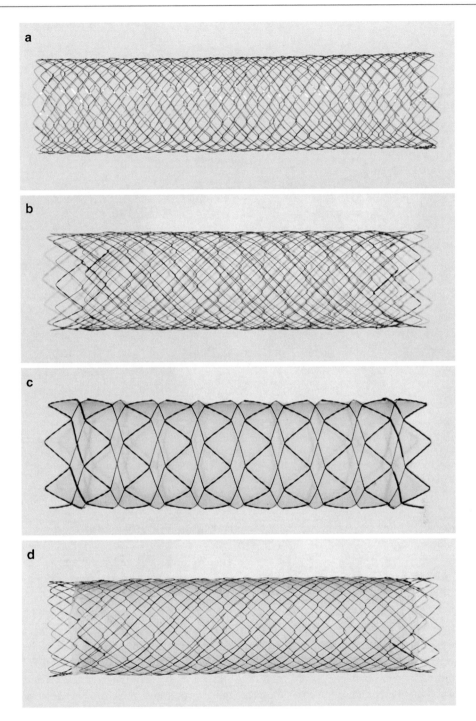

**Fig. 7.10** EGIS pyloric stent. (**a**) EGIS pyloric single bare stent. (**b**) The double-layered structure of EGIS pyloric double bare stent creates a smaller cell size. (**c**) EGIS pyloric single-covered stent is the old model of S&G Biotech. (**d**) Double-covered EGIS pyloric stent is double-layered combination pyloric stent which is made of 2 nitinol-braided stents and a silicone membrane

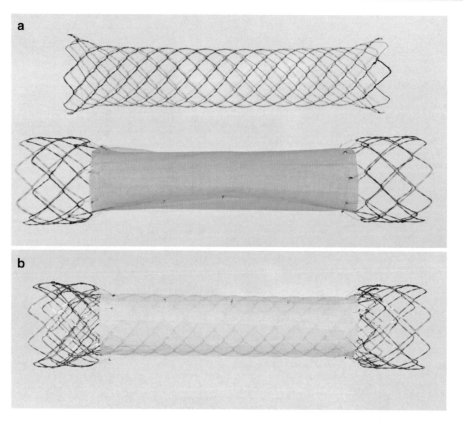

**Fig. 7.11** Hercules SP pyloric stent. This dual stent consists of two stents. (**a**) Inner bare nitinol stent (*top*) and outer stent consist of each end bare nitinol stent and a central Dacron fabric without wire structure (*bottom*). (**b**) Assembly of the two stents consecutively inserted under fluoroscopic guidance of the inner bare nitinol stent after insertion of the outer partially covered stent

single bare and 20% in double bare stents. These stents are not reconstrainable.

## EGIS Pyloric Stent, Single Covered and Double Covered

The covered type of EGIS pyloric stent is available in two models: single covered and double covered (Fig. 7.10c, d). The older model single-covered stent is fully covered with silicone and has 16 gold radiopaque markers (seven each at the ends and two on the midportion). After complete deployment, the stent foreshortens by 25%. EGIS pyloric stent double covered is the double-layered combination pyloric stent made of two nitinol-braided stents and a silicone membrane (Fig. 7.10d). There are 5-mm uncovered portions at the proximal and distal ends of the stent. Other characteristics are the same as EGIS pyloric stent double bare type.

## Hercules SP Pyloric Stent

The Hercules SP pyloric stent is a uniquely designed enteral stent from S&G Biotech designed to prevent tumor ingrowth and stent migration. This dual expandable stent consists of an outer partially covered stent and an inner bare nitinol stent which are inserted consecutively under fluoroscopic guidance (OTW method, Fig. 7.11a, b). The outer partially covered stent consists of three parts – a proximal and distal bare nitinol stent, and a central Dacron fabric without wire structure [23]. Both proximal and distal bare nitinol stent parts are 28 mm in diameter and 25 mm long. The diameter of the central Dacron portion is 18 mm. After the outer partially covered stent is inserted, a bare inner nitinol stent is inserted to expand the wireless Dacron portion of the outer stent and to increase its radial force. There are four gold radiopaque markers – two at each end.

The central Dacron mesh is available in 4-, 6-, 8-, and 10-cm lengths. This stent can only be inserted using OTW method and comes preloaded on a 12-F delivery system with 120 cm length. The distal end of the outer sheath has a radiopaque tungsten marker. After complete deployment, the inner stent foreshortens by 20% and is not reconstrainable.

## SX-ELLA Stent Pyloroduodenal: ENTERELLA

This self-expandable metal uncovered stent is made of braided nitinol and manufactured by ELLA-CS. s.r.o. (Hradec, Czech Republic). It does not have any flares and has a round-edged configuration to reduce trauma (Fig. 7.12). The unconstrained body diameters are 20, 22, and 25 mm, and unconstrained lengths are 8.2, 9.0, 11.3, and 13.5 cm. Three radiopaque markers are placed at each stent end and two markers at the midpoint to improve fluoroscopic visibility and accurate stent positioning (8 in total). A plastic repositioning loop is attached to the proximal stent end and allows repositioning within 5 days after implantation.

This stent can be inserted TTS or OTW with a 10-F delivery system and a standard length of 210 cm, which allows passage through the working channel of an endoscope. The atraumatic tip of the delivery system is radiopaque. It is not possible to recapture the stent once it is partially deployed. The stent foreshortens by approximately 40–50%.

## Endo-Flex Duodenal Stent

The Endo-Flex duodenal stent is an enteral stent from ENDO-FLEX GmbH, Voerde, Germany. This self-expandable metal uncovered stent is made of braided nitinol. It has flared ends (tulip design) to prevent migration and round ends to reduce the risk of tissue injury (Fig. 7.13). The diameter of flared end is 4 mm larger than that of the body, which has an unconstrained diameter of 20 mm. Unconstrained lengths are available in 6, 8, and 10 cm. The length of flares is 10 mm. There are four tantalum radiopaque markers (two for each end) to provide fluoroscopic visualization. This stent can be inserted TTS with a 10-F delivery

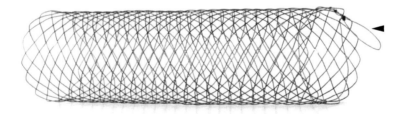

**Fig. 7.12** SX-ELLA Stent Pyloroduodenal – ENTERELLA. A plastic repositioning loop (*arrowhead*) is attached to the proximal stent end

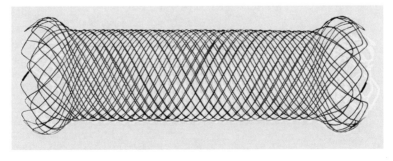

**Fig. 7.13** Endo-Flex duodenal stent. This uncovered stent has a flare at both ends (tulip design) and round ends

system (length 180 cm). There are two stainless steel ring markers (one close to the distal tip, one where the stent is loaded in the system). After complete deployment, the stent foreshortens by approximately 40% (based on a 20-mm stent, nominal expanded length of 60 mm). Both predeployed and expanded lengths are clearly indicated on the product label (i.e., loaded length in applicator 104 mm, length in expanded nominal length 60 mm). Endo-Flex offers both types: reconstrainable (maximum 65%) and standard.

## Aixstent

The Aixstent is a self-expandable metal-uncovered stent made of braided nitinol manufactured by Leufen Medical GmbH, Aachen, Germany. It has a tulip design with flared ends to prevent migration and atraumatic ends to reduce the risk of tissue injury. The diameter of the flared end is 6 mm larger than the 20 mm diameter of the unconstrained body. Unconstrained lengths are 6, 8, and 10 cm. Tantalum radiopaque markers provide excellent fluoroscopic visualization. This stent can be inserted TTS with a 10-F delivery system (length 180 cm).

## Summary

Recent technological advances enable relief of gastroduodenal or proximal small bowel stenosis using self-expandable stents as an alternative and better option to surgery in selected patients. Current enteral stents are flexible for application in angulated anatomy and have large diameters to allow patients to tolerate solid food. Moreover, the long-length and small-diameter slim delivery systems allow through the scope stent placement. Bare stents are the common type of enteral stent provided by all manufacturers. Covered stents were developed to prevent tumor ingrowth, which

**Table 7.1** Characteristics of enteral stents

| | Manufacturer | Covered/ uncovered | Flare on ends | Shortening rates | Reconstrainable point at stent deployment | TTS/ OTW |
|---|---|---|---|---|---|---|
| Wallstent | Boston Scientific Inc., Natick, MA, USA | Uncovered | No flares | Up to 45% | 70% | TTS/ OTW |
| WallFlex | Boston Scientific Inc., Natick, MA, USA | Uncovered | Proximal | Up to 45% | 70% | TTS/ OTW |
| Evolution | Cook Medical Inc., Winston-Salem, NC, USA | Uncovered | Proximal/ distal | Up to 50% | 50% | TTS only |
| Niti-S D/ComVi | Taewoong Medical Inc., Seoul, Korea | Uncovered/ partially covered | No flare | Up to 17% | Nonreconstrainable | TTS/ OTW |
| Niti-S S type | Taewoong Medical Inc., Seoul, Korea | Fully covered | Proximal/ distal | Up to 60% | 70% | TTS/ OTW |
| HANAROSTENT | M.I. Tech, Seoul, Korea | Uncovered/ partially covered | Proximal/ distal | Up to 20% | 80% | TTS/ OTW |
| BONASTENT | Standard Sci-Tech Inc., Seoul, Korea | Uncovered/ partially covered | Proximal/ distal | Up to 30% | 80% | TTS/ OTW |
| BONASTENT M-Duodenal | Standard Sci-Tech Inc., Seoul, Korea | Uncovered | Proximal/ distal | Up to 30% | 80% | TTS/ OTW |
| EGIS single/ double bare | S&G Biotech, Seongnam, Korea | Uncovered | No flare | Up to 32%/20% | Nonreconstrainable | TTS/ OTW |
| EGIS single/ double covered | S&G Biotech, Seongnam, Korea | Fully/partially covered | No flare | Up to 25%/19% | Nonreconstrainable | TTS/ OTW |
| Hercules SP pyloric stent | S&G Biotech, Seongnam, Korea | Partially covered | Proximal/ distal | Up to 20% | Nonreconstrainable | OTW only |
| SX-ELLA stent | ELLA-CS Co, Hradec, Czech Republic | Uncovered | No flare | Up to 50% | Nonreconstrainable | TTS/ OTW |
| Endo-Flex | ENDO-FLEX GmbH, Voerde, Germany | Uncovered | Proximal/ distal | Up to 40% | 65% | TTS/ OTW |

**Table 7.2**  Specifications (diameter and lengths) of stents and delivery systems

| Name | Unconstrained flare diameter/length | Unconstrained body diameter | Unconstrained lengths | Delivery system diameter/length TTS | OTW |
|---|---|---|---|---|---|
| Wallstent | No flare | 20, 22 mm | 6, 9 cm | 3.3 mm/135 and 230 cm | 3.3mm/135 and 230 cm |
| WallFlex | 27 mm/15 mm | 22 mm | 6, 9, 12 cm | 10 Fr/230 cm | 10 Fr/230 cm |
| Evolution | 27 mm/20 mm | 22 mm | 6, 9, 12 cm | 10 Fr/230 cm | N/A |
| Niti-S D type | No flare | 18, 20, 22, 24 mm | 6,8,10,12 cm | 10 Fr/180 cm | 10 Fr/135 cm |
| Niti-S ComVi type | No flare | 18, 20 mm | 6,8,10,12 cm | 10.5 Fr/180 cm | 10.5 Fr/135 cm |
| Niti-S S type | 24 mm/15 mm | 18, 20 mm | 6,8,10,12 cm | 10.5 Fr/180 cm | 10.5 Fr/135 cm |
| HANAROSTENT noncovered | 25 mm/13 mm | 20 mm | 6, 8, 10, 12, 14, 16 cm | 10.2 Fr/230 cm | 10.5 Fr/120 cm |
| HANAROSTENT-covered | 26 mm/13 mm | 20 mm | 6, 8, 10, 12, 14, 16 cm | 10.2 Fr/230 cm | 10.2 Fr/120 cm |
| BONASTENT | 6 mm bigger than body/15 mm | 18, 20 mm | 6,8, 10, 12,14, 16 cm | 10 Fr/180 and 230 cm | 10 Fr/120 cm |
| BONASTENT M-Duodenal | 26 mm/15 mm | 22 mm | 6,8, 10, 12,14, 16 cm | 10 Fr/180 and 230 cm | 10 Fr/120 cm |
| EGIS single/double bare | No flare | 18, 20, 22, 24 mm | 6, 8, 10, 12 cm | 10 Fr/180 cm | 10 Fr/120 cm |
| EGIS single/double covered | No flare | 18, 20, 22, 24 mm | 6, 8, 10, 12 cm | 10 Fr/180 cm | 10 Fr/120 cm |
| Hercules SP pyloric stent | 28 mm/25 mm | 18 mm | 9,11,13,15 cm | N/A | 12 Fr/120 cm |
| SX-ELLA stent | No flare | 20, 22,25 mm | 8.2, 9.0, 11.3, 13.5 cm | 10 Fr/210 cm | 10 Fr/210 cm |
| Endo-Flex | 24 mm/ | 20 mm | 6, 8, 10 cm | 10 Fr/180 cm | 10 Fr/180 cm |

is a disadvantage of bare stents. Several unique designs are used to minimize covered stent migration including uncovered flared ends, multiple-layer design (membrane between wires), and dual stent type (outer-covered, inner bare stent). The characteristics of enteral stents, and their specifications (diameter and lengths) and delivery systems, are summarized in Tables 7.1 and 7.2, respectively. Further technological advancements are expected to lead to improvement in stent design to minimize tumor ingrowth and stent migration.

# References

1. Topazian M, Ring E, Grendell J. Palliation of obstructing gastric cancer with steel mesh, self-expanding endoprostheses. Gastrointest Endosc. 1992;38:58–60.
2. Keymling M, Wagner HJ, Vakil N, et al. Relief of malignant duodenal obstruction by percutaneous insertion of a metal stent. Gastrointest Endosc. 1993;39:439–41.
3. Kozarek RA, Ball TJ, Patterson DJ. Metallic self-expanding stent application in the upper gastrointestinal tract: caveats and concerns. Gastrointest Endosc. 1992;38:1–6.
4. Song HY, Yang DH, Kuh JH, et al. Obstructing cancer of the gastric antrum: palliative treatment with covered metallic stents. Radiology. 1993;187:357–8.
5. Feretis C, Benakis P, Dimopoulos C, et al. Duodenal obstruction caused by pancreatic head carcinoma: palliation with self-expandable endoprostheses. Gastrointest Endosc. 1997;46:161–5.
6. Maetani I, Tada T, Shimura J, et al. Technical modifications and strategies for stenting gastric outlet strictures using esophageal endoprostheses. Endoscopy. 2002;34:402–6.
7. Phillips MS, Gosain S, Bonatti H, et al. Enteral stents for malignancy: a report of 46 consecutive cases over 10 years, with critical review of complications. J Gastrointest Surg. 2008;12:2045–50.
8. Aviv RI, Shyamalan G, Khan FH, et al. Use of stents in the palliative treatment of malignant gastric outlet and duodenal obstruction. Clin Radiol. 2002;57:587–92.
9. Lee JM, Han YM, Lee SY, et al. Palliation of postoperative gastrointestinal anastomotic malignant strictures with flexible covered metallic stents: preliminary results. Cardiovasc Intervent Radiol. 2001;24:25–30.

10. Kim JH, Yoo BM, Lee KJ, et al. Self-expanding coil stent with a long delivery system for palliation of unresectable malignant gastric outlet obstruction: a prospective study. Endoscopy. 2001;33:838–42.

11. Adler DG, Baron TH. Endoscopic palliation of malignant gastric outlet obstruction using self-expanding metal stents: experience in 36 patients. Am J Gastroenterol. 2002;97:72–8.

12. Telford JJ, Carr-Locke DL, Baron TH, et al. Palliation of patients with malignant gastric outlet obstruction with the enteral Wallstent: outcomes from a multicenter study. Gastrointest Endosc. 2004;60:916–20.

13. Soetikno RM, Lichtenstein DR, Vandervoort J, et al. Palliation of malignant gastric outlet obstruction using an endoscopically placed Wallstent. Gastrointest Endosc. 1998;47:267–70.

14. Laasch HU, Martin DF, Maetani I. Enteral stents in the gastric outlet and duodenum. Endoscopy. 2005;37:74–81.

15. Tierney W, Chuttani R, Croffie J, et al. Enteral stents. Gastrointest Endosc. 2006;63:920–6.

16. Baerlocher MO, Asch MR, Dixon P, et al. Interdisciplinary Canadian guidelines on the use of metal stents in the gastrointestinal tract for oncological indications. Can Assoc Radiol J. 2008;59:107–22.

17. Jung GS, Song HY, Kang SG, et al. Malignant gastroduodenal obstructions: treatment by means of a covered expandable metallic stent-initial experience. Radiology. 2000;216:758–63.

18. Katsanos K, Sabharwal T, Adam A. Stenting of the upper gastrointestinal tract: current status. Cardiovasc Intervent Radiol. 2010;33:690–705.

19. van Hooft J, Mutignani M, Repici A, et al. First data on the palliative treatment of patients with malignant gastric outlet obstruction using the WallFlex enteral stent: a retrospective multicenter study. Endoscopy. 2007;39:434–9.

20. Lee SM, Kang DH, Kim GH, et al. Self-expanding metallic stents for gastric outlet obstruction resulting from stomach cancer: a preliminary study with a newly designed double-layered pyloric stent. Gastrointest Endosc. 2007;66:1206–10.

21. Mutignani M, Tringali A, Shah SG, et al. Combined endoscopic stent insertion in malignant biliary and duodenal obstruction. Endoscopy. 2007;39:440–7.

22. Moon JH, Choi HJ, Ko BM, et al. Combined endoscopic stent-in-stent placement for malignant biliary and duodenal obstruction by using a new duodenal metal stent (with videos). Gastrointest Endosc. 2009;70:772–7.

23. Kim JH, Song HY, Shin JH, et al. Metallic stent placement in the palliative treatment of malignant gastroduodenal obstructions: prospective evaluation of results and factors influencing outcome in 213 patients. Gastrointest Endosc. 2007;66:256–64.

# Colonic Prostheses

8

## Tae Il Kim

There are multiple types of commercially available self-expandable metal stents (SEMS) specifically designed for colonic use from various manufacturers. The available stents differ in delivery system, stent material, design, deployed diameter and length, radial force exerted, flexibility, degree of shortening after expansion, and recapturability, which are factors for consideration when selecting a colonic stent model. These many factors might be reflected in developing new types of stents to improve clinical outcomes for patients and/or usability for operators. The detailed features of each stent model, which is available internationally, are summarized in Table 8.1 [1–8].

It might be difficult to make a perfect stent with every desirable attribute that can be passed through the channel of a colonoscope. Therefore, we need to understand the characteristics of each model of colon stent and to select the one best suited for each situation. Broad experience will be helpful in selecting the proper stent model and understanding the delicate details of each model, which are difficult to measure or describe, such as conformability of the deployed stent, flexibility of delivery system, etc.

T.I. Kim, M.D., Ph.D. (✉)
Division of Gastroenterology, Department of Internal Medicine, Institute of Gastroenterology, Severance Hospital, Yonsei University College of Medicine, 250 Seongsanno, Seodaemun-gu, Seoul 120-752, Republic of Korea
e-mail: taeilkim@yuhs.ac

## Delivery System

Delivery systems may vary according to the approach methods for SEMS placement, such as through-the-scope (TTS) and non-TTS stent placements. The delivery system for the TTS method has a longer total working length and smaller predeployment diameter (10 French) to allow the passage of stents directly through the working channel of a therapeutic colonoscope (≥3.8 mm diameter).

The most important point in the delivery system is to deliver excellent sheath pushability and allow for efficient tracking and maneuverability for deployment, especially in difficult anatomical challenges, such as acute and complex angulations. By enhancing flexibility of the delivery system, manufacturers attempt to minimize trauma and to aid in traversing abnormal anatomy without kinking. Moreover, many delivery systems are designed to be reconstrainable by recapturing the stent, when repositioning is desired during deployment. The recapturable ranges of the deployed portion during deployment vary according to the stent models.

For repositioning directly after complete deployment, with a lasso on proximal end of some stent models, it is possible to reposition the stent to the desired area by pulling with forceps on the lasso. In addition, to facilitate accurate stent placement, highly visible endoscopic and/or fluoroscopic markers on the delivery system or

**Table 8.1** Currently available self-expandable metal stents (SEMS) for colorectal obstruction

| Manufacturer model | Delivery system/diameter (Fr) | Stent materials | Deployed diameters/flare (mm) | Deployed length (cm) | Uncovered/covered | Features | Published data (Reference No.) |
|---|---|---|---|---|---|---|---|
| *Boston scientific* | | | | | | | |
| WallFlex enteral colonic | TTS or OTW/10 | Nitinol | 25 (body)/30 (proximal flare) 22 (body)/27 (proximal flare) | 6, 9, 12 | Uncovered | Reconstrainable (at up to 70% of deployment) 30–38% Shortening during expansion Radiopaque markers on delivery system | [1, 3, 4] |
| *Taewoong medical* | | | | | | | |
| Niti-S enteral colonic (D-type) | TTS or OTW/10 | Nitinol | 18, 20, 22, 24/no flare | 6, 8, 10, 12 | Uncovered | Reconstrainable (at up to 1/3 of deployment) 17% Shortening during expansion Radiopaque markers on stent | [2] |
| Niti-S enteral colonic (head type) | TTS or OTW/10, 10.5 | Nitinol | 18, 20/24 (both ends flare) | 6, 8, 10, 12 | Covered (silicone, bare ends) | Reconstrainable (at up to 70% of deployment) 50–60% Shortening during expansion Radiopaque markers on stent | [5] |
| ComVi Niti-S enteral colonic | TTS or OTW/10, 10.5 | Nitinol (double-layer) | 18, 20/no flare | 6, 8, 10, 12 | Covered (PTFE, bare ends) | Reconstrainable (at up to 1/3 of deployment) 17% Shortening during expansion Radiopaque markers on stent | [1, 2] |

*Cook endoscopy*

| | | | | | | | |
|---|---|---|---|---|---|---|---|
| Evolution colonic | TTS or OTW/10 | Nitinol | 25/30 (both ends flare) | 6, 8, 10 | Uncovered | Gun-shaped controlled-release deployment device<br>Reconstrainable (at up to "point of no return")<br>45% Shortening during expansion<br>Radiopaque markers on stent | |
| Colonic Z-stent | Non-TTS/31 | Stainless steel | 25/35 (both ends flare) | 4, 6, 8, 10, 12 | Uncovered | | |
| *M.I.Tech* | | | | | | | |
| Hanarostent colon/rectum (NNN) | TTS or OTW/10.2, 10.5 | Nitinol | 22, 24/26, 28 (both ends flare) | 6, 7, 8, 9, 10, 11, 12, 13, 14, 15, 16 | Uncovered | Reconstrainable (at up to 80% of deployment)<br>20–30% Shortening during expansion<br>Radiopaque markers on stent<br>With or without lasso | [6, 7] |
| Hanarostent colon/rectum (NCN) | TTS or OTW/10.2 | Nitinol | 20/26 (both ends flare) | 7, 8, 9, 10, 11, 12, 13, 14, 15 | Covered (silicone, partial) | Reconstrainable (at up to 80% of deployment)<br>46% Shortening during expansion<br>Radiopaque markers on stent, lasso | |
| Hanarostent colon/rectum (CCC) | Non-TTS/24 | Nitinol | 24/32 (both ends flare) | 7, 8, 9, 10, 11, 12, 13, 14, 15 | Covered (silicone) | 35% Shortening during expansion<br>Radiopaque markers on stent, Two lasso | [8] |
| *ELLA-CS* | | | | | | | |
| SX-ELLA colorectal (Enterella) | Non-TTS/15, 18 (covered) | Nitinol | 20, 22, 25 | 8.2, 9, 11.3, 13.5 | Uncovered or covered (polyurethane) | 35–40% Shortening during expansion<br>Radiopaque markers on stent, lasso | |

*TTS* through-the-scope, *OTW* over-the-wire, *PTFE* polytetrafluoroethylene

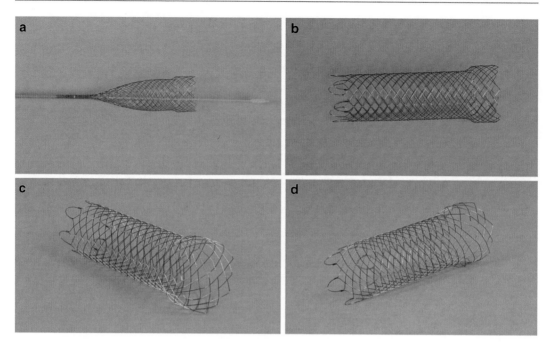

**Fig. 8.1** WallFlex enteral colonic stent (Boston scientific). (**a**) Stent during deployment. (**b–d**) Fully deployed stent

stent define proximal, middle, and/or distal end of the stent.

## Stent Design

As for the stent material, Nitinol (metal alloy of nickel and titanium) exhibits unique properties: shape memory and superelasticity. Because of their ability to conform to anatomical angulations, Nitinol stents now dominate the market. Although the ideal stent diameter for proper radial force is unknown, the postdeployment diameter of colonic SEMS is usually between 18 and 30 mm. The deployed length of colonic stents range from 4 to 16 cm, and the stent chosen should be at least 3–4 cm longer than the obstruction to allow an adequate margin of stent, by at least 1.5–2 cm on either side of the obstruction.

The end portion of most stents is designed to have rounded edges to prevent mucosal injury and complications due to the sharp end of stent wires, and some stents are designed to have a flare in both or the proximal end of stent to potentially reduce the risk of migration (Figs. 8.1, 8.2, 8.3, and 8.4). In addition, radiopaque markers at each end of the stent provide visualization for accurate placement.

Many stent models have improved flexibility, thereby allowing the stent to fully conform to the natural curves of the anatomy while potentially reducing the risk of complications, such as perforation or bleeding. In particular, the D-type stents are constructed with unfixed individual cells, woven with two separated wires, allowing cells to overlap each other over a highly curved area. Compared to the single wire type, this specific construction allows D-type stents to have notable flexibility and conformability, which can prevent abrupt luminal narrowing at flexed areas of the colon (Fig. 8.2). During expansion, most of the stents have shortening in length. The shortening rates will vary between 20% and 45%, contingent upon stent model.

## Uncovered/Covered Stent

One of important factors of stent type utilized, which is directly comparable and related with clinical outcomes, is whether the prosthesis is uncovered/covered. Even though both types of

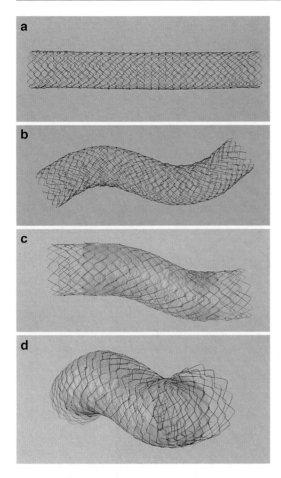

Fig. 8.2 (**a**, **b**) Niti-S enteral colonic (D-type) and (**c**, **d**) ComVi enteral colonic stent (TaeWoong Medical, Gyeonggi-Do, Korea)

stents show similar technical and clinical success rates, they present unique advantages and disadvantages. Covered stents have the advantage of less frequent stent occlusion by tumor ingrowth and the disadvantage of a high risk of stent migration, whereas uncovered stents are associated with less stent migration but are more prone to tumor ingrowth. Although a recent randomized prospective study, comparing the uncovered Wallflex stent and the covered ComVi stent, showed the same results as those mentioned above, neither stent type differed with respect to overall complication rate and stent patency duration, suggesting both types are suitable for relieving malignant colorectal obstruction [1]. Furthermore, the ComVi stent (double-layered combination covered stents) was designed to prevent both tumor ingrowth by incorporation of an interposing membrane and stent migration with the outer uncovered wire designed to embed in the colorectal cancer [2]. However, this new type of colonic stent could not overcome the shortcoming of the covered stent: more frequent stent migration [1, 2].

As for the material of the covered stent membrane, the polytetrafluoroethylene (PTFE) membrane, with its strong physical and chemical resistance, is highly biocompatible and may prevent tumor ingrowth and membrane deformation. Silicone rubber, with nonreactive, stable, and resis-

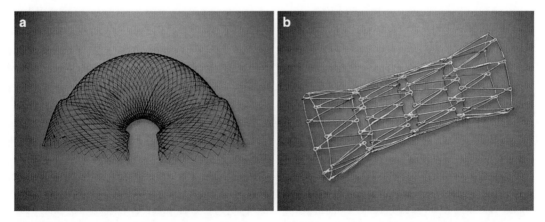

Fig. 8.3 (**a**) Evolution colonic and (**b**) Colonic Z-stent (Cook Endoscopy) (Courtesy of Cook Medical Incorporated, Bloomington, IN)

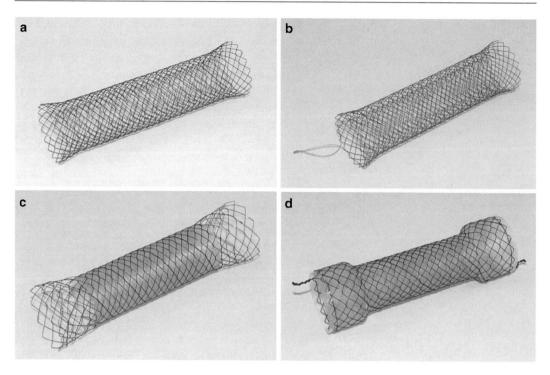

**Fig. 8.4** (**a**, **b**) Hanarostent colon/rectum, uncovered, with/without lasso, (**c**) Hanarostent Colon/rectum, covered, TTS delivery, and (**d**) Hanarostent Colon/rectum, covered, non-TTS delivery (MI Tech). TTS, through-the-scope

tant properties to endure extreme environments and its ease of manufacturing and shaping, is also being used as a membrane in covered stents.

## Conclusion

Several types of colon stents have been developed, and each type and design of stent has unique characteristics. However, it is difficult to prove that these properties make a difference in the outcome of patients or improve maneuverability for its operators. We need to understand the features of each stent through experience, and estimate their effect on clinical outcomes and ease of insertion to develop a new and ideal stent design.

## References

1. Park S, Cheon JH, Park JJ, et al. Comparison of efficacies between stents for malignant colorectal obstruction: a randomized, prospective study. Gastrointest Endosc. 2010;72:304–10.

2. Moon CM, Kim TI, Lee MS, et al. Comparison of a newly designed double-layered combination covered stent and D-weave uncovered stent for decompression of obstructive colorectal cancer: a prospective multicenter study. Dis Colon Rectum. 2010;53:1190–6.

3. Repici A, De Caro G, Luigiano C, et al. Wallflex colonic stent placement for management of malignant colonic obstruction: a prospective study at two centers. Gastrointest Endosc. 2008;67:77–84.

4. van Hooft JE, Fockens P, Marinelli AW, et al. Early closure of a multicenter randomized clinical trial of endoscopic stenting versus surgery for stage IV left-sided colorectal cancer. Endoscopy. 2008;40:184–91.

5. Shim CS, Cho JY, Jung IS, et al. Through-the-scope double colonic stenting in the management of inoperable proximal malignant colonic obstruction: a pilot study. Endoscopy. 2004;36:426–31.

6. Im J, Kim S, Kang H, et al. Clinical outcomes and patency of self-expanding metal stents in patients with malignant colorectal obstruction: a prospective single center study. Int J Colorectal Dis. 2008;23:789–94.

7. Suh J, Kim S, Cho Y, et al. Effectiveness of stent placement for palliative treatment in malignant colorectal obstruction and predictive factors for stent occlusion. Surg Endosc. 2010;24:400–6.

8. Scharf J-G, Ramadori G, Becker H, Muller A. Implantation of a colorectal stent as a therapeutic approach in the treatment of esophageal leakage. BMC Gastroenterol. 2007;7:10.

# Part 4

# Indications and Placement Techniques

# Esophageal Stents: Indications and Placement Techniques

## Andrew S. Ross and Richard A. Kozarek

Since the late nineteenth century, the creation of a new lumen to palliate an obstruction has been pursued on a variety of levels. Though a variety of designs and improvements have been witnessed, perhaps none has been more revolutionary over the past 20 years within the esophagus than the introduction of self-expandable stents, both metal and plastic, into clinical practice. Mounted and constrained onto a delivery catheter, these stents can easily be deployed within the esophagus as a treatment for a variety of conditions, both benign and malignant. This chapter will discuss the indications for esophageal stent placement as well as deployment techniques and postoperative care.

## Malignant Indications

By far, the leading indication for placement of esophageal self-expanding stents, both metal (SEMS) and plastic (SEPS), is palliation of complications related to esophageal malignancies. Owing to a lack of symptoms within the early stages of the disease, up to one-half of patients with esophageal cancer present with stage IV (metastatic) disease; the majority of whom will not survive beyond 12 months [1–4]. Given the poor prognosis in this group of patients, treatment goals are essentially directed toward palliative efforts: maintenance of esophageal luminal patency, optimization of nutrition, and reduction in the risk of aspiration [1].

SEMS are highly efficacious in their ability to palliate dysphagia and close malignant fistulae. Multiple case series and meta-analyses performed over the past 20 years suggest immediate improvement in clinical symptoms in 90–100% of patients [5–25]. Despite the multitude of available SEMS on the market today, there are no data to suggest clinical superiority of one device over another. Whereas the placement of self-expanding esophageal stents is technically feasible in almost all patients in whom it is attempted, they are associated with a risk of associated complications and the need for reintervention in up to one-third of patients due to luminal occlusion from hyperplastic tissue, tumor or solid debris stent-induced fistula, and proximal or distal stent migration [26, 27]. Technical failure of esophageal stent placement is typically related to the inability to pass a wire guide or the stent delivery system beyond the tumor; fortunately, these are both rare events.

The demographics of esophageal cancer have changed significantly over the past three decades [2, 3]. Owing to an increase in obesity, chronic gastroesophageal reflux, and resultant Barrett's esophagus, the majority of esophageal cancers diagnosed are adenocarcinoma. These are typically located in the distal esophagus, in close proximity to or at the level of the gastroesophageal junction (GEJ). Although esophageal stents

A.S. Ross, M.D. (✉) • R.A. Kozarek, M.D.
Digestive Disease Institute, Virginia Mason Medical
Center and University of Washington, 1100 9th Ave.,
C3-GAS, Seattle, WA 98111, USA
e-mail: andrew.ross@vmmc.org

R. Kozarek et al. (eds.), *Self-Expandable Stents in the Gastrointestinal Tract*,
DOI 10.1007/978-1-4614-3746-8_9, © Springer Science+Business Media New York 2013

which cross the GEJ are effective at relieving dysphagia, they are associated with a lower health-related quality of life due to almost universal reflux of gastric contents proximally across a bypassed lower esophageal sphincter [4–28]. Despite the availability of stents with an antireflux mechanism, it is not uncommon that a patient with a stent across the GEJ feels worse after stent placement than before placement [28]. As such, consideration of the severity of clinical symptoms, careful counseling of patients regarding lifestyle modification – upright positioning and the use of proton pump inhibitors – and exhaustive informed consent regarding the associated complications of stents without an antireflux mechanism in this location are required.

Patients with locally advanced esophageal cancers often undergo neoadjuvant chemoradiotherapy. In this group of patients, esophageal stents – both fully covered SEMS and SEPS – have been placed as an alternative to enteral feeding tubes in order to ensure adequate nutrition and palliate dysphagia during this critical phase of treatment [29–32]. In this group of patients, stents are typically left in place for the initial 4 weeks of treatment; after which point, they are removed as most tumors will have responded to treatment by this point and the risk of subsequent stent migration remains high. Although the data suggest that fully covered SEMS or SEPS can be used as an alternative to surgical jejunostomy as a bridge to surgery in patients undergoing neoadjuvant treatment, the rate of endoscopic reintervention can be significant in patients undergoing esophageal stent placement; this must be considered when making a clinical decision in such individuals [29].

The placement of a more "permanent," partially uncovered stent (which until recently has often been far more difficult and risky to remove than FCSEMS or SEPS) as a bridge to surgery in patients with locally advanced esophageal cancer remains controversial [33–36]. From the surgical perspective, stent-induced changes to the stomach (future conduit), occasional difficulty in removing an SEMS at the time of surgery, as well as the risk of bleeding and esophageal perforation related to device insertion in a patient who is

an otherwise good surgical candidate raise significant concerns [37]. In addition, the safety of stent placement in the setting of concurrent radiation therapy – including a possible increased risk of fistula and bleeding – has been questioned although not thoroughly investigated. Although a large observational study involving 200 patients failed to show an increase in major complications following SEMS in this group of patients [38], a retrospective analysis suggested that a history of chemoradiotherapy was associated with major stent complications with an odds ratio of 5.6 [4, 38]. In light of these open questions, the use of partially covered SEMS in the setting of neoadjuvant chemoradiation is largely dictated by local practice bias.

Patients with esophageal cancer may be prone to the formation of malignant tracheoesophageal fistulae (TEF) both from the disease itself as well as the effects of local radiation therapy. Malignant TEF have been reported to be successfully treated by the placement of a covered esophageal stent, alone or in combination with a covered tracheal stent [10, 17, 39–43]. Aside from dysphagia related to obstruction from intrinsic esophageal malignancies, extrinsic compression of the esophageal lumen can be observed in patients with lung cancer, mediastinal masses, and pleural-based malignancies. Self-expandable metal stent (SEMS) placement has been reported to be successful in relieving dysphagia resulting from extrinsic luminal compression [12, 44].

Despite high rates of technical success and initial clinical improvement, esophageal stents placed for malignant indications have a rate of reintervention of up to 30% [4]. Tumor ingrowth, food debris, as well as granulation tissue can all lead to stent occlusion and the need for endoscopic reintervention. Fortunately, endoscopic management of stent occlusion is relatively straightforward; using argon plasma coagulation for treatment of granulation tissue, removal of debris, and additional stent placement can all be employed to relieve obstructive symptoms resulting from stent occlusion. Stent migration can also result in the need for reintervention and has been described in up to 17% of patients undergoing covered (partially or fully) SEMS placement for

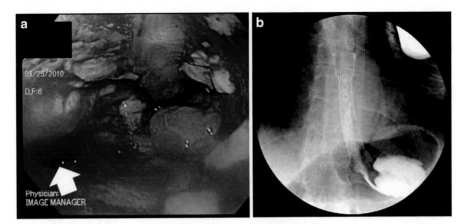

**Fig. 9.1** (a) Endoscopic image demonstrating an iatrogenic esophageal perforation (*arrow*) following esophageal dilation. Recognition of the perforation at the time of endoscopy allowed for the immediate placement of a fully covered SEMS; an esophagram immediately following stent placement demonstrates the absence of a leak (b) This patient was treated nonsurgically and the stent was removed

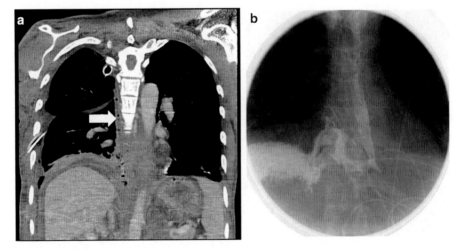

**Fig. 9.2** (a) Pneumomediastinum (*arrow*) in a patient with esophageal rupture secondary to Boerhaave syndrome. (b) An esophagram demonstrates extravasation of contrast into the *right* chest

malignant indications [45]. Most stent designs employ some degree of covering to reduce the risk of tumor ingrowth, a feature which must be balanced with the risk of stent migration due to the lack of tumor intercalation into the struts of the endoprostheses and tissue embedding into surrounding normal tissue. Migrated stents can either be repositioned or removed endoscopically. Endoscopic clips can be employed in an attempt to maintain stent position; though to be effective, the clips must be attached to the esophageal mucosa [46].

## Benign Indications

Benign indications for esophageal stent placement include esophageal perforation, postsurgical anastomotic leaks, and refractory, benign strictures [4]. A number of case series have now demonstrated the clinical efficacy of using SEPS and, more recently, fully covered SEMS and even biodegradable stents for these benign indications [47–61]. Esophageal perforation, which may occur as a result of iatrogenic injury related to

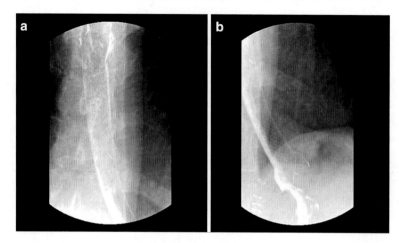

**Fig. 9.3** (**a**) A fully covered SEMS is placed to bridge an esophageal leak in the patient described in Fig. 9.2. An esophagram (**b**) performed following stent deployment demonstrates no further extravasation of contrast into the chest. The stent was removed after approximately 3 months

endoscopic therapy (Fig. 9.1) or spontaneous rupture (Boerhaave syndrome; Figs. 9.2 and 9.3), is often associated with significant morbidity and, in some cases, requires surgical repair [4]. Multiple reports suggest that placement of a completely covered SEMS or SEPS has emerged as an essential part of the management algorithm in these cases [49–52, 62–65] and, in appropriately selected individuals, can result in successful closure of perforations without the need for operative repair.

Esophageal leaks following esophagectomy and anastomotic breakdown following bariatric surgery have been successfully managed using completely covered SEMS or SEPS [53–64]. Though successful in helping to avoid reoperation, the risk of stent migration may be as high as 60% in this group, especially once the anastomosis has healed. As such, vigilance, close clinical follow-up, and prompt stent removal once leak closure has been documented are essential in avoiding additional complications related to migrated stents or the development of stent-induced tracheoesophageal fistula.

Refractory benign esophageal strictures are usually the result of acid-peptic disease, as well as a history of radiation to the head, neck, chest, or mediastinum. Other causes include a history of caustic ingestion and congenital disorders such as esophageal atresia. Temporary placement of a covered SEMS or SEPS or deployment of a biodegradable stent in this population is performed once other management options have been exhausted – including use of proton pump inhibitors, esophageal dilation, as well as steroid injection into the stricture during dilation [47]. Although efficacious in relieving dysphagia in the short-term, the migration rate of covered SEMS and SEPS for refractory benign strictures reaches up to 82% in some series, resulting in dismal rates of long-term symptom relief [66].

## Contraindications

There are very few contraindications to esophageal stent placement. Patients considered for stent placement should have a life expectancy of at least 30 days. Stent placement is contraindicated in patients who are deemed too ill to undergo upper gastrointestinal endoscopy and contraindicated in those with uncontrolled coagulopathy and, possibly, esophageal varices, though temporary placement of fully covered SEMS have been used to control refractory esophageal variceal bleeding [67].

Careful consideration to stent-related compression of the tracheobronchial tree must be given to patients with tumors located in the mid to upper esophagus or in those tumors which involve the airway (Figs. 9.4, 9.5, and 9.6). The radial expansion force associated with SEMS placement across

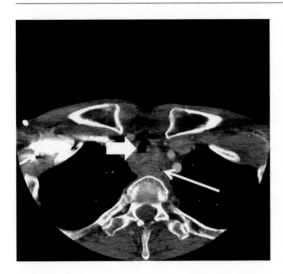

**Fig. 9.4** CT scan in a patient with a proximal squamous esophageal carcinoma. Note the involvement and stenosis of the airway (*arrowhead*) and esophagus (*arrow*)

tumors in this location has the theoretical risk of causing airway obstruction [68–71]. A chest CT scan should be obtained and reviewed with a thoracic surgeon or interventional pulmonologist prior to SEMS placement in patients with mid- to upper esophageal tumors. In selected cases, bronchoscopy with placement of a tracheal or bronchial stent may be indicated prior to or immediately following esophageal stent placement [72]. The use of a bougie or balloon dilator prior to SEMS placement to assess for stridor has also been reported to identify patients at risk for airway obstruction following stent placement [73].

## Technique

The technique for endoscopic placement of esophageal stents, both plastic and metal, is relatively straightforward. Selection of appropriate candidates from the standpoint of medical stability and the ability to tolerate an endoscopic procedure is imperative. As for any endoscopic procedure, patients should be fasting for at least 6 h prior to the procedure. The choice of sedation is based on local practice bias, although our experience suggests that in the majority of patients, esophageal stents can be placed with moderate sedation using an intravenous opiate

and benzodiazepine. Anesthesiology consultation is advisable in patients being considered for esophageal stent placement and who have multiple medical comorbidities (ASA III and IV) or in those with an acute perforation or anastomotic breakdown following bariatric surgery. The latter group is typically acutely ill, obese, and with difficult airways in which endotracheal intubation may be required.

An upper endoscopy to define the proximal and distal margins of stent placement is the first step in esophageal stent placement. For malignant indications, the margins will be determined by the proximal and distal extent of the tumor; for other indications such as refractory strictures, fistulae or anastomotic leaks, margins will be determined by the length of the stricture, size and extent of the fistula as well as total length of the anastomosis to be covered. The distance between the proximal and distal margins to be stented will determine the length of the stent required, though 3–4 cm should be added to the total measured length to allow for an additional 1.5–2 cm of coverage on the proximal and distal ends of the lesion (Fig. 9.7). Stents can be placed within 1–2 cm of the cricopharyngeus for proximal lesions; placement of the endoprosthesis within the cricopharyngeus will usually result in a foreign body sensation and poor patient tolerance. However, patients with prior laryngectomy and very proximal esophageal strictures may tolerate stents placed across the cricopharyngeus [74].

In cases of malignant esophageal obstruction where the upper endoscope cannot be advanced beyond the tumor, careful esophageal dilation can be considered to allow one to choose the correct length of stent. Controlled radial expansion balloon dilators may be preferable to bougies for this purpose as the former allows direct visualization of the stricture and possibly a more "controlled" dilation. The use of fluoroscopy should be strongly considered when dilating malignant esophageal strictures as guidewire passage beyond the tumor may prove difficult in the setting of high-grade obstruction. An alternative approach in this situation is to utilize an ultraslim (≤5.4 mm diameter) pediatric upper endoscope to pass beyond the tumor. In some cases, the use

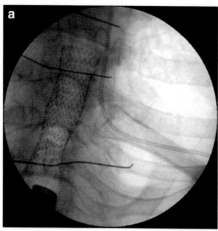
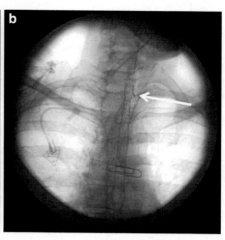

**Fig. 9.5** (**a**) In the patient described in Fig. 9.4, an airway stent was placed first followed in sequence by the placement of an esophageal stent (**b**) Note the use of an endo-

scopic clip (*arrow*) to delineate the proximal margin of the esophageal stricture. A paperclip was used externally to demarcate the distal margin of the stricture

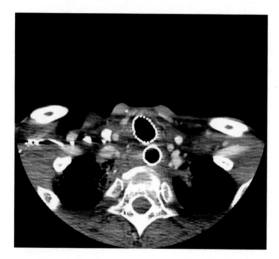

**Fig. 9.6** A CT scan following both airway and esophageal stent deployment demonstrating patency of both passages

of ERCP accessories (catheters, hydrophilic guidewires), retrograde passage of a small caliber endoscope through a mature gastrostomy tract (occasionally using a rendezvous technique with antegrade transoral endoscope passage) may be needed to traverse otherwise impassable strictures.

The distal margin can be measured and a stiff guidewire (e.g., Savary, Cook Endoscopy, Winston-Salem, NC) placed. The esophageal stent is then placed under fluoroscopic (and often

times endoscopic) control. Dilation may also be necessary in cases where the stenosis is too narrow to allow passage of the stent delivery catheter.

The margins of the area to be stented can be marked for fluoroscopic visualization using a variety of methods (Figs. 9.5 and 9.7). Endoscopic clips can be applied or contrast can be injected into the submucosa. Though less desirable, a more cost-effective approach is to mark the margins of the stenosis externally using a radiopaque object (such as a paper clip or hemostat). In some cases, marking of the distal margin of the tumor or stenosis endoscopically is not possible or unnecessary. Lesions or stenoses in the distal esophagus which are located in close proximity to the gastroesophageal junction may not require marking of the distal margin as the distal end of the stent will typically be located in the stomach which is readily visualized fluoroscopically. Once the length of the tumor or stenosis has been measured and appropriately marked, a guidewire is placed across the stenosis into the stomach and the endoscope is removed, leaving the wire in place.

It should be noted that endoscopy is not mandatory for the placement of esophageal stents as they can be placed by fluoroscopy alone. In this setting, a guidewire is manipulated into the

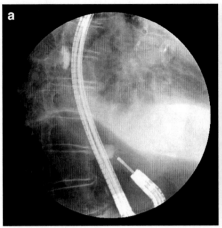 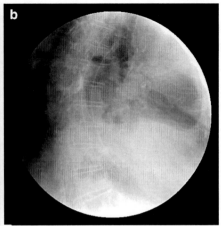

**Fig. 9.7** (**a**) Fluoroscopic image demonstrating submucosal injection of contrast to demarcate the proximal and distal margins of a malignant esophageal stricture. (**b**) A SEMS is placed across the stenosis with the proximal and distal ends of the stent 1.5–2 cm above and below the proximal and distal contrast injections to allow for inevitable foreshortening of the endoprosthesis

stomach and a multilumen balloon catheter is used to delineate stricture length, tightness, and angulation. External markers are placed and an endoprosthesis is selected which is 4–5 cm longer than the measured stricture. Deployment and subsequent assurance of luminal patency are done fluoroscopically. One advantage of this approach over endoscopy is that, in many cases, it can be performed using topical anesthesia only, thus avoiding the need for (and associated risk of) deeper levels of sedation. Conversely, fluoroscopy is not mandatory either as the stent can be placed under direct endoscopic visualization by monitoring the proximal end of the stent, much as when stents are placed across the papilla [75].

For malignant lesions, the type of stent (i.e., covered versus uncovered, with or without an antireflux valve, length, and diameter) will depend on the lesion itself, though our preference is to place the stent with the largest diameter possible. Smaller diameter stents may be used for lesions within the cervical esophagus in order to decrease the possible "foreign body" sensation associated with stent placement in this location. For most malignant lesions, a partially or fully covered SEMS are preferable to an uncovered stent in order to prevent tumor ingrowth and tissue hyperplasia. A covered stent should be also be

utilized for the treatment of malignant tracheoesophageal fistulas. The major drawback to partially or fully covered stents is the increased risk of stent migration. An uncovered stent may be selected for extrinsic compression or in patients with a prior history of stent migration of a partially covered stent.

For benign indications, a self-expanding plastic stent or fully covered metal stent should be selected in order to allow removal at a later date. In some cases, especially in patients with a history of head and neck cancer and cervical esophageal strictures, placement of a covered biliary or tracheobronchial stent may be necessary as the lumen may be too small to accept standard-sized esophageal SEMS; in addition, these smaller diameter SEMS may be better tolerated with less foreign body sensation. Placement of temporary, partially covered stents with the goal of removal is problematic as granulation tissue (Fig. 9.8) within the uncovered portion of the stent makes standard removal techniques difficult, if not impossible. In a recent series, it was shown that placement of a fully covered esophageal stent within the uncovered stent when the latter could not be removed due to tissue embedment allowed subsequent removal [76]. Following 1–2 weeks, both stents can be removed endoscopically. Despite these encouraging data, partially covered stents should

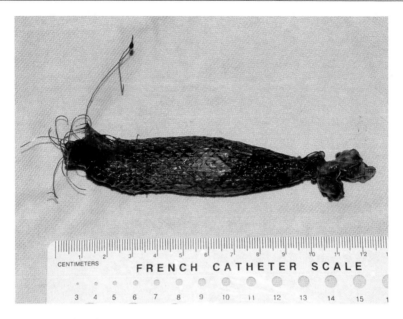

**Fig. 9.8** A partially covered SEMS after endoscopic removal; note the abundance of granulation tissue at the *bottom* of the stent

not be routinely placed for temporary indications outside of centers with considerable experience in their removal. Finally, although not yet approved for use in the United States, biodegradable stents have been described in several series in Europe for treatment of refractory benign esophageal strictures [47].

With regard to length, stents should be long enough to cover the desired lesion. Because endoscopic measurements may be slightly inaccurate, it is best to err on the side of a longer (rather than shorter) stent so as to decrease the risk of failing to palliate the obstructing lesion. The risk of migration is highest in patients with benign indications for esophageal stent placement [4, 66]. Refractory benign esophageal strictures have different characteristics in comparison to their malignant counterparts. Although occasionally problematic (i.e., stent occlusion), ingrowth of tumor into the stent helps to anchor it in position. In addition, malignant strictures tend to be longer than most benign strictures. Several measures can be taken to reduce the risk of stent migration. First, the stent with the largest possible diameter should be selected when placed in the mid or distal esophagus. It should be noted, however, that larger-diameter stents are associated with a high rate of complications [77]. The length of the stent should be long enough to bridge the stenosis, leak, or perforation. Finally, endoscopic clips can be applied to the proximal end of the stent in an attempt to maintain stent position [46, 78].

Once the appropriate stent has been selected, deployment is straightforward. The stent is advanced over the wire guide and the outer markings of the stent aligned with the proximal and distal margins of the stricture, recognizing that braided or knitted SEMS foreshorten by 30–40% with deployment. Foreshortening typically occurs at the end of the stent which is released first. Release of the stent can then proceed under fluoroscopic and, in many cases, endoscopic control with the endoscope placed alongside the prosthesis for direct visualization of the proximal stent margin. Most stents will have the tendency to move distally as the stent is released from the sheath; this can be counteracted by application of gentle traction on the delivery catheter. When stents are placed across the gastroesophageal junction, one should avoid leaving excessive stent within the stomach that can lead to impaction of the distal portion of the stent into the anterior gastric wall since this can cause nausea, vomiting, recurrent dysphagia, and gastric ulceration. In some cases, the SEMS chosen may be too short to fully bridge the stenosis. In such cases, a second, overlapping stent may be placed.

Postdeployment endoscopy can be performed to ensure proper stent positioning, although care should be taken to not advance the endoscope through a tight "waist" in the stent, which can lead to stent dislodgement. In the case of partially and fully covered metal stents, proximal repositioning using a grasping forceps can be accomplished with ease immediately after deployment. However, the same cannot be said for completely uncovered stents, though it is possible. Fully covered SEMS can be proximally repositioned even late after deployment. A grasping forceps (rattooth, shark-tooth) should be readily available to assist with post stent repositioning if necessary. Most stents reach maximal expansion after 24 h. As such, immediate postdeployment dilation of SEMS is typically unnecessary. In some cases, the stent may fail to open, and if the patient remains symptomatic, gentle balloon dilation of the stenosis may be helpful.

## Complications

Early procedure-related complications following esophageal stent placement include aspiration, airway compromise, device malpositioning, and entrapment of the stent delivery system, dislodgement of the stent, hemorrhage, severe chest pain, nausea, regurgitation, and esophageal perforation. These complications occur in up to 10% of individuals [4, 78]. However, many are preventable with careful technique and patient selection. Attention to airway management, including utilization of general anesthesia if necessary, as well as elevation of the patient's head to 30° immediately following the procedure, can reduce the risk of aspiration. In patients with mid- or proximal esophageal tumors, careful review of a chest CT with a thoracic surgeon or interventional pulmonologist, and planning for possible bronchoscopy with airway stent placement can mitigate

the risk of airway compromise in those patients deemed to be at risk.

Late (or delayed) complications include bleeding and fistula formation from stent erosion, severe gastroesophageal reflux, stent migration, and obstruction secondary to tissue ingrowth or food bolus impaction [4, 78, 79]. Some malpositioned or migrated stents can be repositioned or removed using a grasping forceps, inflated balloon catheter or a polypectomy snare. On occasion, migrated stents may be left in the stomach and a new stent placed [4, 80]. The decision to remove a migrated stent should ideally be made based on the patient's performance status as this is not without risk, but leaving a migrated stent within the stomach is associated with a small (but definite) risk of migration into the small intestine with resultant perforation or obstruction. Stents that become occluded secondary to tumor ingrowth can be treated with argon plasma coagulation or revised by placement of a second stent through the first (stent-within-stent deployment). Food bolus impaction can typically be treated endoscopically.

## Postoperative Care

A liquid diet can be resumed immediately for patients with malignant indications for esophageal stent placement. In most patients, diet can then be advanced as tolerated to a goal of mechanical soft diet. Careful nutritional counseling is essential to decrease the risk of stent occlusion by large food particles. Exceptions include patients for whom stents are placed for malignant tracheoesophageal fistulas, esophageal perforation, or anastomotic leaks. In this group, an esophagram (using water-soluble contrast for perforations and leaks and barium for tracheoesophageal fistula) is obtained 24 h following stent deployment to ensure both proper positioning of the stent and closure of the leak. A decision with regard to resumption of oral intake in these patients can then be made within the context of the multidisciplinary care team. In some patients, despite SEMS placement, oral intake may continue to be poor or necessarily restricted. Percutaneous endoscopic gastrostomy in such patients is generally safe, though care should be taken to avoid stent migration [81].

Special consideration should be given to patients in whom stents without an antireflux mechanism are deployed across the EG junction. Regurgitation and gastroesophageal reflux are nearly universal in these patients due to the inadequacy of the lower esophageal sphincter secondary to the endoprosthesis. Consequently, aspiration remains a significant risk in these patients and prokinetic agents are sometimes required. For these individuals, twice-daily proton pump inhibitors are prescribed indefinitely. Elevation of the head of the bed to at least 30° as well as instructions to not eat within 2–3 h of bedtime can help mitigate these stent-related symptoms.

# References

1. Dua KS. Stents for palliating malignant dysphagia and fistula: is the paradigm shifting? Gastrointest Endosc. 2007;65:77–81.
2. Elton E. Esophageal cancer. Dis Mon. 2005;51: 664–84.
3. Enzinger PC, Mayer RJ. Esophageal cancer. N Engl J Med. 2003;349:2241–52.
4. Papachristou GI, Baron TH. Use of stents in benign and malignant esophageal disease. Rev Gastroenterol Disord. 2007;7:74–88.
5. Raijman I, Walden D, Kortan P, et al. Expandable esophageal stents: initial experience with a new nitinol stent. Gastrointest Endosc. 1994;40:614–21.
6. Song HY, Do YS, Han YM, et al. Covered, expandable esophageal metallic stent `tubes: experiences in 119 patients. Radiology. 1994;193:689–95.
7. Fiorini AB, Goldin E, Valero JL, et al. Expandable metal coil stent for treatment of broncho-esophageal fistula. Gastrointest Endosc. 1995;42:81–3.
8. De Palma GD, Galloro G, Sivero L, et al. Self-expanding metal stents for palliation of inoperable carcinoma of the esophagus and gastroesophageal junction. Am J Gastroenterol. 1995;90:2140–2.
9. Moores DW, Ilves R. Treatment of esophageal obstruction with covered, self-expanding esophageal Wallstents. Ann Thorac Surg. 1996;62:963–7.
10. Cook TA, Dehn TC. Use of covered expandable metal stents in the treatment of oesophageal carcinoma and tracheo-oesophageal fistula. Br J Surg. 1996;83: 1417–8.
11. Raijman I, Siddique I, Ajani J, Lynch P. Palliation of malignant dysphagia and fistulae with coated expandable metal stents: experience with 101 patients. Gastrointest Endosc. 1998;48:172–9.
12. Bethge N, Sommer A, Vakil N. Palliation of malignant esophageal obstruction due to intrinsic and extrinsic lesions with expandable metal stents. Am J Gastroenterol. 1998;93:1829–32.
13. Lam YH, Chan A, Lau J, et al. Self-expandable metal stents for malignant dysphagia. Aust N Z J Surg. 1999;69:668–71.
14. Toikkanen VJ, Nemlander AT, Ramo OJ, et al. Expandable metallic stents in the management of malignant oesophageal obstruction. Ann Chir Gynaecol. 2000;89:20–83.
15. Cordero Jr JA, Moores DW. Self-expanding esophageal metallic stents in the treatment of esophageal obstruction. Am Surg. 2000;66:956–8, discussion 958–959.
16. Vakil N, Morris AI, Marcon N, et al. A prospective, randomized, controlled trial of covered expandable metal stents in the palliation of malignant esophageal obstruction at the gastroesophageal junction. Am J Gastroenterol. 2001;96:1791–6.
17. Christie NA, Buenaventura PO, Fernando HC, et al. Results of expandable metal stents for malignant esophageal obstruction in 100 patients: short-term and long-term follow-up. Ann Thorac Surg. 2001;71:1797, discussion 1801–1802.
18. Razzaq R, Laasch HU, England R, et al. Expandable metal stents for the palliation of malignant gastroduodenal obstruction. Cardiovasc Intervent Radiol. 2001;24:313–8.
19. McGrath JP, Browne M, Riordan C, et al. Expandable metal stents in the palliation of malignant dysphagia and oesophageal-respiratory fistulae. Ir Med J. 2001;94:270–2.
20. Kostopoulos PP, Zissis MI, Polydorou AA, et al. Are metal stents effective for palliation of malignant dysphagia and fistulas? Dig Liver Dis. 2003;35:275–82.
21. De Palma GD, Siciliano S, Sivero L, et al. Impact on the quality of remaining life of treatment with self-expandable metal prostheses in patients with inoperable esophago-cardial cancer. Results of a study of 107 consecutive patients treated with Ultraflex-type prostheses. Minerva Gastroenterol Dietol. 1999;45:95–106.
22. Johnson E, Enden T, Noreng HJ, et al. Survival and complications after insertion of self-expandable metal stents for malignant oesophageal stenosis. Scand J Gastroenterol. 2006;41:252–6.
23. Costamagna G, Marchese M, Iacopini F. Self-expanding stents in oesophageal cancer. Eur J Gastroenterol Hepatol. 2006;18:1177–80.
24. Sundelof M, Ringby D, Stockeld D, et al. Palliative treatment of malignant dysphagia with self-expanding metal stents: a 12-year experience. Scand J Gastroenterol. 2007;42:11–6.
25. Xinopoulos D, Dimitroulopoulos D, Tsamakidis K, et al. Palliative treatment of advanced esophageal cancer with metal-covered expandable stents. A cost-effectiveness and quality of life study. J BUON. 2005;10:523–8.
26. Radiology. BSoI. ROST: registry of oesophageal stenting, first report 2004: Hanley-on-Thames: Dendrite Clinical Systems; 2004.

27. Madhusudhan C, Saluja SS, Pal S, et al. Palliative stenting for relief of dysphagia in patients with inoperable esophageal cancer: impact on quality of life. Dis Esophagus. 2009;22:331–6.

28. Blomberg J, Wenger U, Lagergren J, et al. Antireflux stent versus conventional stent in the palliation of distal esophageal cancer. A randomized, multicenter clinical trial. Scand J Gastroenterol. 2010;45:208–16.

29. Pellen MG, Sabri S, Razack A, et al. Safety and efficacy of self-expanding removable metal esophageal stents during neoadjuvant chemotherapy for resectable esophageal cancer. Dis Esophagus. 2012; 25(1):48–53.

30. Bower M, Jones W, Vessels B, et al. Nutritional support with endoluminal stenting during neoadjuvant therapy for esophageal malignancy. Ann Surg Oncol. 2009;16:3161–8.

31. Adler DG, Fang J, Wong R, et al. Placement of Polyflex stents in patients with locally advanced esophageal cancer is safe and improves dysphagia during neoadjuvant therapy. Gastrointest Endosc. 2009;70:614–9.

32. Bower MR, Martin 2nd RC. Nutritional management during neoadjuvant therapy for esophageal cancer. J Surg Oncol. 2009;100:82–7.

33. Kinsman KJ, DeGregorio BT, Katon RM, et al. Prior radiation and chemotherapy increase the risk of life-threatening complications after insertion of metallic stents for esophagogastric malignancy. Gastrointest Endosc. 1996;43:196–203.

34. Siersema PD, Hop WC, Dees J, et al. Coated self-expanding metal stents versus latex prostheses for esophagogastric cancer with special reference to prior radiation and chemotherapy: a controlled, prospective study. Gastrointest Endosc. 1998;47:113–20.

35. Bartelsman JF, Bruno MJ, Jensema AJ, et al. Palliation of patients with esophagogastric neoplasms by insertion of a covered expandable modified Gianturco-Z endoprosthesis: experiences in 153 patients. Gastrointest Endosc. 2000;51:134–8.

36. Ginsberg GG. Palliation of malignant esophageal Dysphagia: would you like plastic or metal? Am J Gastroenterol. 2007;102:2678–9.

37. Siddiqui AA, Loren D, Dudnick R, Kowalski T. Expandable polyester silicon-covered stent for malignant esophageal strictures before neoadjuvant chemoradiation: a pilot study. Dig Dis Sci. 2007;52:823–9.

38. Homs MY, Hansen BE, van Blankenstein M, et al. Prior radiation and/or chemotherapy has no effect on the outcome of metal stent placement for oesophagogastric carcinoma. Eur J Gastroenterol Hepatol. 2004;16:163–70.

39. Kotsis L, Zubovits K, Vadasz P. Management of malignant tracheoesophageal fistulas with a cuffed funnel tube. Ann Thorac Surg. 1997;64:355–8.

40. Kozarek RA, Raltz S, Marcon N, et al. Use of the 25 mm flanged esophageal Z stent for malignant dysphagia: a prospective multicenter trial. Gastrointest Endosc. 1997;46:156–60.

41. Raijman I, Lynch P. Coated expandable esophageal stents in the treatment of digestive-respiratory fistulas. Am J Gastroenterol. 1997;92:2188–91.

42. Chen J, Chen ZM, Pang LW, et al. Deployment of self-expanding metallic stents under fluoroscopic guidance in patients with malignant esophagorespiratory fistula. Hepatogastroenterology. 2011;58:64–8.

43. Rodriguez AN, Diaz-Jimenez JP. Malignant respiratory-digestive fistulas. Curr Opin Pulm Med. 2010;16:329–33.

44. Altemur Karamustafaoglu Y, Yoruk Y. Self-expandable esophageal stents placement for the palliation of dysphagia as a result of lung cancer. Dis Esophagus. 2010;23:561–4.

45. Homs MY, Steyerberg EW, Eijkenboom WM, et al. Single-dose brachytherapy versus metal stent placement for the palliation of dysphagia from oesophageal cancer: multicentre randomised trial. Lancet. 2004;364:1497–504.

46. Vanbiervliet G, Filippi J, Karimdjee BS, et al. The role of clips in preventing migration of fully covered metallic esophageal stents: a pilot comparative study. Surg Endosc. 2012;26:53–9.

47. van Boeckel PG, Vleggaar FP, Siersema PD. A comparison of temporary self-expanding plastic and biodegradable stents for refractory benign esophageal strictures. Clin Gastroenterol Hepatol. 2011;9:653–9.

48. Repici A, Conio M, De Angelis C. Temporary placement of an expandable polyester silicone-covered stent for treatment of refractory benign esophageal strictures. Gastrointest Endosc. 2004;60:513–9.

49. Siersema PD, Homs MY, Haringsma J, et al. Use of large-diameter metallic stents to seal traumatic nonmalignant perforations of the esophagus. Gastrointest Endosc. 2003;58:356–61.

50. Kiernan PD, Sheridan MJ, Hettrick V, et al. Thoracic esophageal perforation: one surgeon's experience. Dis Esophagus. 2006;19:24–30.

51. Radecke K, Lang H, Frilling A, et al. Successful sealing of benign esophageal leaks after temporary placement of a self-expanding plastic stent without fluoroscopic guidance. Z Gastroenterol. 2006;44:1031–8.

52. Freeman RK, Van Woerkom JM, Ascioti AJ. Esophageal stent placement for the treatment of iatrogenic intrathoracic esophageal perforation. Ann Thorac Surg. 2007;83:2003–7, discussion 2007–2008.

53. Hunerbein M, Stroszczynski C, Moesta KT, Schlag PM. Treatment of thoracic anastomotic leaks after esophagectomy with self-expanding plastic stents. Ann Surg. 2004;240:801–7.

54. Yano F, El Sherif A, Filipi CJ, Mittal SK. Use of temporary esophageal stent in management of perforations after benign esophageal surgery. Surg Laparosc Endosc Percutan Tech. 2008;18:283–5.

55. Tuebergen D, Rijcken E, Mennigen R, et al. Treatment of thoracic esophageal anastomotic leaks and esophageal perforations with endoluminal stents: efficacy and current limitations. J Gastrointest Surg. 2008;12: 1168–76.

56. Yano F, Mittal SK. Post-operative esophageal leak treated with removable silicone-covered polyester stent. Dis Esophagus. 2007;20:535–7.

57. Kauer WK, Stein HJ, Dittler HJ, Siewert JR. Stent implantation as a treatment option in patients with thoracic anastomotic leaks after esophagectomy. Surg Endosc. 2008;22:50–3.

58. Profili S, Feo CF, Cossu ML, et al. Effective management of intrathoracic anastomotic leak with covered self-expandable metal stents. Report on three cases. Emerg Radiol. 2008;15:57–60.

59. Schubert D, Scheidbach H, Kuhn R, et al. Endoscopic treatment of thoracic esophageal anastomotic leaks by using silicone-covered, self-expanding polyester stents. Gastrointest Endosc. 2005;61:891–6.

60. Langer FB, Wenzl E, Prager G, et al. Management of postoperative esophageal leaks with the polyflex self-expanding covered plastic stent. Ann Thorac Surg. 2005;79:398–403, discussion 404.

61. Freeman RK, Ascioti AJ, Wozniak TC. Postoperative esophageal leak management with the polyflex esophageal stent. J Thorac Cardiovasc Surg. 2007;133: 333–8.

62. D'Cunha J, Rueth NM, Groth SS, et al. Esophageal stents for anastomotic leaks and perforations. J Thorac Cardiovasc Surg. 2011;142:39–46 e1.

63. Inbar R, Santo E, Subchi Ael A, et al. Insertion of removable self-expanding metal stents as a treatment for postoperative leaks and perforations of the esophagus and stomach. Isr Med Assoc J. 2011;13:230–3.

64. Freeman RK, Vyverberg A, Ascioti AJ. Esophageal stent placement for the treatment of acute intrathoracic anastomotic leak after esophagectomy. Ann Thorac Surg. 2011;92:204–8.

65. Kuppusamy MK, Felisky C, Kozarek RA, et al. Impact of endoscopic assessment and treatment on operative and non-operative management of acute oesophageal perforation. Br J Surg. 2011;98:818–24.

66. Holm AN, de la Mora Levy JG, Gostout CJ, et al. Self-expanding plastic stents in treatment of benign esophageal conditions. Gastrointest Endosc. 2008;67: 20–5.

67. Wright G, Lewis H, Hogan B, et al. A self-expanding metal stent for complicated variceal hemorrhage: experience at a single center. Gastrointest Endosc. 2010;71:71–8.

68. De Olabozal J, Roberts J, Hoeltgen T, Berkelhammer C. Double stenting to prevent airway compression in proximal malignant esophageal strictures. Am J Gastroenterol. 2001;96:2800–1.

69. Kawasaki R, Sano A, Matsumoto S. Long-term outcomes and complications of metallic stents for malignant esophageal stenoses. Kobe J Med Sci. 2003;49:133–42.

70. Farivar AS, Vallieres E, Kowdley KV, et al. Airway obstruction complicating esophageal stent placement in two post-pneumonectomy patients. Ann Thorac Surg. 2004;78:e22–3.

71. Dasgupta A, Jain P, Sandur S, et al. Airway complications of esophageal self-expandable metallic stent. Gastrointest Endosc. 1998;47:532–5.

72. Herth FJ, Peter S, Baty F, et al. Combined airway and oesophageal stenting in malignant airway-oesophageal fistulas: a prospective study. Eur Respir J. 2010;36: 1370–4.

73. Paganin F, Schouler L, Cuissard L, et al. Airway and esophageal stenting in patients with advanced esophageal cancer and pulmonary involvement. PLoS One. 2008;3:e3101.

74. Somani SK, Verma N, Avasthi G, et al. High pharyngoesophageal strictures after laryngopharyngectomy can also be treated by self-expandable plastic stents. Gastrointest Endosc. 2010;71:1304–7.

75. Lazaraki G, Katsinelos P, Nakos A, et al. Malignant esophageal dysphagia palliation using insertion of a covered Ultraflex stent without fluoroscopy: a prospective observational study. Surg Endosc. 2011;25: 628–35.

76. Hirdes MM, Siersema PD, Houben MH, et al. Stent-in-stent technique for removal of embedded esophageal self-expanding metal stents. Am J Gastroenterol. 2011;106:286–93.

77. Sharma P, Kozarek R. Role of esophageal stents in benign and malignant diseases. Am J Gastroenterol. 2010;105:258–73. quiz 274.

78. Baron TH. Minimizing endoscopic complications: endoluminal stents. Gastrointest Endosc Clin N Am. 2007;17:83–104. vii.

79. Siersema PD. New developments in palliative therapy. Best Pract Res Clin Gastroenterol. 2006;20:959–78.

80. Rollhauser C, Fleischer DE. Late migration of a self-expandable metal stent and successful endoscopic management. Gastrointest Endosc. 1999;49:541–4.

81. Adler DG, Baron TH. Endoscopic palliation of malignant dysphagia. Mayo Clin Proc. 2001;76:731–8.

# Biliary and Pancreatic Stents: Indications and Placement Techniques

# 10

Wesley Leung, Mariano Gonzalez-Haba Ruiz, and Irving Waxman

Biliary stent placement was developed as an alternative to established surgical drainage procedures. Stent placement is of intense interest because it has altered the treatment algorithms for many biliary diseases. Until 1979, it was only possible to insert 5 Fr (1.6 mm) diameter plastic stents to treat biliary obstruction. An increase in the diameter of duodenoscope working channels to 4.2 mm allowed for placement of plastic stents up to 11.5 Fr (3.3 mm) in diameter. However, 11.5 and 12 Fr diameter stents are more technically difficult to insert compared to the gold standard large-bore 10 Fr stent and have not been associated with improvement in stent patency. Technologic advances have enabled the development of biliary self-expandable metal stents (SEMS). These stents are passed through the endoscope mounted on small-diameter predeployed delivery systems, yet achieve much larger diameters than plastic stents when fully deployed (up to 30 Fr [10 mm]). Initial biliary SEMS were bare metal (uncovered) and became embedded into the surrounding tumor and normal tissue, making them nearly impossible to remove within a short period after insertion.

With additional technologic advances, covered biliary SEMS have been developed with the coating composed of a variety of materials. Biliary SEMS are now referred to specifically by design as uncovered (UCSEMS), partially covered (PCSEMS), and fully covered (FCSEMS). See Chap. 6 for an overview of available biliary endoprostheses. Indications for placement of stents for pancreatic disease are limited, but supportive data are emerging. In this chapter, the indications for biliary and pancreatic SEMS placement will be reviewed.

## Indications

### Benign Biliary Diseases

Uncovered SEMS imbed into tissue and are nonremovable, whereas covered SEMS do not imbed, allowing removability. This lack of imbedding is based upon both animal and clinical human data [1]. A variety of benign biliary diseases that have been traditionally treated with endoscopic or radiologic placement of plastic stents have recently been treated with temporary placement of PCSEMS and FCSEMS [2]. See Chap. 17 for results and complications of biliary SEMS for benign biliary disorders.

W. Leung, M.D. • M.G.-H. Ruiz, M.D.
• I. Waxman, M.D. (⊠)
Center for Endoscopic Research and Therapeutics,
Section of Gastroenterology, Department of Medicine,
The University of Chicago Medical Center,
5758 South Maryland Avenue, MC 9028, Chicago,
IL 60637-1463, USA
e-mail: Wesley_leung6@hotmail.com; iwaxman@
medicine.bsd.uchicago.edu

R. Kozarek et al. (eds.), *Self-Expandable Stents in the Gastrointestinal Tract*,
DOI 10.1007/978-1-4614-3746-8_10, © Springer Science+Business Media New York 2013

## Benign Biliary Strictures

Benign biliary strictures (BBS) occur as a result of various causes, such as chronic pancreatitis, postsurgical bile duct injury, anastomotic strictures after liver surgery (including liver transplantation), postsphincterotomy, and chole-docholithiasis [3]. Benign biliary strictures may result in chronic cholestasis, jaundice, recurrent cholangitis, and secondary biliary cirrhosis [4, 5]. Thus, proper and prompt management of benign biliary strictures is essential. Although surgery has the theoretical advantage of being definitive [6], endoscopic stent placement has gained acceptance as an initial treatment in patients with BBS and an endoscopically accessible biliary system because of its relative simplicity and low morbidity and mortality. Compared with surgery, endoscopic therapy with dilation and stent placement has similar to lower rates of stricture recurrence [7–9]. In addition, endoscopic treatment preserves the option of surgery if repeated endoscopic attempts fail [10]. Current data favor the use of plastic stents to treat BBS [10–13]. Although UCSEMS were shown to have a longer duration of patency than plastic stents in malignant strictures, their use in benign biliary disease is associated with long-term failure related to mucosal hyperplasia and lack of removability [8, 14–18].

Recently, FCSEMS have been introduced and approved for palliation of malignant biliary strictures but have been recently used to treat benign biliary strictures [19–22]. Placement of FCSEMS has several potential advantages over placement of multiple plastic stents which have become the standard endoscopic treatment of benign biliary strictures. Multiple stent placement requires a number of procedures to achieve the optimal number of plastic stents and for stent exchanges [13]. Multiple endoscopic sessions may be impractical for some patients [12, 21–23]. FCSEMS might offer longer-lasting drainage of the bile duct and dilation of the stricture without the need for preinsertion dilation and without the need for interval procedures to upsize stent diameter and number, and for stent exchanges. PCSEMS have been used for benign disease, but

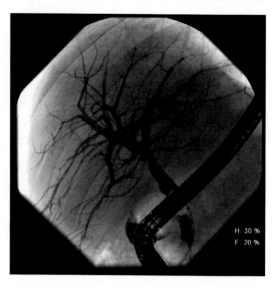

**Fig. 10.1** A fibrotic biliary stricture in a posttransplant donor duct

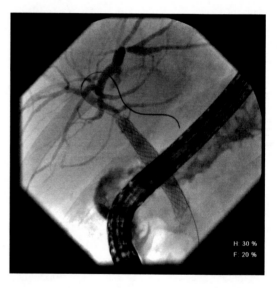

**Fig.10.2** The stricture was treated with placement of a 10 mm × 40 mm fully covered biliary metal stent

tissue hyperplasia and imbedding of the uncovered stent mesh can make these stents difficult to remove and create strictures at the sites of embedding [11, 24, 25]. Primary placement of FCSEMS may therefore be an attractive option for benign biliary strictures (Figs. 10.1 and 10.2). However, early reports suggested a high rate of stent migration [21, 22, 26]. Although FCSEMS with antimigration anchoring fins have become available, these anchoring fins can cause mucosal ulceration and bleeding when extracted [19, 27]. The ideal FCSEMS that allows easy and atraumatic removability while limiting stent migration has not been developed. Several designs for antimigration properties of FCSEMS have been developed [27–30]. A recent study in patients with benign biliary strictures showed that a FCSEMS with an anchoring flap had significantly less stent migration than one with a flared end FCSEM and was easy to remove up to 6 months after insertion [31]. Another alternative to prevent migration of FCSEMS is the placement of an anchoring plastic stent. In recent randomized trial of patients with BBS, patients with FCSEMS were randomized to placement of a long length 5 Fr double pigtail stent inside the FCSEMS immediately after SEMS placement with the proximal end of the plastic stent in the intrahepatic system and the distal end in the duodenum [32]. There was a significant reduction in migration in the anchoring stent group (1/16, 6.3%) than in the nonanchoring group (7/17, 41.2%).

Although placement of covered SEMS across the bifurcation is considered contraindicated because the stent occludes drainage from the contralateral biliary system as well intrahepatic branches, a recent report of two patients with benign hilar strictures showed excellent results when the contralateral side was protected by placement of a traditional plastic stent [33]. Cholangitis did not occur in either patient, and in both patients, subsequent removal of the FCSEMS was successful and resulted in stricture resolution.

## Postoperative Biliary Leaks

Techniques for management of bile leaks include biliary sphincterotomy with or without plastic stent placement. PCSEMS have been used to treat complex bile leaks, but they are associated with induction of tissue hyperplasia at the uncovered ends [34].

Recent studies have shown that FCSEMS are effective to treat a variety of leaks refractory to traditional therapy [2]. Wang et al. examined the efficacy of FCSEMS with anchoring fins for resolving complex bile leaks [35]. Thirteen patients with complex bile leaks underwent ERCP with temporary placement of a FCSEMS following cholecystectomy (n = 8) or liver transplantation (n = 5). All patients had resolution of their bile leaks. Two patients developed a new stricture below the confluence. Three patients died from unrelated causes. Two deaths occurred prior to FCSEMS removal. Ten of eleven patients had evidence of biliary debris at the time of FCSEMS removal. Overall, temporary placement of FCSEMS is effective in resolving bile leaks. FCSEMS are prone to migration and are associated with intraductal ulcerations, choledocholithiasis, and de novo strictures in transplant patients.

## Postsphincterotomy Bleeding

Endoscopic sphincterotomy (ES) is a basic technique for performing various therapeutic interventions during ERCP. Advances in technology and technique have led to improved safety with ES. However, bleeding after ES remains a recognized complication [36]. Minor oozing is relatively common and usually self-limited, but brisk, pulsatile, or continued bleeding may necessitate therapy. However, therapeutic accessories used to endoscopically control of post-ES hemorrhage can be difficult to apply through a side-viewing endoscope. It was recognized that FCSEMS provide mechanical tamponade to treat post-ES bleeding without recurrent hemorrhage at time of removal [37, 38].

## Closure of Sphincterotomy Perforations

Endoscopic sphincterotomy can result also in perforation. Similar to postendoscopic sphincterotomy bleeding, these can be difficult to treat with clip placement using side-viewing endoscopes. Recently, sphincterotomy perforations have been successfully treated using temporary FCSEMS placement [39].

## Difficult or Irretrievable Bile Duct Stones

In approximately 10% of patients, common bile duct stones cannot be removed using standard endoscopic techniques because of the size of stone and/or presence of difficult anatomy (narrowed or strictured distal bile duct). In these cases, drainage is maintained by temporary placement of plastic biliary stents with subsequent repeat ERCP. Recently, temporary placement of partially and fully covered SEMS has been used in such patients with follow-up ERCP, stent removal, and stone extraction. In some cases, extraction and reinsertion of SEMS are needed to achieve complete stone clearance [40].

In summary, biliary SEMS are not approved for use in benign biliary disease in the USA, although one FCSEMS is approved in Europe for temporary placement for treatment of benign biliary strictures. At the present time, placement of uncovered SEMS for benign disease should not be undertaken except in selected circumstances. The use of PCSEMS and FCSEMS for benign biliary disease is controversial and probably best reserved for patients who fail to respond to traditional plastic biliary stent placement.

## Malignant Biliary Obstruction

Within the biliary tree, stents are commonly used to relieve obstruction due to primary pancreaticobiliary malignancy (resectable and unresectable), metastatic disease, and external biliary compression by lymph nodes. See Chap. 17 for results and complications of biliary SEMS for malignant distal biliary disorders.

### Preoperative Biliary Drainage

Placement of a plastic stent or short SEMS in the distal bile duct does not interfere with the ability to perform subsequent pancreaticoduodenectomy. However, the benefit of preoperative endoscopic biliary drainage with regard to postoperative outcomes in patients with resectable pancreaticobiliary disease is debated. Proceeding directly to surgery may limit the number of interventions and

thus decrease costs and potential procedure-related complications. On the other hand, performing preoperative endoscopic biliary drainage may relieve jaundice and prevent complications due to cholestasis. In addition, preoperative stenting may allow time for delivery of neoadjuvant therapy in patients with locally advanced pancreatic cancer. While retrospective studies and meta-analyses have suggested there may be an advantage (or at least no disadvantage) to preoperative biliary drainage, a recent randomized, multicenter study produced contrasting results. In this study, overall and surgical outcomes were compared in patients with potentially resectable pancreatic cancer and malignant obstructive jaundice who underwent either preoperative endoscopic retrograde cholangiopancreatography (ERCP) with biliary drainage for 4–6 weeks followed by attempted pancreaticoduodenectomy, or to surgery alone within 1 week after diagnosis [41]. The overall rate of serious complications was 74% in the preoperative biliary drainage group and 39% in the early surgery group. There was no improvement in any outcome in the biliary drainage group. It is important to note that 10 Fr plastic stents were used in this study, and early stent occlusion occurred in a number of patients. The use of short-length, uncovered SEMS or covered SEMS may have resulted in fewer stent-related complications [42], as data extrapolated from palliation of malignant disease show fewer stent-related complications including death using SEMS as compared to plastic stents [43]. Short-length uncovered SEMS and covered SEMS do not interfere with pancreaticoduodenectomy as UCSEMS are resected with the mass and a covered SEMS can be resected or removed at the time of surgery. If the patient is found to be unresectable, the stent remains for palliation and obviates palliative biliary bypass or need for repeat ERCP for plastic stent exchange.

Preoperative relief of biliary obstruction in patients with potentially resectable cancer of the pancreatic head is recommended in those with acute cholangitis, intense pruritus, or in whom surgery is delayed [42]. Neoadjuvant chemoradiation for resectable adenocarcinoma of the pancreatic head is becoming more common and

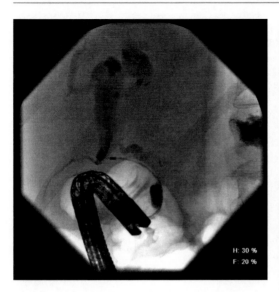

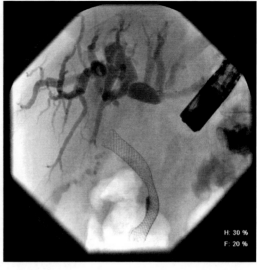

**Fig. 10.3** Adenocarcinoma of the pancreas. Cholangiogram shows a single localized stenosis 20 mm in length on the lower third of the main bile duct

**Fig. 10.4** An 8 mm × 6 cm covered metal stent is placed into the bile duct

results in delay in surgery and a high rate of plastic stent occlusion with subsequent cholangitis. In this situation, preoperative ERCP with the placement of a biliary SEMS is preferred [44].

## Palliation of Unresectable Cancer

*Obstruction of the Distal Bile Duct.* Distal malignant biliary obstruction (i.e., obstruction more than 2 cm distal to the hilum) is often due to pancreatic cancer, cholangiocarcinoma, metastatic disease to the head of the pancreas, or external compression from lymph node metastases. Possible palliative treatments for unresectable malignant biliary obstruction include surgical bypass and either plastic or metal biliary stents placed percutaneously or endoscopically (Figs. 10.3 and 10.4). A large meta-analysis reviewing 2,436 patients compared surgical bypass to endoscopic placement of metal stents and endoscopic placement of plastic stents for palliation of malignant distal bile duct obstruction. Endoscopic metal stents were found to be the treatment of choice due to their prolongation in patency as compared to plastic stents and lower morbidity when compared to surgery [45]. Studies in which plastic and uncovered metal stent placement have been compared for palliation of malignant biliary obstruction have found significantly longer patency

for metal stents [15, 46–48]. Tumor ingrowth is the most common mechanism of stent obstruction with UCSEMS. Covered SEMS were developed to prevent tumor ingrowth and prolong stent patency. A multicenter randomized controlled trial comparing UCSEMS and PCSEMS in palliating distal malignant obstruction revealed no significant difference in time to recurrent biliary obstruction or patient survival between the groups and more serious adverse events (particularly migration) in the PCSEMS group [49]. However, a recent meta-analysis of randomized trials has shown a significantly prolonged patency with CSEMS (partial or full) as compared to UCSEMS with similar rates of adverse events [50]. Therefore, the placement of the type of SEMS (partially, fully, or uncovered) should be based upon personal preference, perceived risk of migration and cholecystitis, potential for need for removal, cost, and anticipated patient survival.

*Obstruction at the Hilum.* Hilar obstruction results from cholangiocarcinoma (Klatskin tumor), gallbladder carcinoma, hepatocellular carcinoma, local extension of pancreatic cancer, solid metastases, or compression from lymph nodes. See Chap. 15 for results and complications of biliary SEMS for malignant hilar obstruction.

The average 5-year survival rate of this type of malignant obstruction in these patients is approximately 10% [51], and endoscopic biliary drainage is the preferred strategy for palliative biliary drainage [52]. However, because of the technical difficulty, endoscopic drainage of hilar obstructions should, in general, be performed by endoscopists with significant case volume and expertise. The optimal extent of drainage achieved by biliary stenting is still controversial. A study by De Palma et al., where 157 patients were randomized to unilateral or bilateral SEMS for malignant hilar biliary obstruction suggested that selective unilateral hilar metal stenting should be performed to avoid the additional risks of complications with bilateral stent placement [53]. However, a more recent retrospective study comparing 46 consecutive patients who received either unilateral or bilateral stents showed that cumulative stent patency was significantly higher in the bilateral stent group [54]. The main determinant for number of stents appears to be related to the volume of liver drained (>50%) and avoiding contamination and drainage of atrophied segments [55].

Our group has used a recently available biliary SEMS with a 6 Fr delivery system that allows two predeployed stents to be passed through the working channel of a standard therapeutic adult endoscope to facilitate for simultaneous side-by-side bilateral deployment in hilar malignant obstruction. Acceptable initial feasibility, safety, and efficacy profiles were demonstrated [56]. Further evaluation is needed to assess definitive patency and outcomes for palliation of malignant hilar obstruction using side-by-side and stent-within-stent (Y configuration) metal stent deployment.

*Unknown Resectability.* In some patients with clinical and radiographically suspected pancreatic cancer, resectability and patient operability may not be definitively known during the initial ERCP and if neoadjuvant chemotherapy is being considered. Options in this setting include placing a plastic (and thus easily removable) stent or a SEMS (which provides longer-term patency, but if uncovered cannot be removed). A Monte Carlo decision analysis compared several strategies in patients with obstructive jaundice from pancreatic cancer with an undetermined surgical plan, and the results suggested that a short-length uncovered SEMS (4–6 cm) is the preferred initial treatment for overall cost minimization [57]. If resectable disease is confirmed at surgery, the stent is removed with the surgical specimen [58]. If subsequent exploration defines unresectable disease, the patient's jaundice is already palliated and does not require major decompressive surgery or an additional ERCP for the placement of SEMS to provide more sustained palliation of biliary obstruction. However, this study was done before the widespread availability of CSEMS. In patients with unknown operative status and/or lack of tissue diagnosis, it is preferable to place a removable stent since some patients may have tumors highly responsive to chemotherapy (e.g., lymphoma) or benign disease that was felt to be malignant (autoimmune pancreatitis) [59].

## Placement Techniques

Biliary SEMS can be placed endoscopically during ERCP or by interventional radiologists under fluoroscopic guidance alone.

## Radiopaque Markers

Radiopaque markers are attached to parts of the stent and delivery system in order to assist with accurate stent placement and to assess stent position by plain abdominal radiography. Markers are composed of gold or platinum and are usually attached to both ends of the stent.

## Stent Delivery System

SEMS are mounted on a delivery catheter, and thus no other accessories (such as a pusher tube used for plastic stent placement) are required apart from a guidewire and, in some cases, dilators. SEMS are constrained on small-diameter delivery systems ($\leq$ 8.5 Fr) and are deployed by retraction of the outer sheath or, in some cases, by unwinding of a constraining thread.

## Endoscopic Placement

After cannulation of the intended duct, the stent length is chosen. The stricture length is assessed in the same way as with plastic stents by comparison of the measured stricture length to a known length such as the endoscope diameter; the stent chosen is approximately 2–4 cm longer than the stricture. For ampullary cancers, a 4-cm stent length is almost always adequate to cross the stricture with approximately 1–1.5 cm of the distal end deployed in the duodenum, and for pancreatic cancers, 4 or 6 cm lengths are most commonly used. For distal cancers with the SEMS exiting the papilla, a biliary sphinctero-tomy is not required and may increase the complication rate (including migration) [60, 61]. Some experts recommend that when placing a covered SEMS, the proximal end is positioned below the cystic duct ostium, when possible, in patients with intact gallbladders to avoid chole-cystitis [62].

If applicable, the SEMS delivery catheter and the constraining sheath are flushed with saline before the delivery catheter is advanced over the guidewire into the desired location. Predilation of the stricture is rarely necessary. The SEMS is deployed under fluoroscopic and endoscopic guidance. While the assistant withdraws the con-straining sheath, the endoscopist lowers the ele-vator slightly to decrease the tension on the outer sheath. Most stents tend to be advanced from the constraining sheath during deployment and move away from the tip of the endoscope. The position of the SEMS is maintained in desired position by the endoscopist pulling back on the delivery cath-eter during deployment. The position can be adjusted distally by traction of the delivery cath-eter and proximally after recapturing the SEMS (only possible with certain stent delivery sys-tems) inside the constraining sheath. After SEMS delivery, the inner catheter that the stent was mounted on is withdrawn. In very tight strictures,

the delivery catheter may become trapped inside the stent which should be suspected when exces-sive resistance is felt during inner catheter removal. To avoid dislodgement of the stent, one should wait, and within a few minutes, the stent should adequately expand to release the catheter.

If the SEMS is placed too proximally, one can attempt to reposition the stent distally in two ways: (1) If a guidewire remains in place, a dilat-ing balloon can be inflated inside the stent and withdrawn. Alternatively, a second overlapping SEMS can be inserted. (2) A rat-tooth forceps or snare can be used to grasp the stent and with-draw it.

If the SEMS protrudes too distally into the duodenum, it can be removed (covered or uncov-ered) or trimmed using argon plasma coagulation (APC) at high wattage to prevent and treat duode-nal ulcers and/or perforation due to impaction of the stent on the opposite duodenal wall [63].

## Specific Situations

### Drainage of Malignant Hilar Obstruction

In malignant hilar strictures, the hepatic region to be drained is usually selected based on preopera-tive imaging (CT or MRI), with the aim of drain-ing more than 50% of the liver volume and avoidance of atrophied segments or lobes [45]. During ERCP, contrast is injected only into the obstructed ducts of interest after they have been entered with a guidewire and catheter using con-trast-free techniques or by limiting contrast injec-tion to the uninvolved bile duct below the bifurcation. If the insertion of bilateral SEMS is undertaken, they can be placed in a "side-by-side" (Figs. 10.5 and 10.6) or a "stent-in-stent" ("Y") configuration. Techniques that may improve successful hilar stent placement include dilating both sides of the hilum using a balloon catheter (usually 6 mm diameter), use of a long, stiff guidewire, insertion of the first SEMS into the more angulated left lobe (insertion in the right lobe is easier due to the straighter trajectory), and selecting the straightest right ductal system.

When the side-by-side technique is used, the distal stent ends should exit into the duodenum

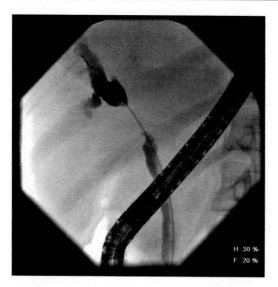

**Fig. 10.5** Cholangiogram of a Bismuth II cholangiocarcinoma containing a single localized stenosis 20 mm in length

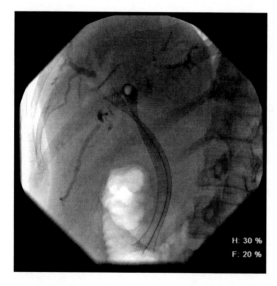

**Fig. 10.6** Bilateral metal stenting of the lesion in Fig. 10.5 (8 mm × 10 cm and 8 mm × 8 mm metal stents placed into the *left* and *right* systems, respectively)

(if possible) or be matched at the same level within the duct so as to facilitate reintervention if occlusion occurs.

When using the stent-in-stent technique or when a unilateral stent is placed, it is best to use stents with a wide cell width (large interstices) to allow a wire and second stent to pass through the

first stent either at the initial procedure or at a later procedure if subsequently needed should jaundice not be relieved with one stent [64].

The other consideration when unilateral stent placement is undertaken for hilar tumors is whether to use a short-length stent that is adequate to cover the length of the stricture yet remain above the level of the papilla. The advantages are the potential decrease in stent-induced hyperplasia as less stent is in contact with the normal duct and potentially an improvement in patency if a sphincterotomy is not performed as this precludes stent occlusion due to reflux of food material.

## Postsurgical Anatomy

In some patients with altered anatomy (e.g., pancreaticoduodenectomy, Roux-en-Y hepaticojejunostomy), the biliary tree can only be reached with colonoscopes. The delivery system of most SEMS is long enough to pass through these endoscopes, and some SEMS have delivery systems with diameters small enough to pass through pediatric colonoscopes [65].

## Stent-in-Stent Placement to Facilitate Uncovered and Partially Covered SEMS Removal

In some cases of UCSEMS or PCSEMS placement, the stent needs to subsequently be removed (examples mentioned above – lymphoma responsive to therapy and unrecognized benign disease). The stent ends of PCSEMS become imbedded, making removal difficult. A recent concept applied to partially covered esophageal SEMS removal has also been applied to partially covered biliary SEMS removal. A fully covered SEMS is placed within the PCSEMS to overlap both ends. Tissue necrosis between the imbedded uncovered portion and the fully covered portion allows the wires of the uncovered stent to then be exposed to the surface. Both SEMS are removed as early as 7 days but up to several weeks later [66, 67]. This technique is likely more effective with PCSEMS than UCSEMS and patients in whom the original stent is exiting the papilla so that the stent can be easily grasped.

## Percutaneous Stent Placement

Percutaneous therapy is performed by interventional radiologists via a transhepatic approach (percutaneous transhepatic cholangiography or PTC). The intrahepatic bile ducts are initially accessed with a skinny needle under ultrasound or fluoroscopic guidance using an antegrade approach. Subsequently, a guidewire is passed into the biliary tree to facilitate catheter placement. In most situations, the stricture is traversed, and the guidewire is passed into the duodenum. In some situations, internal-external drainage is performed temporarily for several days with a plastic catheter, and the SEMS is placed several days later. In some patients, internalization and SEMS placement can be achieved at the initial procedure. More commonly, one procedure is required for initial-external tube placement and another for internalization of a stent, or for removal of a temporary external catheter placed as a precautionary measure at the time of SEMS placement.

Prior to the advent of self-expandable metal stents (SEMS), the percutaneous tract through the liver required aggressive dilation in order to accommodate large-bore plastic stents. This was associated with a higher incidence of postprocedural pain and bleeding. Because SEMS have a small predeployment delivery system, the tract through the liver does not require as large dilation as for SEMS. This is associated with a decreased bleeding risk and the potential of placing a SEMS with a single puncture precluding need of an external catheter.

Percutaneous insertion and internalization of biliary SEMS is achievable in nearly all patients with pancreatic cancer and distal bile duct obstruction. With the advent of endoscopic palliation, however, percutaneous therapy has become less commonly performed and is used when endoscopic techniques are not available, fail, or when the papilla is inaccessible due to duodenal tumor invasion, prior duodenal stent placement across the biliary tree, or because of postsurgical anatomy. There is only one randomized, prospective trial comparing percutaneous and endoscopic therapy for the palliation of distal malignant obstructive jaundice [68]. This landmark study showed that the endoscopic method had a significantly higher success rate for relief of jaundice and significantly lower 30-day mortality. The higher mortality in the percutaneous group was due to complications associated with liver puncture (bleeding and bile leaks). This study is now considered outdated since it was performed using plastic stents prior to the development of expandable metal stents, the insertion of which is less likely to require aggressive dilation of the percutaneous tract through the liver, which in turn decreases bleeding and bile leakage [69, 70]. Nonetheless, more recent studies have shown that major complications following percutaneous SEMS placement are still more common than endoscopic stent placement [71]. Percutaneous stent placement, however, is effective in most patients who have failed attempt at endoscopic stent placement [72]. Additionally, in centers without expertise in ERCP, percutaneous therapy is used as the primary method of nonsurgical palliation of malignant obstructive jaundice. Overall, the technical success rate of percutaneous expandable metal stent placement is high with a high rate of clinical resolution of jaundice [73].

## Combined Percutaneous and Endoscopic Palliation of Obstructive Jaundice: Rendezvous Procedure

In some situations in which endoscopic therapy fails to access the bile duct and/or traverse the stricture, a percutaneous approach can be performed to facilitate the endoscopic procedure. The advantage of this approach versus completion of the entire procedure percutaneously may be realized only when ERCP is undertaken the same day. In this scenario, a guidewire that has been placed transhepatically into the duodenum is grasped endoscopically and used to complete the procedure and without need to dilate the liver or for temporary percutaneous catheter placement [74].

## Combined Malignant Biliary and Duodenal Obstruction

The sequence of biliary and duodenal obstruction, prior intervention for either, and the relationship of the duodenal obstruction anatomically

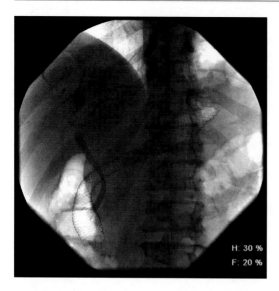

H: 30 %
F: 20 %

**Fig. 10.7** Biliary (8 mm×6 cm) and gastroduodenal (22 mm×120 mm) metal stent placement for malignant biliary and gastric outlet obstruction from gastric cancer

to the papilla determines the strategy one chooses for stent placement in patients with biliary and duodenal obstruction [75]. A complete detailed description of the techniques to manage these patients is presented in Chap. 11. Briefly, the most common scenario is development of a duodenal stricture in a patient with pancreatic cancer and preexisting biliary stent. In this case, if an existing plastic biliary stent is present, it is exchanged for SEMS, and then the duodenal SEMS is inserted. When duodenal and biliary strictures develop simultaneously with the duodenal stricture at or above the papilla, and the papilla cannot be accessed, a duodenal SEMS can be inserted. Biliary cannulation is then attempted (Fig. 10.7). If initial attempts fail, another attempt can be made at 24–48 h (to allow complete duodenal SEMS expansion) to pass the endoscope to the papilla. A biliary SEMS can be inserted as usual if the duodenal stent does not cross the papilla. If the duodenal stent crosses the papilla, cannulation can be performed through the duodenal SEMS mesh. If needed, a window can be created in the side of the duodenal SEMS using argon beam coagulation to expose the papilla and facilitate biliary cannulation [76].

## Endoscopic Ultrasound-Guided Biliary Stent Placement

Endoscopic ultrasound (EUS)-guided cholangiography has evolved from a diagnostic procedure to a therapeutic technique for gaining access to the bile ducts when conventional ERCP fails or is not possible due to altered surgical anatomy. Due to the close proximity to the gastrointestinal tract, the left intrahepatic ducts and common bile ducts are well visualized with EUS and can be accessed through a transgastric or transduodenal approach.

EUS-guided cholangiography is technically feasible and relatively safe in the hands of experienced interventional endoscopists skilled in both ERCP and EUS. This technique offers a potential alternative to surgery and to percutaneous therapy in patients in whom conventional ERCP is unsuccessful or not possible. Currently, this procedure is most often performed in tertiary centers with highly skilled endoscopists using a multidisciplinary approach in these challenging cases.

As a general rule, four EUS-guided approaches have been used to decompress the biliary system:

1. Creation of a choledochoduodenal fistula with stent placement (Figs. 10.8 and 10.9) [77].
2. Creation of a hepatogastric fistula with stent placement into the stomach above the stricture [77].
3. Accessing the left system, passing a guidewire antegrade into the duodenum and passing the stent antegrade through the echoendoscope across the stricture with the distal end below the tumor and the proximal end above the stricture. The entire stent is within the biliary tree, thus creating an internal biliary stent [78].
4. EUS-guided rendezvous by accessing either the left intrahepatic ducts transgastrically or common bile duct transduodenally with passage of a guidewire into the duodenum, removal of the echoendoscope, and passage of a conventional duodenoscope to grasp the wire [79].

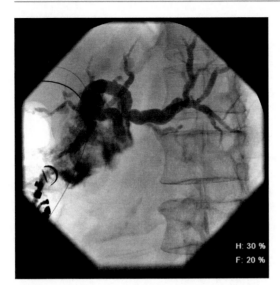

**Fig. 10.8** Patient with a 4.8-cm pancreatic head mass (T3 N1 M0 EUS staging) with biliary and duodenal obstruction of the second portion of duodenum. An EUS-guided transduodenal approach was performed using a 19-gauge needle

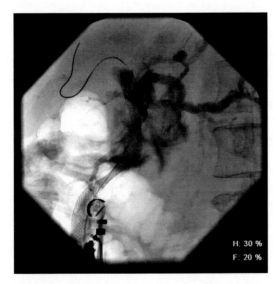

**Fig. 10.9** Wire-guided dilation with the 4-5-7 Fr catheter was successful. An 8 mm×8 cm uncovered metal biliary metal stent was placed across the stricture

The techniques of EUS-guided stent placement will be briefly described. An echoendoscope is passed into the stomach or duodenum depending on the intended approach of access being either transduodenal or transgastric. A diagnostic linear array echoendoscope can be used if the stent has a small delivery system (6 Fr) or if the intent is to not pass the stent through the endoscope. A therapeutic channel endoscope is needed if the intent is to pass stents with larger delivery systems through the endoscope. A 19-gauge fine needle aspiration (FNA) needle is required for passage of a 0.035″ guidewire, whereas a 22-gauge needle accepts a 0.018″ wire. If the goal is to pass the wire through the papilla, the trajectory of the puncture is important such that it is directed toward the distal bile duct and not toward the intrahepatic system, if possible. Color Doppler is used to prevent inadvertent puncture of vessels. Once the duct of interest is identified, the FNA needle is used to puncture through the gastric or duodenal wall. Aspiration of bile and injection of contrast under fluoroscopy confirms entry into the biliary tree. The needle is flushed with water and a guidewire is passed deeply into the duct. The FNA needle is withdrawn and the tract dilated. Tapered catheters often pass easily through duodenal wall to then allow dilation (4 mm) to permit stent passage. The gastric wall is thick, and creation of a tract usually requires the use of electrocautery (triple lumen needle knife, cystenterotome) over the wire and into the bile duct followed by balloon dilation of the tract. The stent is passed through the echoendoscope into the duct and deployed as outlined in options 1, 2, or 3 above. If a rendezvous approach (option 4) is chosen, then a traditional long length biliary guidewire (400 cm) wire is passed across the papilla and the echoendoscope withdrawn. A duodenoscope is advanced alongside the guidewire and passed into the duodenum where the wire is grasped and withdrawn thorough the working channel. The stent is then deployed as per the usual transpapillary approach.

Complications of EUS-guided puncture include bile leakage, pneumoperitoneum (usually self-limited), perforation, bleeding, and cholangitis. One must also be aware that the tip of the guidewire can be sheared off within the biliary tree if withdrawn into the needle. Hydrophilic wires are especially useful to negotiate strictures and to pass tortuous areas but are more difficult to exchange accessories and to maintain stability with removal of the endoscope.

## Pancreatic Applications

There are several potential applications for the use of SEMS in the treatment of pancreatic diseases though the data for these indications is limited and controversial.

## Pancreatic Duct Strictures

Painful chronic pancreatitis with a dominant main pancreatic duct (PD) stricture is usually managed with endoscopic placement of one or more plastic stents [80–85]. The majority of patients with chronic pancreatitis who respond to pancreatic stent placement experience sustained clinical improvement after stent removal [86–88]. A subset of patients experience recurrent pain caused by recurrent or persistent stricture of the main pancreatic duct [79, 81, 82, 85–87]. For these refractory strictures in patients with advanced chronic pancreatitis, placement of the maximally permitted number of large-diameter (8.5–11 Fr) plastic stents has been shown to be effective in allowing durable stricture resolution and preventing recurrent pain in a majority of patients [82].

As an alternative to plastic stents, SEMS have been used to treat benign pancreatic strictures. It must be emphasized that the use of SEMS in the main pancreatic duct is highly controversial and should be undertaken with caution if at all. Placement of UCSEMS for benign pancreatic duct strictures is associated with epithelial hyperplasia, tissue embedding, and lack of removability and should not be used in benign disease but may be acceptable for palliation of intractable pain or recurrent pancreatitis in patients with unresectable periampullary and pancreatic malignancies and underlying ductal obstruction.

The use of removable CSEMS in patients with benign pancreatic strictures is controversial and not advocated because of potential for occlusion of side branches and induction of new strictures. Additionally, the relative oversize of

the stent to the duct is a concern since traditional biliary SEMS are 8 and 10 mm in diameter. In one study, FCSEMS were placed in patients with chronic pancreatic duct strictures for 3 months with a high rate of recurrent pain after removal. After another 3-month period of FCSEMS placement, improvement was sustained [20]. This raises the question of the optimal duration of stent placement [89]. A longer duration of stenting may be needed to induce sufficient remodeling [21]. More prolonged placement of FCSEMS, however, may increase the risk of stent occlusion or disintegration of the covering membrane with embedding and lack of removability.

In a study by Park et al., FCSEMS were placed for 2 months to treat benign PD strictures with good efficacy and relative safety, but the greatest problem was frequent stent migration [31]. The same group recently showed temporary 3-month placement of modified FCSEMS with antimigration features was effective in resolving pancreatic duct strictures in chronic pancreatitis, with an acceptable safety profile and limited stent migration [31]. A minority of the patients developed asymptomatic focal de novo pancreatic strictures. More robust, long-term studies using removable FCSEMS in chronic pancreatitis patients with dominant strictures are needed before CSEMS can be recommended.

## Pancreatic Fluid Collections

Pancreatic fluid collections (PFCs) develop secondary to either fluid leakage or pancreatic necrosis after acute pancreatitis, chronic pancreatitis, surgery, or abdominal trauma [90–93]. The presence of underlying ductal damage, the severity of acute pancreatitis, and the maturation of the collection in relation to the onset of acute pancreatitis are factors that influence the formation and composition of the PFC [94–97]. Indications for PFC drainage include infection, pain, gastric outlet or biliary obstruction, leakage, fistulization, and enlargement [94–98]. Therapeutic options for PFCs include surgical, percutaneous, and endoscopic drainage. Over the last decade, endoscopic drainage of PFCs has been the procedure of choice in many tertiary-care institutions [94, 99, 100]. Clinical success rates of 70–87% have been reported, with complication rates of 11–34% [100, 101].

Endoscopic drainage of PFCs may be achieved by transmural or transpapillary placement of plastic endoprostheses [94, 102]. The evolution of EUS has extended the indications for transmural drainage to include pancreatic abscesses, organized liquefied necrosis, and nonbulging PFCs [31, 103].

A major area of interest is the type of stent used for endoscopic transmural drainage. The conventional technique is placement of one or more 10 Fr plastic stents but with the need for multiple revisions in 17.7–27% of cases [104, 105]. The use of biliary FCSEMS to create a temporary access fistula as a conduit for endoscopic drainage of liquefied fluid collections has been studied in small case series and has shown to be effective [106].

## Pancreatic Necrosis

Endoscopic drainage of symptomatic sterile or infected walled-off (organized pancreatic necrosis) is difficult because the solid debris needs to be evacuated, which cannot be achieved with small-diameter plastic or metal stents. A study by Belle et al. described temporary use of a specially designed large-diameter PCSEMS to keep the gastrostomy tract open for drainage of walled-off necrosis and allow passage of the endoscope into the necrosis for endoscopic necrosectomy [107]. The stent had a diameter of 20–25 mm and a length of 50 mm and was placed following the first transgastric necrosectomy. After a treatment period of 7–11 days involving 2–3 endoscopic procedures, clinical success was achieved, defined as complete removal of necrosis, in all cases without major complications. The stent was subsequently removed.

Another use of large-diameter metal stents was recently described. A fully covered esophageal SEMS was placed through a percutaneously created tract into a retroperitoneal necrotic collection to allow a portal for direct endoscopic necrosectomy [108].

## Pancreatolithiasis

Endoscopic clearance of large or impacted stones in the main pancreatic duct remains a clinical challenge in patients with chronic pancreatitis and pancreatic strictures. In a study by Yang and colleagues, a technically modified uncovered self-expandable metallic pancreatic stent was implanted in the pancreatic duct in four patients and was removed for 4–7 days later after the stent allowed stricture dilation [109]. The calculi were endoscopically removed in all four patients without severe complications. At a follow-up of 9–15 months, no major complications or stone recurrence occurred. This small study suggests that this technique could be an alternative to extracorporeal shock wave lithotripsy in the management of large pancreatic duct stones.

## Conclusion

Significant improvements in SEMS design and the evolution of EUS have spawned newer indications and placement techniques that previously could only be imagined. A variety of new stents are in the developmental phase including drug-eluting SEMS covered with antitumor agents, biodegradable stents, and a new lumen-apposing stent that has been shown in animals to be effective for transluminal drainage of nonadherent extraintestinal fluid collections. Although SEMS are an exciting development in the management of several hepatobiliary and pancreatic disorders, other options are possible in some patients, and these are best explored within multidisciplinary teams that include surgeons, radiologists, and oncologists.

# References

1. Bakhru MR, Foley PL, Gatesman J, et al. Fully covered self-expanding stents placed temporarily in the bile duct: safety profile and histologic classification in a porcine model. BMC Gastroenterol. 2011;11:76.

2. Baron TH. Covered self-expandable metal stents for benign biliary tract diseases. Curr Opin Gastroenterol. 2011;27:262–7.

3. Judah JR, Draganov PV. Endoscopic therapy of benign biliary strictures. World J Gastroenterol. 2007;13:3531–9.

4. Hammel P, Couvelard A, O'Toole D, et al. Regression of liver fibrosis after biliary drainage in patients with chronic pancreatitis and stenosis of the common bile duct. N Engl J Med. 2001;344:418–23.

5. Warshaw AL, Schapiro RH, Ferrucci JT, et al. Persistent obstructive jaundice, cholangitis, and biliary cirrhosis due to common bile duct stenosis in chronic pancreatitis. Gastroenterology. 1976; 70: 562–7.

6. Quintero GA, Patino JF. Surgical management of benign strictures of the biliary tract. World J Surg. 2001;25:1245–50.

7. Smits ME, Rauws EA, van Gulik TM, et al. Long-term results of endoscopic stenting and surgical drainage for biliary stricture due to chronic pancreatitis. Br J Surg. 1996;83:764–8.

8. Dumonceau JM, Deviere J, Delhaye M, et al. Plastic and metal stents for postoperative benign bile duct strictures: the best and the worst. Gastrointest Endosc. 1996;47:8–17.

9. Tocchi A, Mazzoni G, Liotta G, et al. Management of benign biliary strictures: biliary enteric anastomosis vs endoscopic stenting. Arch Surg. 2000;135: 153–7.

10. Frattaroli FM, Reggio D, Guadalaxara A, et al. Benign biliary strictures: a review of 21 years of experience. J Am Coll Surg. 1996;183:506–13.

11. Berkelhammer C, Kortan P, Haber GB. Endoscopic biliary prostheses as treatment for benign postoperative bile duct strictures. Gastrointest Endosc. 1989;35:95–101.

12. Draganov P, Hoffman B, Marsh W, et al. Long-term outcome in patients with benign biliary strictures treated endoscopically with multiple stents. Gastrointest Endosc. 2002;55:680–6.

13. Costamagna G, Pandolfi M, Mutignani M, et al. Long-term results of endoscopic management of postoperative bile duct strictures with increasing numbers of stents. Gastrointest Endosc. 2001;54: 162–8.

14. Davids PH, Groen AK, Rauws EA, et al. Randomised trial of self-expanding metal stents versus polyethylene stents for distal malignant biliary obstruction. Lancet. 1992;340:1488–92.

15. Kaassis M, Boyer J, Dumas R, et al. Plastic or metal stents for malignant stricture of the common bile duct? Results of a randomized prospective study. Gastrointest Endosc. 2003;57:178–82.

16. Knyrim K, Wagner HJ, Pausch J, et al. A prospective, randomized, controlled trial of metal stents for malignant obstruction of the common bile duct. Endoscopy. 1993;25:207–12.

17. Wagner HJ, Knyrim K, Vakil N, et al. Plastic endoprostheses versus metal stents in the palliative treatment of malignant hilar biliary obstruction. A prospective and randomized trial. Endoscopy. 1993;25:213–8.

18. Katsinelos P, Paikos D, Kountouras J, et al. Tannenbaum and metal stents in the palliative treatment of malignant distal bile duct obstruction: a comparative study of patency and cost effectiveness. Surg Endosc. 2006;20:1587–93.

19. Mahajan A, Ho H, Sauer B, et al. Temporary placement of fully covered self-expandable metal stents in benign biliary strictures: midterm evaluation (with video). Gastrointest Endosc. 2009;70:303–9.

20. Sauer B, Talreja J, Ellen K, et al. Temporary placement of a fully covered self-expandable metal stent in the pancreatic duct for management of symptomatic refractory chronic pancreatitis: preliminary data (with videos). Gastrointest Endosc. 2008;68:1173–8.

21. Park DH, Kim MH, Moon SH, et al. Feasibility and safety of placement of a newly designed, fully covered self-expandable metal stent for refractory benign pancreatic ductal strictures: a pilot study (with video). Gastrointest Endosc. 2008;68:1182–9.

22. Cahen DL, Rauws EA, Gouma DJ, et al. Removable fully covered self-expandable metal stents in the treatment of common bile duct strictures due to chronic pancreatitis: a case series. Endoscopy. 2008;40:697–700.

23. Catalano MF, Linder JD, George S, et al. Treatment of symptomatic distal common bile duct stenosis secondary to chronic pancreatitis: comparison of single vs. multiple simultaneous stents. Gastrointest Endosc. 2004;60:945–52.

24. Kahaleh M, Behm B, Clarke BW, et al. Temporary placement of covered self-expandable metal stents in benign biliary strictures: a new paradigm? (with video). Gastrointest Endosc. 2008;67:446–54.

25. Park DH, Kim MH, Choi JS, et al. Covered versus uncovered Wallstent for malignant extrahepatic biliary obstruction: a cohort comparative analysis. Clin Gastroenterol Hepatol. 2006;4:790–6.

26. Traina M, Tarantino I, Barresi L, et al. Efficacy and safety of fully covered elf-expandable metallic stents in biliary complications after liver transplantation: a preliminary study. Liver Transpl. 2009;15:1493–8.

27. Wang AY, Ellen K, Berg CL, et al. Fully covered self-expandable metallic stents in the management of complex biliary leaks: preliminary data – a case series. Endoscopy. 2009;41:781–6.

28. Eloubeidi MA, Lopes TL. Novel removable internally fully covered self-expanding metal esophageal stent: feasibility, technique of removal, and tissue

response in humans. Am J Gastroenterol. 2009;104:1374–81.

29. Park DH, Koo JE, Oh J, et al. EUS-guided biliary drainage with one-step placement of a fully covered metal stent for malignant biliary obstruction: a prospective feasibility study. Am J Gastroenterol. 2009;104:2168–74.

30. Park DH, Song TJ, Eum J, et al. EUS-guided hepaticogastrostomy with a fully covered metal stent as the biliary diversion technique for an occluded biliary metal stent after a failed ERCP (with videos). Gastrointest Endosc. 2010;71:413–9.

31. Park DH, Lee SS, Lee TH, et al. Anchoring flap versus flared end, fully covered self-expandable metal stents to prevent migration in patients with benign biliary strictures: a multicenter, prospective, comparative pilot study (with videos). Gastrointest Endosc. 2011;73:64–70.

32. Park JK, Moon JH, Choi HJ, et al. Anchoring of a fully covered self-expandable metal stent with a 5F double-pigtail plastic stent to prevent migration in the management of benign biliary strictures. Am J Gastroenterol. 2011;106:1761–5. doi:10.1038/ajg.2011.212.

33. Poley JW, Van Tilburg AJ, Kuipers EJ, Bruno MJ. Breaking the barrier: using extractable fully covered metal stents to treat benign biliary strictures. Gastrointest Endosc. 2011;74:916–20.

34. Baron TH, Poterucha JJ. Insertion and removal of covered expandable metal stents for closure of complex biliary leaks. Clin Gastroenterol Hepatol. 2006;4:381–6.

35. Wang AY, Ellen K, Berg CL, Schmitt TM, Kahaleh M. Fully covered self-expandable metallic stents in the management of complex biliary leaks: preliminary data – a case series. Endoscopy. 2009; 41: 781–6.

36. Ferreira LE, Baron TH. Post-sphincterotomy bleeding: who, what, when, and how. Am J Gastroenterol. 2007;102:2850–8.

37. DiPisa M, Tarantino I, Barresi L, et al. Placement of covered self-expandable metal biliary stent for the treatment of severe post-sphincterotomy bleeding: outcomes of two cases. Gastroenterol Res Pract. 2010;2010:138748.

38. Itoi T, Yasuda I, Doi S, et al. Endoscopic hemostasis using covered metallic stent placement for uncontrolled post-endoscopic sphincterotomy bleeding. Endoscopy. 2011;43:369–72.

39. Jeon HJ, Han JH, Park S, et al. Endoscopic sphincterotomy-related perforation in the common bile duct successfully treated by placement of a covered metal stent. Endoscopy. 2011; 43(Supl 2) UCTN:E295–E96.

40. Cerefice M, Sauer B, Javaid M, et al. Complex biliary stones: treatment with removable self-expandable metal stents: a new approach (with videos). Gastrointest Endosc. 2011;74:520–6.

41. van der Gaag NA, Rauws EA, van Eijck CH, et al. Preoperative biliary drainage for cancer of the head of the pancreas. N Engl J Med. 2010;362:129–37.

42. Baron TH, Kozarek RA. Preoperative biliary stents in pancreatic cancer—proceed with caution. N Engl J Med. 2010;362:170–2.

43. Baron TH, Petersen BT, Mergener K, et al. Quality indicators for endoscopic retrograde cholangiopancreatography. Am J Gastroenterol. 2006;101:892–7.

44. Bonin EA, Barton TH. Preoperative biliary stents in pancreatic cancer. J Hepatobiliary Pancreat Sci. 2011;18:621–9.

45. Moss AC, Morris E, Leyden J, MacMathuna P. Malignant distal biliary obstruction: a systematic review and meta-analysis of endoscopic and surgical bypass results. Cancer Treat Rev. 2007;33:213.

46. Saleem A, Leggett CL, Murad MH, Baron TH. Meta-analysis of randomized trials comparing the patency of covered and uncovered self-expandable metal stents for palliation of distal malignant bile duct obstruction. Gastrointest Endosc. 2011;74:321–7. e1-3.

47. Davids PH, Groen AK, Rauws EA, et al. Randomised trial of self-expanding metal stents versus polyethylene stents for distal malignant biliary obstruction. Lancet. 1992;340(8834–8835):1488–92.

48. Knyrim K, Wagner HJ, Pausch J, Vakil N. A prospective, randomized, controlled trial of metal stents for malignant obstruction of the common bile duct. Endoscopy. 1993;25:207–12.

49. Soderlund C, Linder S. Covered metal versus plastic stents for malignant common bile duct stenosis: a prospective, randomized, controlled trial. Gastrointest Endosc. 2006;63:986–95.

50. Telford JJ, Carr-Locke DL, Baron TH, et al. A randomized trial comparing uncovered and partially covered self-expandable metal stents in the palliation of distal malignant biliary obstruction. Gastrointest Endosc. 2010;72:907–14.

51. Bismuth H, Castaing D, Traynor O. Resection or palliation: priority of surgery in the treatment of hilar cancer. World J Surg. 1988;12:39–47.

52. Larghi A, Tringali A, Lecca PG, et al. Management of hilar biliary strictures. Am J Gastroenterol. 2008;103:458.

53. De Palma GD, Galloro G, Siciliano S, et al. Unilateral versus bilateral endoscopic hepatic duct drainage in patients with malignant hilar biliary obstruction: results of a prospective, randomized, and controlled study. Gastrointest Endosc. 2001;53:547–53.

54. Naitoh I, Ohara H, Nakazawa T, et al. Unilateral versus bilateral endoscopic metal stenting for malignant hilar biliary obstruction. J Gastroenterol Hepatol. 2009;24:552–7.

55. Vienne A, Hobeika E, Gouya H, et al. Prediction of drainage effectiveness during endoscopic stenting of malignant hilar strictures: the role of liver volume assessment. Gastrointest Endosc. 2010;72:728–35.

56. Chennat J, Waxman I. Initial performance profile of a new 6F self-expanding metal stent for palliation of malignant hilar biliary obstruction. Gastrointest Endosc. 2010;72:632–6.

57. Chen VK, Arguedas MR, Baron TH. Expandable metal biliary stents before pancreaticoduodenectomy for pancreatic cancer: a Monte-Carlo decision analysis. Clin Gastroenterol Hepatol. 2005;3:1229–37.

58. Lawrence C, Howell DA, Conklin DE, et al. Delayed pancreaticoduodenectomy for cancer patients with prior ERCP-placed, nonforeshortening, self-expanding metal stents: a positive outcome. Gastrointest Endosc. 2006;63:804–7.

59. Bakken JC, Baron TH. Metal stents and biliary obstruction secondary to lymphoma: a tale of caution. Dig Dis Sci. 2010;55:3636.

60. Artifon EL, Sakai P, Ishioka S, et al. Endoscopic sphincterotomy before deployment of covered metal stent is associated with greater complication rate: a prospective randomized controlled trial. J Clin Gastroenterol. 2008;42:815–9.

61. Banerjee N, Hilden K, Baron TH, Adler DG. Endoscopic biliary sphincterotomy is not required for transpapillary SEMs placement for biliary obstruction. Dig Dis Sci. 2011;56:591–5.

62. Suk KT, Kim HS, Kim JW et al. Risk factors for cholecystitis after metal stent placement in malignant biliary obstruction. Gastrointest Endosc. 2006;64(4):522–9.

63. Ishii K, Itoi T, Sofuni A, et al. Endoscopic removal and trimming of distal self-expandable metallic biliary stents. World J Gastroenterol. 2011;17:2652–7.

64. Chahal P, Baron TH. Expandable metal stents for endoscopic bilateral stent-within-stent placement for malignant hilar biliary obstruction. Gastrointest Endosc. 2010;71:195–9.

65. Saleem A, Baron TH. Small diameter delivery system allows expandable metal biliary stent placement using a pediatric colonoscope in surgically altered anatomy. Endoscopy. 2011;43(Suppl 2):UCTN:369–70.

66. Tan DM, Lillemoe KD, Fogel EL. A new technique for endoscopic removal of uncovered biliary self-expandable metal stents: stent-in-stent technique with a fully covered biliary stent. Gastrointest Endosc. 2012;75:923–5.

67. Arias Dachary FJ, Chioccioli C, Deprez PH. Application of the "covered-stent-in-uncovered-stent" technique for easy and safe removal of embedded biliary uncovered SEMS with tissue ingrowth. Endoscopy. 2010;42(Suppl 2):E304–5.

68. Speer AG, Cotton PB, Russell RC, et al. Randomised trial of endoscopic versus percutaneous stent insertion in malignant obstructive jaundice. Lancet. 1987;2:57–62.

69. Inal M, Aksunger E, Akgul E, et al. Percutaneous placement of metallic stents in malignant biliary obstruction: one-stage or two-stage procedure? Predilate or not? Cardiovasc Intervent Radiol. 2003;26:40–5.

70. Beissert M, Wittenberg G, Sandstede J, et al. Metallic stents and plastic endoprostheses in percutaneous treatment of biliary obstruction. Z Gastroenterol. 2002;40:503–10.

71. Pinol V, Castells A, Bordas JM, et al. Percutaneous self-expanding metal stents versus endoscopic polyethylene endoprostheses for treating malignant biliary obstruction: randomized clinical trial. Radiology. 2002;225:27–34.

72. Doctor N, Dick R, Rai R, et al. Results of percutaneous plastic stents for malignant distal biliary obstruction following failed endoscopic stent insertion and comparison with current literature on expandable metallic stents. Eur J Gastroenterol Hepatol. 1999;11:775–80.

73. Kaskarelis IS, Papadaki MG, Papageorgiou GN, et al. Long-term follow-up in patients with malignant biliary obstruction after percutaneous placement of uncovered Wallstent endoprostheses. Acta Radiol. 1999;40:528–33.

74. Wayman J, Mansfield JC, Matthewson K, et al. Combined percutaneous and endoscopic procedures for bile duct obstruction: simultaneous and delayed techniques compared. Hepatogastroenterology. 2003;50:915–8.

75. Baron TH. Management of simultaneous biliary and duodenal obstruction: the endoscopic perspective. Gut Liver. 2010;4(Suppl1):S50–6.

76. Topazian M, Baron TH. Endoscopic fenestration of duodenal stents using argon plasma to facilitate ERCP. Gastrointest Endosc. 2009;69:166–9.

77. Itoi T, Isayama H, Sofuni A, et al. Stent selection and tips on placement technique of EUS-guided biliary drainage: transduodenal and transgastric stenting. J Hepatobiliary Pancreat Sci. 2011;18:664–72.

78. Nguyen-Tang T, Binmoeller KF, Sanchez-Yague A, Shah JN. Endoscopic ultrasound (EUS)-guided transhepatic anterograde self-expandable metal stent (SEMS) placement across malignant biliary obstruction. Endoscopy. 2010;42:232–6.

79. Kim YS, Gupta K, Mallery S, et al. Endoscopic ultrasound rendezvous for bile duct access using a transduodenal approach: cumulative experience at a single center. A case series. Endoscopy. 2010;42:496–502.

80. Smits ME, Badiga SM, Rauws EA, et al. Long-term results of pancreatic stents in chronic pancreatitis. Gastrointest Endosc. 1995;42:461–7.

81. Adler DG, Lichtenstein D, Baron TH, et al. The role of endoscopy in patients with chronic pancreatitis. Gastrointest Endosc. 2006;63:933–7.

82. Costamagna G, Bulajic M, Tringali A, et al. Multiple stenting of refractory pancreatic duct strictures in severe chronic pancreatitis: long-term results. Endoscopy. 2006;38:254–9.

83. Delhaye M, Arvanitakis M, Bali M, et al. Endoscopic therapy for chronic pancreatitis. Scand J Surg. 2005;94:143–53.

84. Testoni PA. Endoscopic stenting in benign pancreatic diseases. JOP. 2007;8:141–50.

85. Topazian M, Aslanian H, Andersen D. Outcome following endoscopic stenting of pancreatic duct strictures in chronic pancreatitis. J Clin Gastroenterol. 2005;39:908–11.

86. Binmoeller KF, Jue P, Seifert H, et al. Endoscopic pancreatic stent drainage in chronic pancreatitis and a dominant stricture: long-term results. Endoscopy. 1995;27:638–44.

87. Eleftherladis N, Dinu F, Delhaye M, et al. Long-term outcome after pancreatic stenting in severe chronic pancreatitis. Endoscopy. 2005;37:223–30.

88. Farnbacher MJ, Muhldorfer S, Wehler M, et al. Interventional endoscopic therapy in chronic pancreatitis including temporary stenting: a definitive treatment? Scand J Gastroenterol. 2006;41:111–7.

89. Ostroff JW. Pain and chronic pancreatitis: are we really ready for metal in the pancreatic duct? Gastrointest Endosc. 2008;68:1179–81.

90. Baillie J. Pancreatic pseudocysts (part I). Gastrointest Endosc. 2004;59:873–9.

91. Yeo CL, Cameron JL, Sohn TA, et al. Six hundred fifty consecutive pancreaticoduodenectomies in the 1990s: pathology, complications, and outcomes. Ann Surg. 1997;226:248–60.

92. Arvanitakis M, Delhaye M, Chamlou R, et al. Endoscopic therapy for main pancreatic duct rupture after silastic-ring vertical gastroplasty. Gastrointest Endosc. 2005;62:143–51.

93. Kloppel G. Pseudocysts and other non-neoplastic cysts of the pancreas. Semin Diagn Pathol. 2000;17: 7–15.

94. Baron TH, Harewood GC, Morgan DE, et al. Outcome differences after endoscopic drainage of pancreatic necrosis, acute pancreatic pseudocysts, and chronic pancreatic pseudocysts. Gastrointest Endosc. 2002;56:7–17.

95. Baron TH, Morgan DE. The diagnosis and management of fluid collections associated with pancreatitis. Am J Med. 1997;102:555–63.

96. Yeo CJ, Bastidas JA, Lynch-Nyhan A, et al. The natural history of pancreatic pseudocysts documented by computed tomography. Surg Gynecol Obstet. 1990;170:411–7.

97. Bradley EL, Clements Jr JL, Gonzalez AC. The natural history of pancreatic pseudocysts: a unified concept of management. Am J Surg. 1979;137: 135–41.

98. Gouyon B, Levy P, Ruszniewski P, et al. Predictive factors in the outcome of pseudocysts complicating alcoholic chronic pancreatitis. Gut. 1997;41:821–5.

99. Binmoeller KF, Seifart H, Walter A, et al. Transpapillary and transmural drainage of pancreatic pseudocysts. Gastrointest Endosc. 1995;42: 219–24.

100. Cahen D, Rauws E, Fockens P, et al. Endoscopic drainage of pancreatic pseudocysts; long-term outcome and procedural factors associated with safe and successful treatment. Endoscopy. 2005;37: 977–83.

101. Hookey LC, Debroux S, Delhaye M, et al. Endoscopic drainage of pancreatic fluid collections in 116 patients: a comparison of etiologies, drainage techniques, and outcomes. Gastrointest Endosc. 2006;63:635–43.

102. Delhaye M, Matos C, Deviere J. Endoscopic management of chronic pancreatitis. Gastrointest Endosc Clin N Am. 2003;13:717–42.

103. Arvanitakis M, Delhaye M, Bali MA, et al. Pancreatic fluid collections: a randomized controlled trial regarding stent removal after endoscopic transmural drainage. Gastrointest Endosc. 2007;65:609–19.

104. Kruger M, Schneider AS, Manns MP, et al. Endoscopic management of pancreatic pseudocysts or abscesses after an EUS-guided 1-step procedure for initial access. Gastrointest Endosc. 2006;63:409–16.

105. Lopes CV, Pesenti C, Bories E, et al. Endoscopic-ultrasound-guided endoscopic transmural drainage of pancreatic pseudocysts and abscesses. Scand J Gastroenterol. 2007;42:524–9.

106. Talreja JP, Shami VM, Ku J, et al. Transenteric drainage of pancreatic-fluid collections with fully covered self-expanding metallic stents (with video). Gastrointest Endosc. 2008;68:1199–203. AS 91.

107. Belle S, Collet P, Post S, Kaehler G. Temporary cystogastrostomy with self-expanding metallic stents for pancreatic necrosis. Endoscopy. 2010;42:493–5.

108. van Sonnenberg E, Wittich GR, Casola G, et al. Percutaneous drainage of infected and noninfected pancreatic pseudocysts: experience in 101 cases. Radiology. 1989;170:757–61.

109. Yang XJ, Lin Y, Zeng X, et al. A minimally invasive alternative for managing large pancreatic duct stones using a modified expandable metal mesh stent. Pancreatology. 2009;9:111–5.

# Enteric Stents: Indications and Placement Techniques

# 11

## Todd Baron

Self-expandable metal biliary stents (SEMS), first used outside of the USA, became commercially available in the USA approximately 20 years ago because of their prolonged patency when compared to plastic biliary stents [1]. Esophageal SEMS were introduced soon after expandable biliary stents, and SEMS specifically designed for gastroduodenal use were developed several years later. However, both esophageal and biliary SEMS have been used for relief of gastroduodenal obstruction. The indications and placement techniques for enteric stents, defined as gastric and small bowel stents for the purposes of this chapter, will be reviewed.

## Basic Concepts

Self-expandable stents placed for enteric use are composed of a variety of materials ranging from plastic to stainless steel to nitinol. Stents vary based upon type of material that they are composed of, lattice width (if any), configuration, length and diameter, and presence and degree of covering. More importantly, in order for precise placement to be achieved, the degree of shortening (if any) that occurs with expansion and the nuances of the delivery and release systems must be known. There are a number of stents available from a

T. Baron, M.D. (✉)
Department of Medicine, Mayo Clinic,
200 First Street SW, Rochester, MN 55905, USA
e-mail: baron.todd@mayo.edu

variety of manufacturers around the world. The principles of all expandable stents are similar, and the concepts presented here can be applied to all expandable stents.

It is extremely helpful to have nursing assistants who are comfortable with complex therapeutic endoscopic procedures to include expandable stent placement. Moreover, an understanding of the complexities of stent placement will assure that complications are minimized [2].

## Indications for and Contraindications to Enteric Stent Placement

### Indications

There are several indications for placement of enteric stents (Table 11.1). These can be divided into benign and malignant conditions, although indications for placement in malignant disease are much more common than for benign disease. In Table 11.1, indications are divided into location and type of disease process. Indications for enteric stent placement in benign diseases are generally due to postoperative complications that include strictures, leaks, and fistula. Post-bariatric surgery, historically Roux-en-Y gastric bypass, and more recently, sleeve gastrectomy can be associated with postoperative leaks, fistula, and strictures and can be managed using temporary stent placement [3–11] (Fig. 11.1). Similarly, occasional patients who have had prior Billroth II operations and pancreaticoduodenectomy may

R. Kozarek et al. (eds.), *Self-Expandable Stents in the Gastrointestinal Tract*,
DOI 10.1007/978-1-4614-3746-8_11, © Springer Science+Business Media New York 2013

**Table 11.1** Indications for placement of enteric stents

| Benign |
| --- |
| *Gastric* |
| Postoperative fistula/leaks – gastric (sleeve gastrectomy) and gastrojejunal anastomosis (Roux-en-Y gastric bypass, post-Whipple and Billroth II) |
| Gastric stricture (sleeve gastrectomy) |
| *Duodenal* – stricture due to peptic ulcer disease; duodenal fistula (rare) |
| *Small bowel* – postoperative strictures – anastomotic, Crohn's disease (rare) |
| Malignant |
| *Gastric obstruction* |
| Primary and recurrent gastric cancer |
| Gastrojejunal anastomosis (afferent and efferent limb obstruction) |
| Gastric stricture (sleeve gastrectomy) |
| *Duodenal obstruction* |
| Periampullary cancer |
| Pancreatic cancer/metastatic disease to the head of the pancreas |
| Cholangiocarcinoma |
| Gallbladder cancer |
| Locally invasive tumors (colon cancer) |
| *Small bowel* – metastatic disease (particularly ligament of Treitz), distal terminal ileum (pelvic cancers, metastatic disease) |
| Other (uncommon) |
| Perforation of the duodenum or jejunal limbs of anastomoses (within reach of endoscope and stent delivery system) |
| Bridge to surgery |
| Transgastric or transduodenal placement for drainage or debridement of pancreatic necrosis |

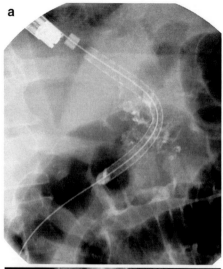

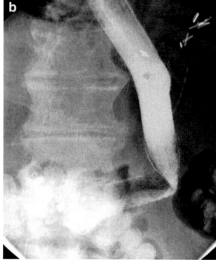

**Fig. 11.1** Use of a fully covered stent for treatment of complete gastric outlet obstruction due to a benign stricture following sleeve gastrectomy. (**a**) Endoscope is positioned above the predeployed stent. (**b**) Postdeployment upper gastrointestinal series shows persistent narrowing. The stent was removed 3 months later, and the patient remains well 5 years later

develop benign anastomotic complications that can be managed with stents [12]. Crohn's disease with small bowel stricture is an uncommon indication for stent placement, although recent data on the use of SEMS [13], as well biodegradable stents [14], show promise for these patients. In most patients with benign strictures, stent placement should only be considered after the patient has failed an adequate trial of serial endoscopic dilation.

Malignant disease is a much more common cause of luminal obstruction and needs palliative enteric stent placement. Rarely, enteric stents are placed as a *bridge* to surgery (e.g., primary small bowel lymphoma), although there are no published data for this indication.

Before offering stent placement for relief of gastric outlet obstruction (GOO), the degree of oral intake should be assessed. A gastric outlet obstruction scoring system (GOOSS), adapted from the dysphagia scoring system, was introduced by Adler and Baron in 2002 [15] and has become accepted as a measure of oral intake (Table 11.2). Patients with GOOSS scores <2 are candidates for stent placement. Alternatively, palliative gastrojejunostomy, increasingly performed laparoscopically, should be considered an alternative to stent placement in patients with anticipated survival longer than 3–4 months [16, 17], potentially predictable by a WHO (World Health Organization) score. The WHO score is based upon a scale of 0–5, with 0 being healthy and 5 being dead. A recent study showed that patients

**Table 11.2** Gastric outlet obstruction scoring system (GOOSS)

| Level of oral intake | Score |
| --- | --- |
| No oral intake | 0 |
| Liquids only | 1 |
| Soft solids | 2 |
| Low-residue or full diet | 3 |

with a WHO score of 0–1 may be managed with gastrojejunostomy, while those with a WHO score of 3–4 should be considered for stent placement [18] as a consequence of the longer survival and more durable duration of palliation in the surgical group. The type of malignancy that causes lumen obstruction (Table 11.1) varies throughout the world. For example, in the East, primary and recurrent gastric cancer with resultant GOO is more common, whereas in the West, pancreatic cancer is the most common cause of GOO.

Occasional patients have distal small bowel obstruction that does not involve the colon, but only be reached retrograde via colonoscopy (Fig. 11.2). Free luminal perforation, usually iatrogenic, is a rare indication for enteric stent placement [19] (Fig. 11.3).

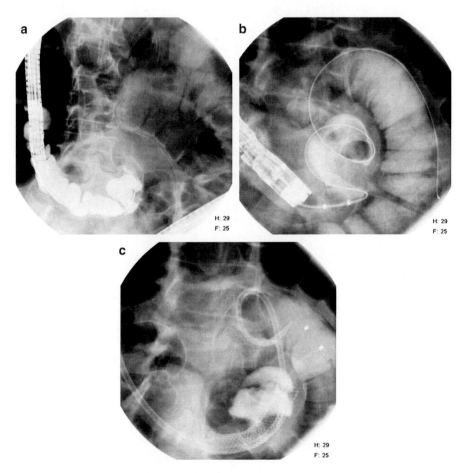

**Fig. 11.2** Placement of fully covered biliary stent for treatment of a benign postoperative distal ileal anastomotic stricture. (**a**) Colonoscope has been passed through the ileocecal valve to the site of obstruction. Injected contrast does not pass the obstruction. (**b**) After traversing the stricture with a guidewire, the upstream dilated ileum is seen. (**c**) Note placement of a fully covered biliary stent and 10-Fr nasojejunal tube inserted for safety and decompression. The stent passed spontaneously 1 month after resolution of obstruction

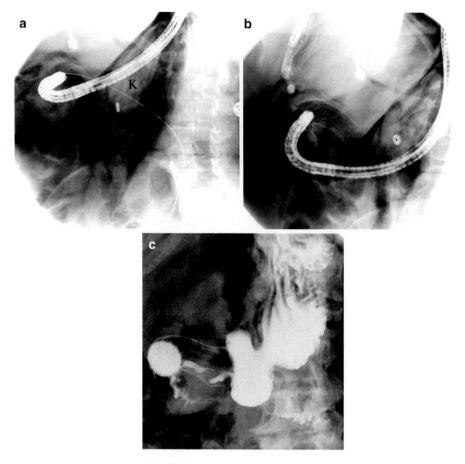

**Fig. 11.3** Closure of a large lateral wall duodenal perforation during ERCP for obstructive jaundice. (**a**) The duodenoscope has been removed and a Savary wire advanced beyond the ligament of Treitz using a forward-viewing endoscope. Free air outlines the kidney (K). (**b**) Immediately after placement of a covered non-TTS esophageal stent. (**c**) Upper GI 2 days later shows no leak

## Contraindications

There are relatively few contraindications to placing self-expandable, enteric metal stents. Free perforation, although considered a contraindication to most endoscopic procedures, may, in fact, be an indication for perforation closure (Fig. 11.3).

Peritoneal carcinomatosis is a relative contraindication to enteric stent placement because many patients have multifocal areas of obstruction and encasement of the small bowel and may not respond to stent placement for palliation of obstruction; moreover, if clinically successful, the improvement is often short-lived. Patients with peritoneal carcinomatosis are identified by the presence of underlying malignant ascites

and/or peritoneal thickening on abdominal CT imaging. There are two morphologic types of peritoneal implants. Layered implants (higher grade, nonmucinous, and invasive lesions) conform to the normal shape of abdominal structures and are not well seen on computed tomography (CT), whereas nodular implants (lower grade, mucinous, and noninvasive lesions) are more readily apparent (Fig. 11.4a) [20]. In one recent study, patients with peritoneal carcinomatosis were found to have similar results to those without [21]. This is in contrast to this author's experience, although I believe that selected patients with peritoneal carcinomatosis and what appears to be a single, dominant obstructive stricture with marked upstream dilation and a clear-cut

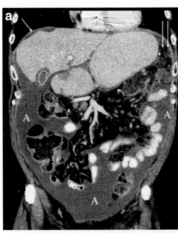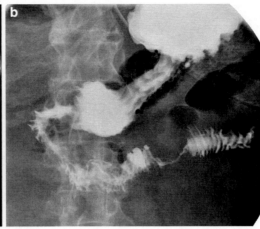

**Fig. 11.4** Peritoneal carcinomatosis in the setting of SEMS placement. (**a**) CT shows typical features with ascites and nodularity around the liver (*single arrow*) and nodules in the left upper quadrant adjacent to the colon (*double arrows*). Ascites (marked by A) is present throughout. (**b**) Upper gastrointestinal series in same patient shows high-grade lesion. Despite successful stent placement and patency confirmed by upper gastrointestinal series, the patient did not clinically improve, and distal lesions were identified

transition point on CT may respond to stent therapy (Fig. 11.4b). In such cases, where stent placement is technically successful, yet clinically unsuccessful, placement of additional stents is usually futile and other means of palliation should be undertaken (such as nasogastric or decompressive gastrostomy tube placement).

## Stent Selection

Selection of the appropriate stent is based upon the indication for placement and stent availability. For documented, unresectable disease, uncovered stents are most commonly used because of their low rate of migration compared to covered stents, although the latter are associated with a decrease in tumor ingrowth [22]. Covered stents for enteric use are available outside of the USA. In the USA, the only available, dedicated enteric stents are uncovered [23]. The advantage of these dedicated stents is that their delivery systems are long enough and small enough in diameter to pass through the scope (TTS), including adult colonoscopes. The lack of removability, however, makes them unsuitable for treatment of benign disease or closure of fistula. Thus, within the USA, stent options for benign disease and for closure of fistula are limited to the use of esophageal and biliary stents.

Esophageal stents are available as fully and partially covered self-expandable metal (SEMS) or plastic (SEPS) but are limited by their short, non-TTS delivery systems. The only available SEPS (see Chap. 3) has a particularly rigid delivery system that limits their use to placement in lesions that are close to the mouth and are relatively straight in the projected pathway (e.g., treatment of a Roux-en-Y gastrojejunal anastomotic stricture or leak).

Esophageal SEMS are more flexible, but their relatively short delivery systems generally limit transoral placement in patients with nonsurgically altered anatomy to the first and second portion of the duodenum in best-case scenarios. However, novel placement techniques include placement through gastrostomy tracts – either after maturation [24] or through fresh tracts created with introducer systems (Fig. 11.5), *extension* of delivery systems [25], and use of overtubes [26].

Biliary SEMS are available as partially and fully covered stents and are long enough to pass through a colonoscope and for benign strictures of the small bowel, either antegrade or retrograde. The disadvantage to these stents is a luminal diameter of 8–10 mm. However, side-by-side

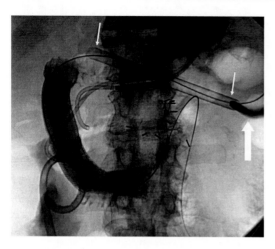

**Fig. 11.5** Closure of a large duodenal fistula (at site of percutaneous pigtail drain) using overlapping covered (partially and fully) esophageal stents. A gastrostomy sheath (*small arrows*) was placed percutaneously immediately before stents were passed through the sheath. Note small-caliber endoscope (*large arrow*) could also be passed through sheath to assess stent position after deployment

placement is possible to achieve luminal diameters of 20 mm (Fig. 11.6).

## Gastroduodenal Stent Placement

### Preparation, Sedation, and Positioning

Obtaining a pre-procedural radiographic contrast study is not essential, and often not performed, although such imaging allows determination of the anatomy and stricture length (Figs. 11.4 and 11.6a) and precludes need for passage of the endoscope beyond the lesion to determine their length and angulation. It is most helpful if it is unclear whether the patient's symptoms are due to obstruction or other cancer-related processes (neural invasion by tumor with delayed gastric emptying, peritoneal carcinomatosis). Most patients will have had a recent abdominal CT scan which provides information on degree of obstruction, location, length of stricture, and presence or absence of fistula.

Before undertaking stent placement in patients with malignant gastroduodenal obstruction, it is important to first assess the status of the biliary tree, since placement of an expandable stent across the papilla may make subsequent endo-scopic access to the papilla difficult, if not impossible. In addition, in patients with proximal duodenal strictures, the stent does not necessarily have to cross the papilla to achieve palliation. Thus, a stent should be chosen that is adequate to cross the lesion, but not excessively long so as to prevent access to the papilla, if potentially required in the future. A recent review of combined gastroduodenal and biliary obstruction has been published [27], and a technical approach to combined obstruction will be discussed later in this chapter.

Not unexpectedly, patients with complete gastric outlet obstruction have retained liquids and/or solids and are at risk for aspiration during stent placement unless precautions are taken. Patients with complete obstruction are already nil per os, hospitalized, and often have nasogastric suction for decompression. Nonetheless, solid food may not be adequately evacuated and remain in place. Outpatients with subtotal obstruction should consume clear liquids for at least 24 h prior to their procedure, but may have retained solid food. Sedation with airway protection (endotracheal intubation), large-bore evacuation, type of endoscope, and patient positioning all play a role in the prevention of aspiration and optimization of endoscopic visualization. Large-bore evacuation tubes can be used, if necessary, to allow endoscopic visualization, but are best reserved for patients who have airway protection. Large working channel (6 mm) endoscopes, such as those designed for removal of blood clots during gastrointestinal bleeding, can be used to evacuate semisolid material.

Fluoroscopy, although not always necessary when stents are placed using endoscopic techniques, especially for nonobstructive indications, should be readily available and is mandatory when stents are placed using interventional radiologic techniques alone. Placing the patient in the left lateral decubitus position prevents aspiration, but the fluoroscopic image is less than ideal for gastroduodenal stent placement. Thus, placement in the prone or supine position is preferred. When moderate or monitored anesthesia care is used, I place the patient in the left lateral decubitus position and remove all gastric contents, if possible. The patient is

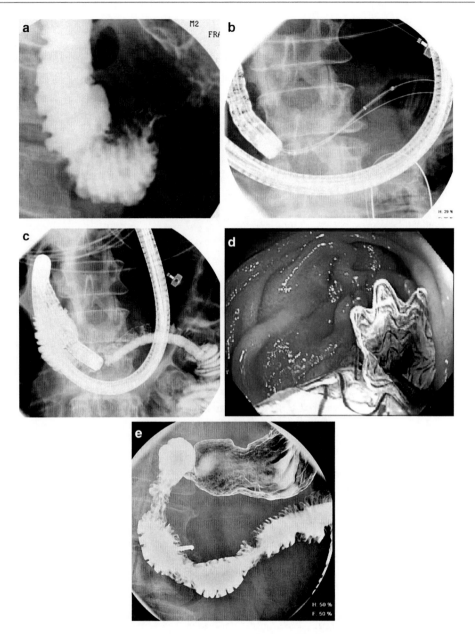

**Fig. 11.6** Treatment of a benign duodenojejunal anasto-motic stricture with side-by-side covered biliary stents. (**a**) Upper GI contrast series showing stricture. (**b**) Two guidewires are passed alongside each other. The first stent is predeployed in position across the stricture. (**c**) Radiograph taken immediately after deployment of both stents. Contrast is injected through the inferior stent. (**d**) Endoscopic photo of side-by-side covered expandable metal biliary stents. (**e**) Follow-up upper gastrointestinal series after removal of both stents shows resolution of stricture

subsequently placed supine and the airway carefully monitored and suctioned with the head of the bed elevated (if possible). In addition, one may consider endotracheal intubation in these patients to prevent aspiration.

## Choice of Endoscope

The choice of endoscope for gastroduodenal stent placement depends on the site of the lesion (stomach versus duodenum), type of stent, and whether an ERCP will be done at the same setting. Small-caliber endoscopes (5.4-mm outer diameter or less) can be used for gastric lesions and those with a disease process at or near a gastrojejunal anastomosis. These endoscopes allow easy traversal of tight strictures for endoscopic inspection and may obviate fluoroscopy to determine stricture length. However, the working channel is small, suction capability is suboptimal, and the scopes do not permit passage of accessories (catheters), and essentially, only guidewires can be passed. However, once a guidewire is passed, the endoscope can be removed, and a therapeutic channel endoscope can be backloaded over the wire for TTS delivery [28].

Standard adult endoscopes are intermediate in terms of flexibility and use of accessories, but the working channel does not allow TTS stent placement. Therapeutic channel endoscopes (working channel ≥3.8 mm) are most often used when TTS stents with predeployment delivery systems of 10 Fr are placed.

Duodenoscopes also allow passage of TTS stents and are advantageous when ERCP with biliary stent placement and gastroduodenal stents are placed in the same session, precluding the need to change endoscopes. The side-viewing duodenoscope may be helpful in those patients in whom the stricture cannot be traversed with a forward endoscope and may allow an en face view of the stricture.

Upper endoscopes and duodenoscopes are usually limited to lesions proximal to the second duodenum in patients with GOO since the often dilated stomach creates looping that consumes the length of the endoscope. Thus, even for proximal duodenal lesions, it may be useful to use adult caliber colonoscopes for TTS placement. These scopes are essential for lesions beyond the second to third duodenum, to include the proximal jejunum in patients with intact anatomy. Moreover, they are often used for patients with afferent limb obstructions far from the origin of the anastomoses.

Finally, balloon enteroscopes may be useful in selected cases, not only because of the ability to pass deep into the bowel but also because of their flexibility. Following wire passage beyond the stenosis, the endoscope can either be removed

and a therapeutic endoscope backloaded over the wire, or the stent can be passed through the overtube [29]. Similar placement techniques have been used with spiral overtubes [30].

## Insertion Techniques

Stents can be placed using endoscopic techniques with or without fluoroscopy and can be TTS or non-TTS. Alternatively, stents can be placed using interventional radiologic techniques alone. TTS and non-TTS endoscopic techniques will be discussed separately, but the rate-limiting step that is common to all techniques for successful placement is passage of a guidewire across the intended site of placement. This can be technically difficult in patients whose primary problem is obstruction, particularly complete obstruction. Thus, techniques to traverse the lesion are especially important. This chapter will focus primarily on endoscopic approaches.

### Through-the-Scope Insertion

Since therapeutic channel endoscopes (working channel ≥3.8 mm) are needed to place TTS stents and are large in caliber, it is frequently not possible to traverse the stricture with the endoscope and is not necessary to achieve placement. Thus, aggressive dilation of the stricture in order to traverse it (unless a duodenoscope is needed to pass through the stricture to reach the papilla) should be avoided to minimize perforation risks. Occasionally, however, small-caliber endoscopes are useful to pass guidewires; however, the working channel only accepts 0.035–038″ guidewires and not standard diameter biliary catheters. This requires removal of the endoscope and backloading of a therapeutic endoscope to place the stent in TTS fashion [28], although at times, a second guidewire can be inserted through a therapeutic scope alongside the initial wire without the need to backload the wire.

The usual approach is to pass the endoscope to the site of the lesion. In the presence of subtotal obstruction, water-soluble contrast can be injected through the working channel of the endoscope to define stricture characteristics and a flexible 0.025–0.035″ long-length biliary wire passed through the stricture *freehand* or through a catheter. The stent is passed through the lesion and deployed across the stricture. In complete obstruction or more difficult, tortuous strictures, a biliary occlusion (stone retrieval) balloon preloaded with a hydrophilic wire is inflated to 18 mm with its tip positioned against the lesion to provide pressure for injection across the stricture in an attempt to obtain a *"strictureogram"* (Fig. 11.7a). If this is unsuccessful, a biliary sphincterotome may be useful (Fig. 11.7b) when an en face view of the stricture cannot be obtained since they can be bowed to change direction and orientation, especially those that are rotatable. Once the stricture has been traversed with the catheter, contrast is injected to confirm bowel entry and to define the stricture length (Fig. 11.7c). The stent length can be confirmed by inflating the occlusion balloon once it is beyond the stricture. The inflated balloon is pulled snugly against the distal end of the stricture. The catheter is grasped at the biopsy port, and the balloon is deflated and withdrawn until it is visible endoscopically on the proximal side of the stricture. The distance between the operators' fingers and the biopsy cap corresponds to the length of the stricture.

A stent is chosen with a final length after deployment about 4 cm longer than the measured stricture. The stent is passed through the channel of the endoscope and across the lesion. Predeployment stent placement is rarely needed because of the small diameter delivery systems.

It is important to note that most gastroduodenal stents foreshorten up to 40% during deployment and all deploy from the distal end. Thus, a key to optimal stent placement is to position the endoscope about three to four centimeters proximally from the proximal end of the stricture while endoscopically monitoring the proximal end. The stent will appear to move away from the tip of the endoscope as it is pushed out of the delivery system as it shortens during expansion; thus, the endoscopist usually needs to pull back on the delivery system during deployment. Most dedicated enteral stents are recapturable up to 70–80% of complete deployment, and thus, if the process is not progressing as planned, the stent can be recaptured and redeployed after appropriate adjustments are made.

After deployment of the stent, the delivery system is withdrawn, but the guidewire should not be removed until one is certain that the stricture has been adequately covered by the stent. In extremely tight strictures, the delivery system may not be easily withdrawn as it may be constrained by the unexpanded stent. In addition, the WallFlex stent has a shelf on the distal end of the delivery system, which may *catch* on the wires. The assistant should place the stent in the predeployment position to match the sheath against the distal end of the stent and resolve this shelf. The endoscopist simultaneously needs to advance the delivery catheter as this maneuver tends to pull the distal nose proximally and may dislodge the stent proximally.

Proper positioning of the stent within the stricture is confirmed fluoroscopically by a waist within the stent (Fig. 11.7d). Contrast can be injected through the working channel and into the stent to assess complete patency. Leaving the wire in place allows additional stent(s) to be deployed in overlapping fashion, if needed or for postdeployment balloon dilation. If overlapping stents are required, it is essential to have at least 2 cm overlapping after deployment, since with further expansion after placement, the stents may shorten and separate. Balloon dilation is usually not needed as the stent will expand on its own and postdeployment dilation has been shown to induce perforation.

For strictures in the second duodenum, there is some debate about whether or not the proximal end of the stent should remain in the duodenum or in the gastric antrum because of the potential difference in functional result. Stent-induced perforation may occur when the proximal end of a stent with sharp wires remains in the duodenum [19]. Newer stents with rounded edges may reduce this complication and allow for more physiologic gastric emptying.

## Non-Through-the-Scope Stent Insertion

Non-TTS stent placement is most often used when placed by interventional radiologists and when endoscopists use stents that cannot be placed TTS (e.g., use of esophageal stents). The difficulty with non-TTS placement is the lack of mechanical advantage in lesions distal to the

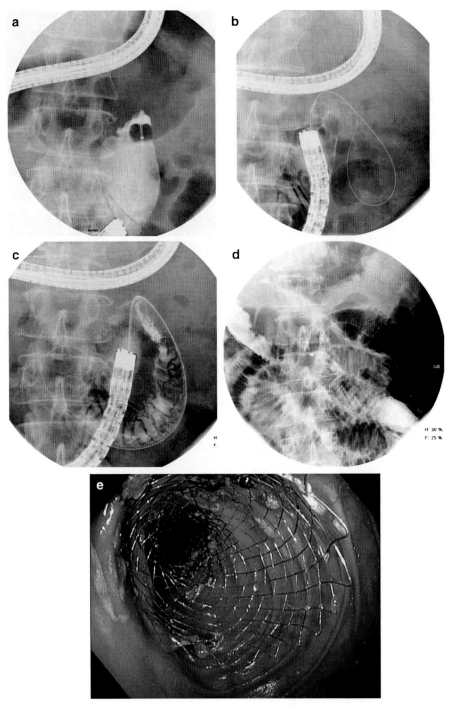

**Fig. 11.7** Palliation of malignant obstruction near the ligament of Treitz due to gastric cancer. (**a**) A colonoscope is in position at the lesion. An occlusion balloon is inflated and contrast injected under pressure. No contrast passes. (**b**) A rotatable biliary sphincterotome with small diameter hydrophilic wire is passed across the stricture. (**c**) Contrast is injected confirming passage into small bowel. (**d**) Radiographic image immediately after stent deployment. (**e**) Endoscopic photo of deployed stent

stomach. This is often accentuated by a dilated gastric lumen whereby the delivery system loops within the stomach. However, since a large diameter endoscope is not needed, small-caliber endoscopes can be used, which may be more easily passed in patients with strictures in the setting of proximal lesions (gastric or gastrojejunal). Since the stent does not pass through the endoscope, a much stiffer guidewire (e.g., Savary, Cook Endoscopy, Amplatz Super Stiff, BSCI) is useful, especially for passage of esophageal stents into the second duodenum. For transoral placement of esophageal stents into the duodenum, I prefer to use colonic-length Savary wires (inserted well beyond the ligament of Treitz) passed through a pediatric colonoscope. This may require dilation of the stricture not only to pass the endoscope across the lesion but also to allow passage of the delivery system across the stricture, since esophageal stents have larger diameters than TTS stents. The predeployed stents are passed over the guidewire and across the lesion. A small diameter endoscope can be passed alongside the stent to monitor the deployment. Additionally, use of therapeutic caliber rat-tooth or pelican forceps can be used to grasp the stent and advance it across the lesion when looping occurs in the stomach.

## Distal Small Bowel Stent Placement

Obstructive lesions in the distal small bowel (distal terminal ileum) are often within reach of an adult colonoscope in patients with native anatomy. In patients with a history of partial or complete colectomy, lesions more proximally can be reached. It is worth noting that the endoscope may need to be passed through existing stoma tracts. The principles of insertion are the same as previously mentioned.

## Miscellaneous Tips and Considerations

In patients who have an existing nasogastric or nasojejunal feeding tube in place across the site of an obstructing lesion, the tube can be removed

after inserting a guidewire. Small diameter delivery systems (as in TTS stents) can then be placed over the wire transnasally and across the lesion. The endoscope can be passed alongside the stent to monitor deployment. Alternatively, the wire could be rerouted from the nose to the mouth and the endoscope backloaded over the wire for TTS delivery.

When non-TTS esophageal stents are used for duodenal use, one available stent (Ultraflex, BSCI), which is available with a proximal delivery system, may be particularly useful. This is because the stent does not need to passed as distally (often a limitation due to the short delivery system) since almost all of the shortening occurs from the proximal end. Also, by cutting the distal *olive* plastic tip just below the string allows additional length of stent advancement.

In patients with Billroth II and Whipple anatomy where an obstruction of one or both limbs is close to the origin of the afferent and the efferent limbs, a stent may need to be placed in both limbs. This can be done by passing wires side by side and delivering the stents sequentially (Fig. 11.8). Alternatively, a stent can be placed in the afferent limb with the proximal end in the stomach. The efferent stent can be passed through the interstices of the afferent limb with the proximal end positioned more proximally than the first stent so that food preferentially passes into the efferent limb yet still allows bile to pass from the afferent stent through the efferent stent.

## Combined Biliary and Duodenal Stent Placement

Patients with gastroduodenal obstruction often have both biliary and duodenal obstruction during their disease process, but one usually precedes the other and is separated temporally. The approach to combined gastroduodenal and biliary stent placement for palliation varies on the location of the duodenal obstruction to the papilla, presence of prior biliary or gastroduodenal stents, and types of indwelling biliary stent (plastic or SEMS). A thorough review on this subject is available [27] and is summarized below.

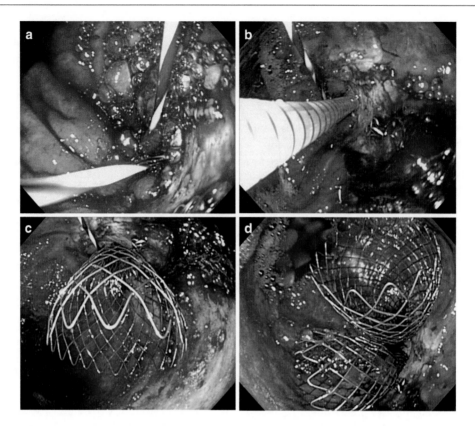

**Fig. 11.8** Stent placement into the afferent and efferent limbs of a Billroth II patient with recurrent gastric cancer. (**a**) Endoscopic photo of guidewires passed into the afferent and efferent limbs. (**b**) A guidewire remains in the efferent limb while the predeployed stent is passed into the afferent limb. (**c**) Fully deployed stent across the afferent limb stricture. Note guidewire in place in efferent limb. (**d**) Final endoscopic image of both deployed stents

- The gastroduodenal obstruction may be proximal to the papilla (type I), at the level of the papilla (type II), or distal to the papilla (type III).
- For type I lesions, the endoscope is passed to the papilla after dilating the obstruction and ERCP with biliary SEMS is performed. A gastroduodenal stent is then placed. If the endoscope cannot be passed to the papilla despite dilating the stricture, a gastroduodenal SEMS is placed with the distal end above the papilla and the duodenoscope advanced through the stent to perform ERCP, either at the same session or a later session after the stent expands. Aggressive dilation of the stent to allow passage of the duodenoscope may result in complications [31].
- Type II lesions are the most difficult since the papilla may not be identifiable due to tumor invasion. If the duodenoscope can be passed to the papilla and it can be identified, then ERCP with biliary SEMS is performed followed by duodenal stent placement. If the papilla cannot be identified, there are several options. A rendezvous can be preformed either by EUS guidance (Fig. 11.9a–c) or percutaneously to place a biliary stent followed by placement of a duodenal stent (Fig. 11.9d), either at the same or different sessions. A duodenal stent could be placed with the biliary tree managed by EUS or percutaneous rendezvous or by EUS or percutaneous biliary stent placement alone. Finally, a biliary stent could be placed by EUS or percutaneous techniques followed by duodenal stent placement.
- For type III lesions, the order of placement of the duodenal and biliary SEMS is not crucial as long as the duodenal SEMS does not cross the papilla.

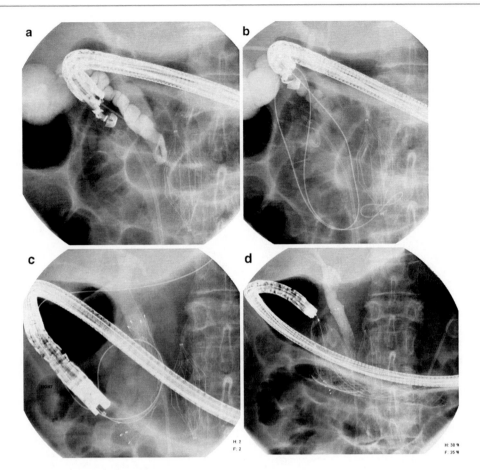

**Fig. 11.9** Endoscopic management of biliary and duodenal obstruction in a type II lesion. The papilla could not be identified due to tumor invasion. (**a**) EUS puncture into the biliary tree. (**b**) A guidewire is passed into the duodenum. (**c**) A duodenoscope has been passed to grasp the wire and to place an expandable biliary stent. (**d**) Placement of expandable duodenal stent across the duodenal stricture and over the lumen of the biliary stent

• In patients who need relief of biliary obstruction in a patient with an indwelling gastroduodenal stent that crosses the papilla (whether type I, II, or III lesions), an attempt can be made at endoscopic identification of the papilla through the interstices of the duodenal stent, followed by cannulation and placement of a biliary stent. Creation of a window in the duodenal stent using argon plasma coagulation (APC) to identify the papilla is also possible. Alternatively, a percutaneously placed or endoscopic ultrasound (EUS)-placed stent (with or without rendezvous) can be performed.

## Magnetic Anastomosis and Stent Placement

Recently, the combination of magnets and expandable stent has been used to create a gastrojejunostomy to allow bypass of obstructing lesions of the stomach and duodenum [32–34]. Briefly, the gastric outlet or duodenal stricture is dilated to allow passage of an endoscope. A guidewire is passed through the endoscope channel into the jejunum. A strong rare earth magnet is advanced under fluoroscopic guidance to the distal duodenum with a 10-Fr catheter advanced over the guidewire.

A gastric magnet is placed in the stomach using the same technique and maneuvered using the endoscope and a foreign-body forceps under fluoroscopic and endoscopic guidance so that it mates transmurally with the duodenal magnet. The coupled magnet buttons are withdrawn 7–10 days after placement using an extractor magnet. The fistula created by the two magnets is cannulated, and a guidewire is passed through the anastomosis into the distal jejunum. A variety of stents (covered and uncovered) can be passed across the anastomosis to maintain patency. Covered stents can potentially be removed at a later date without need of reinsertion. Unfortunately, such devices are not commercially available.

## Key Issues

- A variety of stents are available for enteric use.
- Optimal stent placement can be achieved by having knowledge of basic stent principles, proper patient preparation, and familiarity with the deployment and physical characteristics of the various stents.
- Having assistants that are comfortable with performing complex procedures is extremely helpful in achieving optimal stent placement.
- Knowledge of the precise anatomy and prior surgery is mandatory.
- Expandable stent technology continues to evolve, although the basic principles of stent placement are unlikely to change.
- Covered stents for gastroduodenal use may be limited to non-TTS esophageal stents.

## References

1. Baron TH. Expandable gastrointestinal stents. Gastroenterol. 2007;133:1407–11.
2. Baron TH. Minimizing endoscopic complications: endoluminal stents. Gastrointest Endosc Clin N Am. 2007;17:83–104.
3. Eisendrath P, Cremer M, Himpens J, et al. Endotherapy including temporary stenting of fistulas of the upper gastrointestinal tract after laparoscopic bariatric surgery. Endoscopy. 2007;39:625–30.
4. Kriwanek S, Ott N, Ali-Abdullah S, et al. Treatment of gastro-jejunal leakage and fistulization after gastric bypass with coated self-expanding stents. Obes Surg. 2006;16:1669–74.
5. Merrifield BF, Lautz D, Thompson CC. Endoscopic repair of gastric leaks after Roux-en-Y gastric bypass: a less invasive approach. Gastrointest Endosc. 2006;63:710–4.
6. Nguyen NT, Nguyen XM, Dholakia C. The use of endoscopic stent in management of leaks after sleeve gastrectomy. Obes Surg. 2010;20:1289–92.
7. Trelles N, Gagner M, Palermo M, et al. Gastrocolic fistula after re-sleeve gastrectomy: outcomes after esophageal stent implantation. Surg Obes Relat Dis. 2010;6:308–12.
8. Eubanks S, Edwards CA, Fearing NM, et al. Use of endoscopic stents to treat anastomotic complications after bariatric surgery. J Am Coll Surg. 2008;206:935–8. discussion 938–39.
9. Serra C, Baltasar A, Andreo L, et al. Treatment of gastric leaks with coated self-expanding stents after sleeve gastrectomy. Obes Surg. 2007;17:866–72.
10. Edwards CA, Bui TP, Astudillo JA. Management of anastomotic leaks after Roux-en-Y bypass using self-expanding polyester stents. Surg Obes Relat Dis. 2008;4:594–9. discussion 599–600.
11. Swinnen J, Eisendrath P, Rigaux J, et al. Self-expandable metal stents for the treatment of benign upper GI leaks and perforations. Gastrointest Endosc. 2011;73:890–9.
12. Wu G, Li YD, Han XW, Ding PX. An integrated, self-expanding, Y-shaped, metallic stent for patients with complex obstruction after gastrojejunostomy (Billroth II): initial experience. Radiol Med. 2011;116:759–65.
13. Levine RA, Wasvary H, Kadro O. Endoprosthetic management of refractory ileocolonic anastomotic strictures after resection for Crohn's disease: report of nine-year follow-up and review of the literature. Inflamm Bowel Dis. 2012;18:506–12.
14. Rejchrt S, Kopacova M, Brozik J, Bures J. Biodegradable stents for the treatment of benign stenoses of the small and large intestines. Endoscopy. 2011;43:911–7.
15. Adler DG, Baron TH. Endoscopic palliation of malignant gastric outlet obstruction using self-expanding metal stents: experience in 36 patients. Am J Gastroenterol. 2002;97:72–8.
16. Jeurnink SM, van Eijck CH, Steyerberg EW, et al. Stent versus gastrojejunostomy for the palliation of gastric outlet obstruction: a systematic review. BMC Gastroenterol. 2007;7:18.
17. Jeurnink SM, Steyerberg EW, van Hooft JE, et al. Surgical gastrojejunostomy or endoscopic stent placement for the palliation of malignant gastric outlet obstruction (SUSTENT study): a multicenter randomized trial. Gastrointest Endosc. 2010;71:490–9.
18. Jeurnink SM, Steyerberg EW, Vleggaar FP, et al. Predictors of survival in patients with malignant gastric outlet obstruction: a patient-oriented decision approach for palliative treatment. Dig Liver Dis. 2011;43:548–52.
19. Small AJ, Petersen BT, Baron TH. Closure of a duodenal stent-induced perforation by endoscopic stent removal and covered self-expandable metal stent placement (with video). Gastrointest Endosc. 2007;66:1063–5.

20. González-Moreno S, González-Bayón L, Ortega-Pérez G, González-Hernando C. Imaging of peritoneal carcinomatosis. Cancer J. 2009;15(3):184–9.

21. Mendelsohn RB, Gerdes H, Markowitz AJ, et al. Carcinomatosis is not a contraindication to enteral stenting in selected patients with malignant gastric outlet obstruction. Gastrointest Endosc. 2011; 73:1135–40.

22. Kim CG, Choi IJ, Lee JY, et al. Covered versus uncovered self-expandable metallic stents for palliation of malignant pyloric obstruction in gastric cancer patients: a randomized, prospective study. Gastrointest Endosc. 2010;72(1):25–32.

23. Tierney W, Chuttani R, Croffie J, et al. Enteral stents. Gastrointest Endosc. 2006;63:920–6.

24. Sharma VK, Xie QY, Hassan HA, Howden CW. Placement of a covered metal stent via gastrostomy for management of malignant duodenocolic fistula with duodenal obstruction. Gastrointest Endosc. 2002;55(7):937–40.

25. Maetani I, Tada T, Shimura J. Technical modifications and strategies for stenting gastric outlet strictures using esophageal endoprostheses. Endoscopy. 2002;34:402–6.

26. Ikeda T, Ueda N, Yonemura Y. Peroral placement of a self-expandable covered metallic stent using an overtube for malignant gastroduodenal obstructions. Surg Today. 2011;41:637–42.

27. Baron TH. Management of simultaneous biliary and duodenal obstruction: the endoscopic perspective. Gut Liver. 2010;4(Suppl 1):S50–6.

28. García-Cano J. Use of an ultrathin gastroscope to allow endoscopic insertion of enteral Wallstents without fluoroscopic monitoring. Dig Dis Sci. 2006;51:1231–5.

29. Ross AS, Semrad C, Waxman I, Dye C. Enteral stent placement by double balloon enteroscopy for palliation of malignant small bowel obstruction. Gastrointest Endosc. 2006;64:835–7.

30. Lennon AM, Chandrasekhara V, Shin EJ, Okolo 3rd PI. Spiral-enteroscopy-assisted enteral stent placement for palliation of malignant small-bowel obstruction (with video). Gastrointest Endosc. 2010;71:422–5.

31. Saleem A, Bakken J, Baron TH. Early massive bleeding after duodenal self-expandable metal stent placement for palliation of malignant gastric outlet obstruction (with video). Gastrointest Endosc. 2011;74:1426–7.

32. Cope C, Clark TW, Ginsberg G, Habecker P. Stent placement of gastroenteric anastomoses formed by magnetic compression. J Vasc Interv Radiol. 1999;10:1379–86.

33. Cope C, Ginsberg GG. Long-term patency of experimental magnetic compression gastroenteric anastomoses achieved with covered stents. Gastrointest Endosc. 2001;53:780–4.

34. van Hooft JE, Vleggaar FP, Le Moine O, et al. Endoscopic magnetic gastroenteric anastomosis for palliation of malignant gastric outlet obstruction: a prospective multicenter study. Gastrointest Endosc. 2010;72:530–5.

# Colonic Self-Expandable Metal Stents: Indications and Placement Techniques

**12**

Jesús García-Cano

Self-expandable metal stents (SEMS) in the colon and rectum can be employed in malignant colorectal obstruction (MCRO), benign colorectal obstruction (BCRO), and rectocolonic fistulae or leaks (RCF) with or without obstruction. MCRO is by far the most frequent scenario for colonic SEMS. The majority of stents are placed in the left side of the colon. Currently, technical improvement allows SEMS to be placed in the entire large bowel. Low rectal lesions close to the anal margin are challenging for stenting because they can cause an unpleasant tenesmus and incontinence.

## SEMS in Malignant Colorectal Obstruction

In 1990, Dohmoto et al. [1] first reported the use of SEMS for the treatment of neoplastic rectal obstruction. Afterward, Spinelli et al. in 1992 [2] published the placement of stents in the colon to treat large bowel obstruction. Since then, dedicated enteral or specific colorectal stents have been manufactured and an increasing use of SEMS for MCRO has been reported. However, prior to 2004 [3], SEMS were inserted by endoscopists in

published series [4–14] less than once monthly (0.77 in the quoted articles).

This procedure allows, with minimal intervention, resolution of colonic obstruction. Patients can then either undergo scheduled surgery or have the stent left in place as a definitive palliative treatment. In patients with acute MCRO and who are candidates for surgery, placement of a preoperative stent can prevent most colostomies, because patients can be stabilized, and the large bowel can be adequately cleaned before elective operation and have one-stage surgery late (Fig. 12.1).

Moreover, this procedure has now spread into general endoscopic practice [15]. As a result, the accumulating experience suggests that stent placement has positive outcomes compared with surgery, including shorter hospital stays and lower rates of adverse events. Positive outcomes of SEMS for MCRO are especially prominent when SEMS are used as a bridge to surgery [16].

Some objections have been raised for long-term palliation, and it has been proposed that, because of less effectiveness than previously suggested in patients with incurable obstructing colorectal cancer eligible for chemotherapy and a long life expectancy, palliative treatments other than SEMS should be considered [17]. However, recent studies comparing SEMS and surgery as long-term palliation found stents to be effective and acceptable as initial palliative therapy for malignant colorectal obstruction because of an earlier recovery, shorter hospital stay, lower rate of early complications, and no need for colostomy compared with palliative surgery. Moreover,

J. García-Cano, M.D., Ph.D. (✉)
Department of Digestive Diseases,
Hospital Virgen de La Luz, C/Hermandad Donantes
de sangre n. 1, Cuenca 16002, Spain
e-mail: j.garcia-cano@terra.es

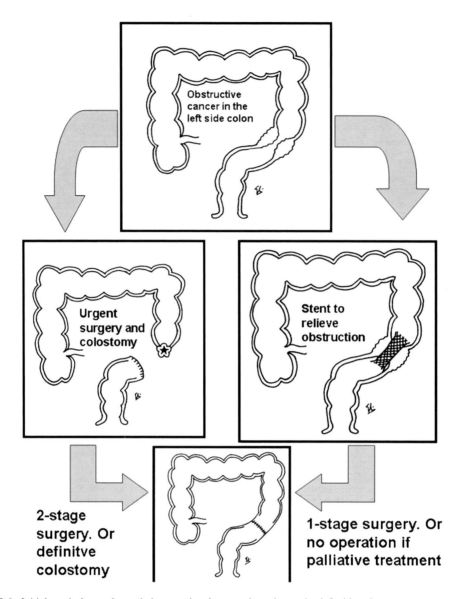

**Fig. 12.1** Initial surgical or endoscopic interventional approach to obstructive left-side colon cancer

long-term outcomes and complications of SEMS were comparable to those of surgery, and most stent-related complications during follow-up were manageable with endoscopic treatment. Therefore, SEMS could be recommended not only to patients with malignant colorectal obstruction and short life expectancy but also to those with a longer life expectancy [18]. Further, in nonresectable metastasis and obstructing colon cancer, SEMS allows chemotherapy to be administered earlier and has no detrimental effect on morbidity and survival [19], although several studies have indicated that palliative chemotherapy might increase the risk of complications (such as perforation) by inducing tumor shrinkage and tissue necrosis [20].

The current available data support that implantation of SEMS is an effective, safe, and cost-effective [21] palliative therapy in MCRO, either as a bridge to scheduled surgery [22] or for noncurable obstructive colorectal cancer [23], and, when possible, should replace surgery as the therapy of choice for these indications. For MCRO in the left colon, stents represent the best option when skills are available [24].

## From the Emergency Room to Endoscopic Placement of SEMS in Malignant Colorectal Obstruction

Patients with colonic obstruction are admitted to the emergency room for abdominal pain, bloating, and vomiting. As in other parts of medicine, history and physical exam are the cornerstones of patient management [25]. Most malignant obstructions remain partial, but increasing abdominal distention, worsening nausea, and obstipation over 1–2 weeks suggest progression to complete obstruction. Plain radiography of the abdomen (kidney, ureter, bladder views) has only modest specificity and sensitivity in detecting bowel obstruction, but is usually the first imaging test carried out when colonic obstruction is suspected. A surgical consult is typically done. In some hospitals, the next step is to call the endoscopist to perform both diagnostic and, if possible, therapeutic endoscopy [15].

However, an abdominal computed tomography (CT) scan should be performed as the primary imaging study for patients with obstructive symptoms and especially with a palpable abdominal mass. It has a specificity of 100% and a sensitivity of 94% and plays a major role in decision-making regarding surgery, endoscopy, or palliative interventions [26] as it locates the obstruction and differentiates benign from malignant causes with a fair degree of precision [27]. Furthermore, MCRO can be secondary to a noncolonic neoplasm, such ovarian cancer.

It is not entirely necessary, but may be helpful, to obtain a retrograde radiographic study with water-soluble contrast to assess the anatomy, length of stricture, and degree of obstruction (Fig. 12.2). A barium enema examination provides greater mucosal details, but there is risk of impaction and it is generally not necessary in this setting [28]. After MCRO is confirmed, intravenous fluids should be administered for volume resuscitation and correction of electrolytes, and intermittent nasogastric suction may be performed for bowel decompression [29].

Placement of SEMS in MCRO is an interventional procedure not as complex as, for instance, ERCP, but special procedural skills are needed by the physician and the entire endoscopic team. Therefore, in the majority of hospitals, if the patient is diagnosed out of working hours, he or she can generally be managed with supportive care until the next morning. In larger centers, it is possible to perform such procedure at all times, even late in the night.

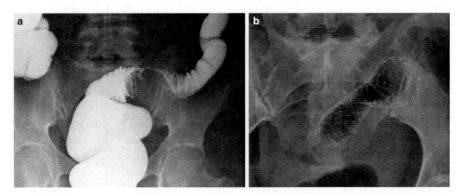

**Fig. 12.2** Water-soluble contrast retrograde study of the colon. (**a**) Characteristics of the neoplastic stricture are clearly delineated and helped to solve the obstruction by means of an Ultraflex Precision stent (**b**)

## Patient Preparation for SEMS in Malignant Colorectal Obstruction

As in all other digestive interventions, written informed consent must be obtained from each patient before the endoscopic procedure. Outcomes and possible complications should be also explained to close relatives. Absolute contraindications to stenting are colonic or tumor perforation with peritonitis, or patient refusal to undergo the procedure. A relative contraindication is a rectal tumor within 2 cm of the anal margin [30].

In general, patients can undergo bowel cleansing by means of enemas. But oral preparation can be sometimes used when the clinical situation appears less severe and in cases where obstruction is located in the right colon. During colonoscopy, insufflation must be used as little as possible to prevent further pneumatic damage to the obstructed bowel. Prophylactic antibiotics should be considered in patients with complete obstruction and a markedly dilated colon because introduction of air during the procedure may promote microperforation and bacteremia [5].

## Choosing the Appropriate Stent for Malignant Colorectal Obstruction

### Through-the-Scope Stents

Most published data relate to patients treated with enteral or dedicated colonic stents that can be inserted through the therapeutic working channel (>3.7 mm) of the scope (also called TTS) (Table 12.1). Initially, the enteral Wallstent (Boston Scientific, Natick, Massachusetts, USA) was one of the most inserted SEMS [31]. This is a stainless-steel woven stent that is preloaded on a delivery system that can be introduced through the working channel of a therapeutic endoscope with subsequent deployment up to an 18-mm to 22-mm internal diameter controlled by both fluoroscopic and endoscopic views. The limited flexibility of the metal wire mesh of the Wallstent might contribute to stent migration. Also, the sharp ends of the metal meshes of the Wallstent may injure the intestinal wall and could lead to ulceration with the associated risk of bleeding and perforation. Recently, the same manufacturer has launched a new dedicated colonic stent, WallFlex, which is made of nitinol (a nickel-titanium alloy material with *shape memory* that facilitates expansion inside the bowel to a predesigned configuration) instead of stainless steel and includes a proximal flare to minimize risk of migration. This new stent has been constructed to provide an improved flexibility while maintaining lumen integrity and has looped ends to reduce risk of mucosal injury (Fig. 12.3). The WallFlex stent (like almost all SEMS) undergoes partial foreshortening during deployment, which the endoscopist must take into account during positioning. The delivery system is designed to permit recapture and repositioning of the stent [32]. This SEMS is uncovered (bare) over the mesh, and this allows the tumor to penetrate the metal cells, thus decreasing migration. However, the tumor can grow into the stent and obstruct it over time.

The Niti-S colorectal Stent (Taewoong Medical, Seoul, Korea) is also made of nitinol and designed to solve obstructions in the large bowel and rectum. According to the manufacturer, its TTS delivery catheter allows easy approach to ascending, transverse, or descending colon. It is also available with stepped heads (28 mm) to prevent migration and is available either covered or uncovered. The same company has launched the Niti-S colonic stent, D-type. The D-Weave feature contributes to the flexibility to adjust properly with curved anatomy. It has also blunt ends to avoid mucosal damage. Furthermore, a newly designed double-layered covered stent (Niti-S D-Weave combination covered stent or Comvi) could be useful in preventing both stent migration and tumor ingrowth after stent insertion [33].

The Hanaro stent (M. I. Tech Co., Ltd., Seoul, Korea) is also available in some countries [34]. It is made of nitinol and has a variety of lengths and designs (covered, uncovered, flared ends).

Evolution colonic stent is a recently marketed Cook colorectal stent, available in Europe. It is

**Table 12.1** Colonic self-expandable metal stents

| Manufacturer | Model | Material | Type of insertion | Deployed diameters (mm) and lengths (cm) | Features |
|---|---|---|---|---|---|
| Boston Scientific | Enteral Wallstent | Uncovered stainless-steel alloy | TTS | 20 or 22 mm 6, 9 cm | Reconstrainable foreshortening up to 49% |
| Boston Scientific | Colonic WallFlex | Uncovered woven nitinol | TTS | 22- or 25-mm proximal flare 27 or 30 mm 6, 9, 12 cm | Reconstrainable foreshortening up to 38% |
| Boston Scientific | Ultraflex Precision | Uncovered woven nitinol | OTW | 25-mm proximal flare 30 mm 5.7, 8.7, 11.7 cm | No reconstrainable foreshortening 23% |
| Taewoong Medical | Colorectal D-weave double layered | Covered or uncovered nitinol | TTS or OTW related to model | 20-, 22-, 24-mm proximal and distal flares 28 and 30 mm 6,8,10,12 cm | Reconstrainable |
| M.I. Tech | Hanaro stent colorectal | Uncovered nitinol | TTS | 22 mm 8, 11, 14 cm | Partly reconstrainable |
| Cook endoscopy | Evolution colonic stent | Uncovered single-weave nitinol | TTS | 25-mm proximal and distal flares 30 mm 6, 8, 10 cm | Reconstrainable foreshortening 45% |
| Cook endoscopy | Colonic Z-stent | Stainless steel | OTW | 25 mm 4, 6, 8, 10, 12 cm | No foreshortening |
| Standard SciTech | Colonic Bonastent uncovered or partially covered | Nitinol | TTS or OTW related to model | 22, 24, 26 mm 6, 8, 10 cm | Reconstrainable foreshortening |
| Ella-CS | Enterella | Uncovered or covered braided nitinol | OTW | 20, 22, 25 mm 8.2, 9, 1.13, 1.35 cm | Foreshortening |

Not all the stents are available in all countries. TTS means insertion through the working channel of a therapeutic endoscope. OTW is a non-TTS stent that does not fit into the working channel (usually delivery system >10 French) and has to be inserted over a wire previously placed beyond the stricture. Almost all commercial stents shorten after deployment; this is called foreshortening. Reconstrainability is the property of re-sheathing completely a partially deployed stent

**a**                                                          **b**

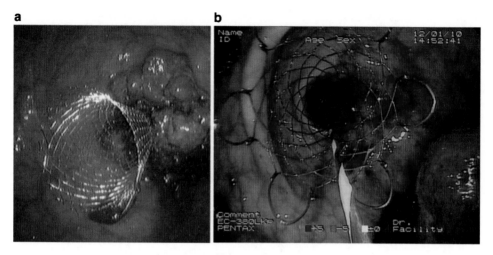

**Fig. 12.3** Wallstent (**a**) and WallFlex (**b**) after complete deployment in a tumor stricture causing obstruction. Wallstent is a stainless-steel woven stent with sharp ends, while WallFlex is made of nitinol and has looped ends to reduce risk of mucosal injury

constructed of thin gauge, single-weave nitinol. To reduce the risk of migration, the Evolution colonic stent has proximal and distal flanges. Four radiopaque markers at each end of the stent provide visualization for accurate placement. It is now undergoing an international trial (NCT01102283).

Bonastent colorectal stents are designed with a patented nitinol hook and cross wire structure (Polygon Mesh surface) that, according to the manufacturer, allows the stent to adapt and conform to the human anatomy, resulting in reduced migration and tumor ingrowth. The stents are provided preloaded on an ergonomically designed delivery device and are offered both covered and uncovered. However, they are not yet available in many countries.

### Non-Through-the-Scope or Over-the-Wire Stents

SEMS with delivery systems unable to pass undeployed through the therapeutic working channel of an endoscope are also called OTW (over-the-wire). In this way, many esophageal stents have been and continue to be used in the rectum and sigmoid areas.

Rectocolonic dedicated SEMS are the Z-Stent (Cook), the Ultraflex Precision (Boston Scientific),

and some designs of Niti-S, Bonastent, and Ella colorectal stent (Enterella). The Z-Stent is constructed of a series of cages of stainless steel, depending of the length of the stent. The Ultraflex Precision colonic stent has a mesh construction of nitinol. The wire strands are arrayed in a diamond configuration and welded at the ends. This design is intended to resist radial compression and allow compliance in bends in the colorectum without collapsing [35].

### Placement Techniques of SEMS in Malignant Colorectal Obstruction

Because a variety of prostheses are marketed throughout the world that vary in construction, material, and design [36], on practical grounds, the election of the manufacturer and type of stent usually is contingent upon availability, ease of use, and previous experience for all the endoscopic team (physicians and endoscopy assistants). Few studies comparing one stent to another have been made. For instance, uncovered WallFlex and double-layered covered Niti-S Comvi stents were compared, and they were both found suitable for relieving MCRO. Tumor ingrowth was more common in the WallFlex group, but stent migration was more common in the Comvi group [37].

It was also found that insertion of either an uncovered or covered stent is similarly an effective treatment modality of MCRO for preoperative purposes, and there are no advantages of covered over uncovered stents during the follow-up period when used palliatively [38]. However, stent dysfunction, stent-related complications, and need for reintervention were found to be higher in a comparison between the "old" Wallstent and the Ultraflex Precision colonic stent. In addition, the latter appears to be better suited for palliation of left-sided MCRO [39].

## Standard Through-the-Scope Procedure

Stent placement is usually done with the patient using conscious sedation (midazolam and/or fentanyl), but deep sedation (propofol) or no sedation can be also employed. A therapeutic endoscope (working channel ≥ 3.7 mm), either forward (gastroscope, colonoscope) or side viewing (duodenoscope), is used for placement of the TTS colonic stent. For the majority of occasions, even beyond the splenic angle, a therapeutic gastroscope is suitable. Experience with instruments used for ERCP, such as catheters and guidewires, is very useful for successful insertion of colonic and other digestive stents. If the patient is in the supine position, anatomical orientation is improved (Fig. 12.4). However, usually the procedure is started in the left lateral decubitus as in most of the colonoscopies; later the patient can be turned.

The most critical step for SEMS insertion is the passage of a guidewire through the malignant stricture and to place it beyond the tumor, in healthy tissue (Fig. 12.5). The undeployed stent is then pushed over this guidewire and may then be opened inside the tumor solving the obstruction. Fluoroscopic guidance is the best method to ensure that the guidewire has been properly positioned. In addition, events beyond the stricture, such as stent opening, can be appropriately monitored with fluoroscopy. Malignant stricture dilation should be undertaken carefully because of the possible risk of perforation.

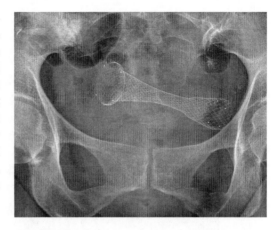

**Fig. 12.4** Evolution colonic stent inserted in a tumor stricture in the sigmoid. With the patient in the supine position, anatomical orientation is improved

The procedure starts with advancing an endoscope with a therapeutic working channel to the proximal part of the tumor. A guidewire of 0.035 in. (0.875 mm) in diameter fitted with an atraumatic hydrophilic tip is passed through the working channel to make it through the whole stenosed segment. This passage is confirmed by fluoroscopy. A biliary catheter used for endoscopic retrograde cholangiopancreatography (ERCP) is then introduced over the guidewire, and the obstruction is delineated by contrast injection. The length of the stricture is also assessed. The catheter is then withdrawn, and the undeployed stent is inserted over the guidewire. Ideally, the length of the stent has to exceed the stricture length for at least 2 cm. If one single stent does not cover the entire stricture, they can be overlapped (Fig. 12.6). Once the SEMS is inside the stricture, it is gradually opened up to place it correctly with proximal and distal ends located in healthy areas. During stent release, the distal end (seen in the endoscopic view) shortens toward the stricture; therefore, continuous adjustment is necessary. It is not advisable to advance a partially deployed stent, but it may be pulled back if placed too distally. Care must be taken not to release the stent by accident. It is safer to re-sheath the stent and start again.

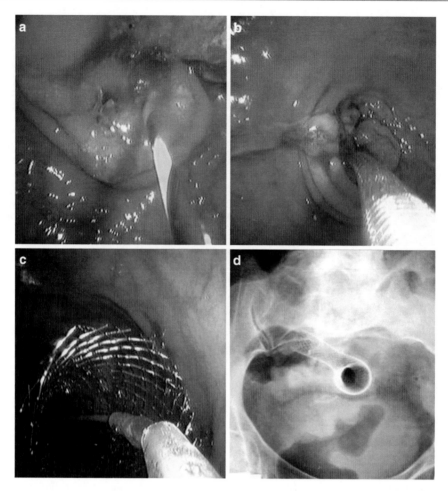

**Fig. 12.5** Through-the-scope (TTS) insertion technique of a self-expanding metal stent to palliate a malignant colonic obstruction. (**a**) Guidewire "cannulation" of the tumor. This guidewire is placed far beyond the stricture. (**b**) The unde-ployed stent is slid over the guidewire. (**c**) Stent release bridging the entire stricture. This maneuver is monitored endoscopically and upstream ones fluoroscopically. (**d**) Final stent position after the procedure

## Standard Over-the-Wire Procedure

Sedation is administered like in the TTS procedure. The patient is initially placed in the left lateral decubitus position, and rotation of the patient into the supine position can be done, as needed, to improve the anatomic view under fluoroscopy. The stricture is gently cannulated with a guidewire through the working channel of a gastroscope. Sometimes, it is necessary to exchange the initial floppy guidewire for a stiffer one. The scope is withdrawn and the OTW stent slid over the guidewire. The procedure can be performed only under fluoroscopic control, but many endoscopists prefer to also use endoscopic control passing a gastroscope beside the delivery catheter. Furthermore, endoscopy is very useful in low rectal strictures to avoid deployment next to the anus. After longitudinal centering of the stent in relation to the stricture, deployment is commenced.

Ideally in TTS and OTW insertion techniques, the deployed stent should have an hourglass configuration. This means the stricture is in the SEMS center (Fig. 12.7).

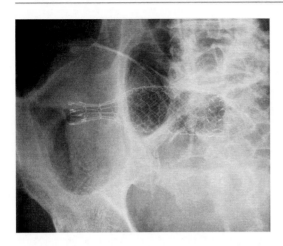

**Fig. 12.6** The Ultraflex Precision proximal (*upper*) end is not completely opened after deployment. This is because the stent had not bridged the entire stricture and is within the tumor. Another coaxial stent must be inserted to properly solve the obstruction

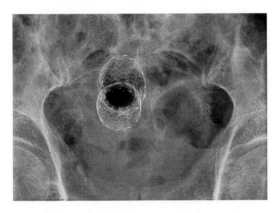

**Fig. 12.7** Ultraflex Precision located just in the middle of the stricture has an hourglass configuration

## Placement of SEMS in the Rectosigmoid Area Without Fluoroscopy

If fluoroscopy facilities are not accessible, other techniques can be used. Currently, several models of very small caliber endoscopes (ultrathin endoscopes [UTE]) are available. They are able to pass through many strictures in the digestive tract. According to a previously described technique [40–41], once the tumor is traversed by a 6-mm-diameter endoscope (for instance, Pentax EG-1870 K), a guidewire is left in place through the UTE working channel (Fig. 12.8).

Subsequently, the UTE is removed, leaving the guidewire in place beyond the stenosis. This guidewire is then inserted in a retrograde manner in the therapeutic endoscope working channel, and a SEMS is placed over it. This technique is riskier because only downstream events (in the endoscopic view) are properly monitored, whereas upstream maneuvers are done blindly.

The small caliber endoscope can also be used together with fluoroscopy to negotiate difficult strictures and serve as an aid for either TTS or OTW techniques. At the end of the procedure, the position of the stent must be confirmed endoscopically and fluoroscopically or with radiographs (Fig. 12.9). The patient can be admitted to surgical or medical ward (including oncology department). Once obstructive symptoms ameliorate, tolerance to liquids can be tried.

## Outcomes of SEMS for Malignant Colorectal Obstruction

Evaluation of results achieved with endoscopic SEMS insertion to palliate MCRO must focus on several issues:
1. Technical success (adequate placement of the stent bridging the entire stricture)
2. Clinical success (improving of symptoms related with colonic obstruction)
3. Occurrence of complications, early or late, related to stent insertion
4. Comparison with the previous standard surgical care for MCRO
5. Improving global quality of life of patients
Sebastian et al. reported a review of published series until 2003. There were a total of 791 patients. Technical success was 93%, clinical success 89%. As it is shown in Table 12.2 [42–47], a plethora of endoscopic studies have been published since then. Rates are similar to those reported by Sebastian et al. [48] which also included interventional radiology series. It is interesting to underline that most series come from specialized hospitals; sometimes, they are single-center studies. In 2006, initial treatment of MCRO with SEMS in general endoscopic practice was reported [15]. Figures for clinical

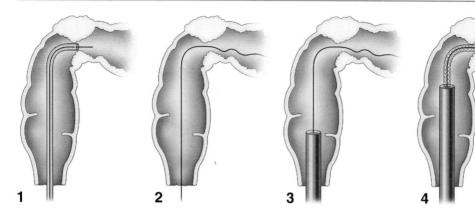

**Fig. 12.8** Use of an ultrathin endoscope to insert SEMS in the rectosigmoid without fluoroscopy. (*1*) An ultrathin gastroscope (Pentax EG-1870 K, outer diameter 6 mm) is employed to pass severe tumor strictures in the rectosigmoid and place a guidewire beyond the stenosis. (*2*) The ultrathin endoscope is removed, leaving the guidewire in place. During withdrawal, characteristics of the stricture (*length, shape*) were assessed. (*3*) The guidewire is then backloaded into a therapeutic endoscope. (*4*) Insertion of a through-the-scope (TTS) stent is then performed. If a non-TTS SEMS was chosen, insertion and deployment were monitored with the endoscope side to side

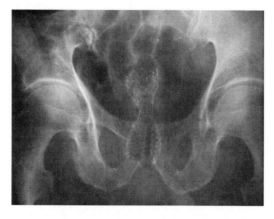

**Fig. 12.9** Ultraflex Precision located in the rectosigmoid junction, immediately after the procedure. The radiograph confirms its proper position, both ends are opened, and the waist is in the middle of the stent

success were slightly under the mean (78.8%), while technical success (92.6%) was comparable to other series.

It is difficult to compare series because different types of stents were used, and in some series, only the left colon was stented. SEMS insertion for MCRO is an interventional procedure not as complex as ERCP or pancreatic fluid collection drainage, but special therapeutic endoscopic skills are needed. At present, insertion techniques for the majority of cases have been standardized [49, 50]. In a certain arbitrary way, ten left-side procedures have been considered as adequate training for straightforward noncomplicated obstructions [51]. With increasing experience, the right colon can be stented with similar success as the left one [52] and difficult cases solved [53].

Placement of SEMS in patients with malignant rectal obstruction within 5 cm of the anal verge (or 2 cm between the SEMS and the anal canal) may cause problems such as anal pain and tenesmus. Song et al. [54] reported insertion of three types of retrievable OTW stents. Ten of 16 patients with obstruction within 5 cm of the anal verge and 1 of 14 patients with obstruction beyond 5 cm complained of pain after placement of SEMS; the pain was tolerable to the patients with or without the use of analgesics and provided preoperative decompression of obstruction symptoms. Perhaps in low rectal lesions, deployment of OTW can be better controlled endoscopically than TTS stents (Fig. 12.10).

The most feared complication is perforation. This untoward event ranged from 0% to 9% in series after year 2000. The patient must undergo an urgent operation, or in case of extreme fragility, only palliative measures can be undertaken. The most frequent late complications are migration and obstruction by tumor growth into mesh cells. They can be solved endoscopically by the

**Table 12.2** Experience with endoscopically placed self-expanding metal stents in malignant colorectal obstruction in some published series with at least 20 patients

| Author (reference) | Year of publication | n | Insertion success | Clinical success | Perforation rate |
|---|---|---|---|---|---|
| Baron [5] | 1998 | 27 | 25 (94%) | 23 (85%) | 4 (15%) |
| Spinelli [8] | 2001 | 37 | 36 (97%) | 28 (75.6%) | 2 (5.4%) |
| Smedh [68] | 2003 | 23 | 19 (82%) | 18 (78.2%) | 0 |
| Lambertini [11] | 2003 | 22 | 20 (91%) | 20 (91%) | 2 (9%) |
| Meisner [12] | 2004 | 89 | 84 (94.3%) | 76 (85.3%) | 0 |
| Suzuki [13] | 2004 | 42 | 36 (85.7%) | 35 (83.3%) | 2 (4.7%) |
| Law [7] | 2004 | 52 | 51 (98%) | 50 (96.1%) | 1 (1.9%) |
| Carne [69] | 2004 | 25 | 22 (88%) | 20 (80%) | 0 |
| García-Cano [15] | 2006 | 175 | 162 (92.6%) | 138 (78.8%) | 7 (4%) |
| Ptok [43] | 2006 | 48 | 44 (92%) | 44 (92%) | 0 |
| Soto [46] | 2006 | 62 | 58 (93.54%) | 56 (90.3%) | 3 (4.8%) |
| Karoui [19] | 2007 | 31 | 30 (97%) | 27 (87%) | 0 |
| Lee KM [38] | 2007 | 80 | 78 (97,5%) | 77 (96.2%) | 0 |
| Repici [35][a] | 2007 | 44 | 42 (95.4%) | 41 (93.1%) | 0 |
| Repici [32] | 2008 | 42 | 40 (95.2%) | 40 (95.2%) | 1 (2.38%) |
| Im [34] | 2008 | 51 | 51 (100%) | 43 (84.3%) | 1 (1.9%) |
| Fernández-Esparrach [17] | 2010 | 47 | 44 (94%) | 44 (94%) | 3 (7%) |
| Small [31] | 2010 | 233 | 224 (96.1%) | 222 (95.2%) | 18 (7.7%) |
| Park [37] | 2010 | 151 | 149 (98.6%) | 140 (92.7%) | 0 |
| Branger [42] | 2010 | 93 | 86 (92.5%) | 80 (86%) | 3 (3.2%) |
| Donnellan [44] | 2010 | 43 | 40 (93%) | 40 (93%) | 2 (4.6%) |
| Lee JH [45] | 2010 | 46 | 46 (100%) | 39 (84.8%) | 2 (4.3%) |
| Lee HJ [18] | 2011 | 71 | 68 (95.8%) | 68 (94%) | 4 (5.6%) |
| Luigiano [47] | 2011 | 39 | 36 (92,3%) | 35 (89.7%) | 2 (5.1%) |

Success and perforation rates are calculated according to the initial number (n) of attempted procedures. Perforation rate is during insertion or early after the intervention
[a]Repici's 2007 article is related to Ultraflex Precision and 2008 using the WallFlex. The same author published in 2000 [6] another study placing the esophageal Ultraflex

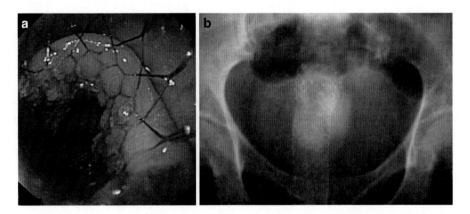

**Fig. 12.10** Ultraflex Precision immediately above the anal canal (**a**) endoscopy, (**b**) radiograph. The patient complained of tenesmus and pain. However, the bowel could be properly cleaned before scheduled surgery

insertion of new stents or by trimming the obstructed one, for instance, with argon plasma coagulation.

In the largest series published to date [31] which comprise patients for palliation and as a bridge to surgery, complication rates in successfully inserted SEMS were 24% in both groups, including perforation (7.7%), occlusion (7.7%), migration (6.9%), and erosion/ulcer (1.7%). Additional complications included hematochezia (0.9%), bacteremia/fever (3%), and tenesmus (2.1%).

Gender (males), degree of obstruction (complete), stent diameter (≤22 mm), stricture dilation prior to stent insertion, and operator experience were significant risk factors for these adverse events. In the palliative group, intraluminal lesions, chemotherapy with bevacizumab, and distal colon placement of the stent were also associated with higher complication rates as compared to extraluminal lesions. Patients on bevacizumab therapy nearly tripled the risk of perforation. In the palliation group, the long-term (6 months) clinical success rate was 77.2% with a mean in situ period of 128 days. Stent patency until death was achieved in 88.5% of patients.

After relief of acute colonic obstruction by SEMS insertion, a scheduled second colonoscopy before surgical resection has been shown to be feasible and perhaps, should be recommended to exclude synchronous lesions. The cecum can be reached through the fully open stent [55].

There is currently vast evidence in favor of SEMS as initial decompression for acute MCRO. Nevertheless, according to variability in biological events, there are some studies against this practice. For instance, van Hooft et al. [56] found a high rate of perforations and Pirlet et al. [57] in a randomized trial failed to demonstrate that emergency preoperative SEMS for patients presenting with acute left-sided malignant colonic obstruction could significantly decrease the need for stoma placement. Nevertheless, in this latter study, the failure rate in stent insertion was very high, 53.3%.

The amount of knowledge about SEMS as first treatment for MCRO is increasing rapidly. In the best-results scenario for surgery, although the technical and clinical outcomes for colostomy

and stent placement appear comparable [58], stent placement is less costly and associated with shorter length of hospital stay and fewer complications. Furthermore, colon stent placement is associated with improved overall quality-of-life scores and gastrointestinal symptoms – specifically quality-of-life scores [59].

In addition, SEMS serve as a safe and effective bridge to subsequent laparoscopic surgery in patients with obstructing left-sided colon cancer. This endolaparoscopic approach makes a one-stage operation more feasible, is associated with reduced incidence of stoma creation, and allows patients with MCRO to benefit from the advantage of minimally invasive surgery [60]. For unresectable MCRO, stent therapy is effective, safe, and feasible [61]. As SEMS appear to be the modern initial treatment of colonic obstruction [62], dissemination of stent placement beyond large teaching hospitals located in urban areas as a treatment for MCRO is important given its implications for patient care and resource use [15, 58].

## SEMS in Benign Colorectal Obstruction and Fistulae

For benign colorectal obstruction (BCRO) conditions, SEMS should be preferably retrievable unless further surgical management is contemplated. Ease of retrieval usually implies use of a fully or partially covered prosthesis to avoid becoming embedded, making endoscopic extraction almost impossible. Some of these stents have not been specifically designed for the colon but for other anatomic locations such as the esophagus (Fig. 12.11). With these, SEMS migration almost invariably occurs. Sometimes, the duration of the inserted stent (days or weeks) allows benign strictures (such as postoperative) to undergo a permanent dilation with the healing of a concomitant fistula. However, repeat surgery will be necessary in a considerable number of patients due to primary or secondary failure of stenting [63]. Stents should be avoided in acute diverticular disease because of a higher incidence of complications [64, 65]. In general, if noncovered SEMS are employed, they can effectively

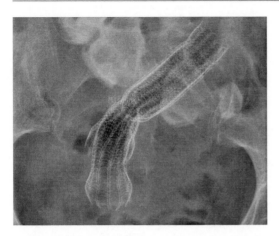

**Fig. 12.11** Postsurgical benign stricture in the sigmoid. Two non-TTS esophageal stents (partially covered Ultraflex) were inserted in a coaxial manner to solve the obstruction. After several weeks in place, they were spontaneously expelled

decompress high-grade, benign colonic obstructions and offer medium-term symptom relief, allowing later, elective surgery. The operation should not be retarded for the high rate of delayed complications [66]. The majority of SEMS for BCRO and fistulae have been placed in the left colon. In addition, inventive endoscopists are continuously developing new techniques, for instance, insertion of a transverse colon covered OTW stent through the overtube of a double balloon enteroscope [67].

## Conclusions

Insertion of SEMS for rectocolonic obstructions takes part in advanced therapeutic endoscopy, and interventional skills for all the members of the endoscopic team are necessary. Currently, a large number of dedicated colonic SEMS are available either in TTS or OTW insertion forms. Scientific literature is rapidly increasing to confirm that the best way to initially relieve MCRO is SEMS insertion, especially in the left colon. Afterward, patients can undergo scheduled surgery or have the stent for long-term palliation. Despite complications inherent to all interventional procedures, both strategies have been shown to compare favorably with surgery. The

use of SEMS in BCRO and fistulae should be approached with caution. The best results are achieved when, like in MCRO, after reaching colonic decompression and patient stabilization, resective surgery is undertaken.

## References

1. Dohmoto M, Rupp KD, Hohlbach G. Endoscopically-implanted prosthesis in rectal carcinoma. Dtsch Med Wochenschr. 1990;115:915 (German).
2. Spinelli P, Dal Fante M, Mancini A. Self-expanding mesh stent for endoscopic palliation of rectal obstructing tumors: a preliminary report. Surg Endosc. 1992;6:72–4.
3. Garcia-Cano J. Endoscopic insertion of self-expanding metal stents as first step to treat malignant colorectal obstruction. Am J Gastroenterol. 2005;100:1203–4.
4. García-Cano J, González Martín JA, Redondo-Cerezo E, et al. Treatment of malignant colorectal obstruction by means of endoscopic insertion of self-expandable metallic stents. An Med Interna. 2003;20:515–20 (Spanish).
5. Baron TH, Dean PA, Yates 3rd MR, Canon C, Koehler RE. Expandable metal stents for the treatment of colonic obstruction: techniques and outcomes. Gastrointest Endosc. 1998;47:277–86.
6. Repici A, Reggio D, DeAngelis C, et al. Covered metal stents for management of inoperable malignant colorectal strictures. Gastrointest Endosc. 2000;52:735–40.
7. Law WL, Chu KW, Ho JWC, et al. Self-expanding metallic stent in the treatment of colonic obstruction caused by advanced malignancies. Dis Colon Rectum. 2000;43:1522–7.
8. Spinelli P, Mancini A. Use of self-expanding metal stents for palliation of rectosigmoid cancer. Gastrointest Endosc. 2001;53:203–6.
9. Ben Sousan E, Savoye G, Hochain P, et al. Expandable metal stents in palliative treatment of malignant colorectal stricture. A report of 17 consecutive patients. Gastroenterol Clin Biol. 2001;25:463–7.
10. Xinopoulos D, Dimitroulopoulos D, Tsamakidis K, et al. Treatment of malignant colonic obstructions with metal stents and laser. Hepatogastroenterology. 2002;49:359–62.
11. Lambertini M, Tamburini A, Corinaldesi F, et al. Metal endoprosthesis in the treatment of acute neoplastic occlusion of the colon. Our experience. Tumori. 2003;89(4 Suppl):86–9.
12. Meisner S, Hensler M, Knop FK, et al. Self-expanding metal stents for colonic obstruction: experiences from 104 procedures in a single center. Dis Colon Rectum. 2004;47:444–50.
13. Suzuki N, Saunders BP, Thomas-Gibson S, et al. Colorectal stenting for malignant and benign disease: outcomes in colorectal stenting. Dis Colon Rectum. 2004;47:1201–7.

14. Tamim WZ, Ghellai A, Couniham TC, et al. Experience with endoluminal colonic Wall Stents for benign and malignant disease. Arch Surg. 2000;135:434–8.

15. García-Cano J, González-Huix F, Juzgado D, et al. Use of self-expanding metal stents to treat malignant colorectal obstruction in general endoscopic practice (with videos). Gastrointest Endosc. 2006;64:914–20.

16. Watt AM, Faragher IG, Griffin TT, et al. Self-expanding metallic stents for relieving malignant colorectal obstruction: a systematic review. Ann Surg. 2007;246:24–30.

17. Fernández-Esparrach G, Bordas JM, Giráldez MD, et al. Severe complications limit long-term clinical success of self-expanding metal stents in patients with obstructive colorectal cancer. Am J Gastroenterol. 2010;105:1087–93.

18. Lee HJ, Hong SP, Cheon JH, et al. Long-term outcome of palliative therapy for malignant colorectal obstruction in patients with unresectable metastatic colorectal cancers: endoscopic stenting versus surgery. Gastrointest Endosc. 2011;73:535–42.

19. Karoui M, Charachon A, Delbaldo C, et al. Stents for palliation of obstructive metastatic colon cancer: impact on management and chemotherapy administration. Arch Surg. 2007;142:619–23.

20. Khot UP, Lang AW, Murali K, et al. Systematic review of the efficacy and safety of colorectal stents. Br J Surg. 2002;89:1096–102.

21. Targownik LE, Spiegel BM, Sack J, et al. Colonic stent vs. emergency surgery for management of acute left-sided malignant colonic obstruction: a decision analysis. Gastrointest Endosc. 2004;60:865–74.

22. Martinez-Santos C, Lobato RF, Fradejas JM, et al. Self-expandable stent before elective surgery vs. emergency surgery for the treatment of malignant colorectal obstructions: comparison of primary anastomosis and morbidity rates. Dis Colon Rectum. 2002;45:401–6.

23. Bittinger M, Messman H. Self-expanding metal stents as nonsurgical palliative therapy for malignant colonic obstruction: time to change the standard of care? (Editorial). Gastrointest Endosc. 2007;66:928–9.

24. Ansaloni L, Andersson R, Bazzoli F, et al. Guidelines in the management of obstructing cancer in the left colon: consensus conference of the world society of emergency surgery (WSES) and peritoneum and surgery (PnS) society. World J Emerg Surg. 2010;5:29.

25. Böhner H, Yang Q, Franke C, et al. Simple data from history and physical examination help to exclude bowel obstruction and to avoid radiographic studies in patients with acute abdominal pain. Eur J Surg. 1998;164:777–84.

26. Ripamonti CI, Easson AM, Gerdes H. Management of malignant bowel obstruction. Eur J Cancer. 2008;44:1105–15.

27. Ha HK, Shin BS, Lee SI, et al. Usefulness of CT in patients with intestinal obstruction who have undergone abdominal surgery for malignancy. AJR Am J Roentgenol. 1998;171:1587–93.

28. Baron TH, Harewood GC. Technological review. Enteral self-expandable stents. Gastrointest Endosc. 2003;58:421–33.

29. Fanelli DR, Fisher L, Fukami N, et al. ASGE guideline. The role of endoscopy in the management of patients with known and suspected colonic obstruction and pseudo-obstruction. Gastrointest Endosc. 2010;74:669–79.

30. Turner J, Cummin T, Bennett A, et al. Stents and stentability: treatment for malignant bowel obstruction. Br J Hosp Med (Lond). 2008;69:676–80.

31. Small AJ, Coelho-Prabhu N, Baron TH. Endoscopic placement of self-expandable metal stents for malignant colonic obstruction: long-term outcomes and complication factors. Gastrointest Endosc. 2010;71:560–72.

32. Repici A, De Caro G, Luigiano C, et al. WallFlex colonic stent placement for management of malignant colonic obstruction: a prospective study at two centers. Gastrointest Endosc. 2008;67:77–84.

33. Moon CM, Kim TI, Lee MS, et al. Comparison of a newly designed Niti-S D-Weave combination covered stent and Niti-S D-Weave uncovered stent for decompression of obstructive colorectal cancer: a randomized prospective controlled multicenter study. Gastrointest Endosc. 2009;69:AB379.

34. Im JP, Kim SG, Kang HW, et al. Clinical outcomes and patency of self-expanding metal stents in patients with malignant colorectal obstruction: a prospective single center study. Int J Colorectal Dis. 2008;23:789–94.

35. Repici A, Fregonese D, Costamagna G, et al. Ultraflex precision colonic stent placement for palliation of malignant colonic obstruction: a prospective multicenter study. Gastrointest Endosc. 2007;66:920–7.

36. Kozarek R. Making sense out of colonic stents (Editorial). Gastrointest Endosc. 2008;67:85–7.

37. Park S, Cheon JH, Park JJ, et al. Comparison of efficacies between stents for malignant colorectal obstruction: a randomized, prospective study. Gastrointest Endosc. 2010;72:304–10.

38. Lee KM, Shin SJ, Hwang JC, et al. Comparison of uncovered stent with covered stent for treatment of malignant colorectal obstruction. Gastrointest Endosc. 2007;66:931–6.

39. Small AJ, Baron TH. Comparison of Wallstent and Ultraflex stents for palliation of malignant left-sided colon obstruction: a retrospective, case-matched analysis. Gastrointest Endosc. 2008;67:478–88.

40. García-Cano J. Use of an ultrathin gastroscope to allow endoscopic insertion of enteral Wallstents without fluoroscopic monitoring. Dig Dis Sci. 2006;51:1231–5.

41. García-Cano J, Sánchez-Manjavacas N, Viñuelas M, et al. Use of an ultrathin endoscope to insert self-expanding metal stents in tumoral strictures of the Rectosigmoid without fluoroscopy. Gastrointest Endosc. 2007;65:AB258.

42. Branger F, Thibaudeau E, Mucci-Hennekinne S, et al. Management of acute malignant large-bowel obstruction

with self-expanding metal stent. Int J Colorectal Dis. 2010;25:1481–5.

43. Ptok H, Meyer F, Marusch F, et al. Palliative stent implantation in the treatment of malignant colorectal obstruction. Surg Endosc. 2006;20:909–14.

44. Donnellan F, Cullen G, Cagney D, et al. Efficacy and safety of colonic stenting for malignant disease in the elderly. Int J Colorectal Dis. 2010;25:747–50.

45. Lee JH, Ross WA, Davila R, et al. Self-expandable metal stents (SEMS) can serve as a bridge to surgery or as a definitive therapy in patients with an advanced stage of cancer: clinical experience of a tertiary cancer center. Dig Dis Sci. 2010;55:3530–6.

46. Soto S, López-Rosés L, González-Ramírez A, et al. Endoscopic treatment of acute colorectal obstruction with self-expandable metallic stents: experience in a community hospital. Surg Endosc. 2006;20:1072–6.

47. Luigiano C, Ferrara F, Fabbri C, et al. Through-the-scope large diameter self-expanding metal stent placement as a safe and effective technique for palliation of malignant colorectal obstruction: a single center experience with a long-term follow-up. Scand J Gastroenterol. 2011;46:591–6.

48. Sebastian S, Johnston S, Geoghegan T, et al. Pooled analysis of the efficacy and safety of self-expanding metal stenting in malignant colorectal obstruction. Am J Gastroenterol. 2004;99:2051–7.

49. Keymling M. Colorectal stenting. Endoscopy. 2003;35:234–8.

50. Baron TH. Colonic stenting: a palliative measure only or a bridge to surgery? Endoscopy. 2010;42:163–8.

51. García-Cano J, Sánchez-Manjavacas N, Gómez Ruiz CJ, et al. Endoscopic insertion of self-expanding metal stents in malignant colonic obstructions. Gastroenterol Hepatol. 2006;29:610–5 (Spanish).

52. Repici A, Adler DG, Gibbs CM, et al. Stenting of the proximal colon in patients with malignant large bowel obstruction: techniques and outcomes. Gastrointest Endosc. 2007;66:940–4.

53. López-Roses L, González Ramírez A, Lancho Seco A, et al. A new use for the rotatable sphincterotome as an aid for stenting malignant gastroduodenal tract stenosis. Endoscopy. 2004;36:1132.

54. Song H-Y, Kim JH, Kim KR, et al. Malignant rectal obstruction within 5 cm of the anal verge: is there a role for expandable metallic stent placement? Gastrointest Endosc. 2008;68:713–20.

55. Vitale MA, Villotti G, d'Alba L, et al. Preoperative colonoscopy after self-expandable metallic stent placement in patients with acute neoplastic colon obstruction. Gastrointest Endosc. 2006;63:814–9.

56. van Hooft JE, Fockens P, Marinelli AW, Dutch Colorectal Stent Group. Early closure of a multicenter randomized clinical trial of endoscopic stenting versus surgery for stage IV left-sided colorectal cancer. Endoscopy. 2008;40:184–91.

57. Pirlet IA, Slim K, Kwiatkowski F, et al. Emergency preoperative stenting versus surgery for acute left-sided malignant colonic obstruction: a multicenter randomized controlled trial. Surg Endosc. 2011;25:1814–21.

58. Varadarajulu S, Roy A, Lopes T, Drelichman ER, et al. Endoscopic stenting versus surgical colostomy for the management of malignant colonic obstruction: comparison of hospital costs and clinical outcomes. Surg Endosc. 2011;25:2203–9.

59. Nagula S, Ishill N, Nash C, et al. Quality of life and symptom control after stent placement or surgical palliation of malignant colorectal obstruction. J Am Coll Surg. 2010;210:45–53.

60. Cheung HY, Chung CC, Tsang WW, et al. Endolaparoscopic approach vs conventional open surgery in the treatment of obstructing left-sided colon cancer: a randomized controlled trial. Arch Surg. 2009;144:1127–32.

61. Inaba Y, Arai Y, Yamaura H, et al. Phase II clinical study on stent therapy for unresectable malignant colorectal obstruction (JIVROSG-0206). Am J Clin Oncol. 2012;35(1):73–6.

62. Feo L, Schaffzin DM. Colonic stents: the modern treatment of colonic obstruction. Adv Ther. 2011;28:73–86.

63. Dai Y, Chopra SS, Wysocki WM, Hünerbein M. Treatment of benign colorectal strictures by temporary stenting with self-expanding stents. Int J Colorectal Dis. 2010;25:1475–9.

64. Forshaw MJ, Sankararajah D, Stewart M, Parker MC. Self-expanding metallic stents in the treatment of benign colorectal disease: indications and outcomes. Colorectal Dis. 2006;8:102–11.

65. Keränen I, Lepistö A, Udd M, et al. Outcome of patients after endoluminal stent placement for benign colorectal obstruction. Scand J Gastroenterol. 2010;45:725–31.

66. Small AJ, Young-Fadok TM, Baron TH. Expandable metal stent placement for benign colorectal obstruction: outcomes for 23 cases. Surg Endosc. 2008;22:454–62.

67. Fähndrich M, Sandmann M, Heike M. A new method for placement of covered colorectal stents in the proximal colon using double balloon enteroscopy. Endoscopy. 2011;43(Suppl 2):E23.

68. Smedh K, Birgisson H, Raab Y, et al. Self-expanding stent in obstructing colorectal cancer. A new technique to avoid abdominal surgery. Lakartidningen. 2003;100:1982–6 [Swedish].

69. Carne PW, Frye JN, Robertson GM, et al. Stents or open operation for palliation of colorectal cancer: a retrospective, cohort study of perioperative outcome and long-term survival. Dis Colon Rectum. 2004;47:1455–61.

# Part 5
# Results to Include Complications

# Esophageal Stents: Malignancy

13

## Peter D. Siersema

Dysphagia due to malignant esophageal obstruction is frequently encountered. Malignant strictures are generally caused by primary esophageal cancer but can also be due to extrinsic compression, often as a result of a malignant mediastinal mass or lung cancer. Over the past 30 years, esophageal stents have rapidly evolved from rigid, plastic tubes to partially or fully covered self-expandable metal stents (SEMS) in the 1990s and self-expanding plastic stents (SEPS) in the beginning of twenty-first century. While the first SEMS were made of stainless steel, SEMS are now composed of nitinol. This nickel titanium alloy increases its flexibility and reduces the risk for esophageal injury. The process of developing specific stent characteristics to reduce complications of stent placement, such as migration, reflux esophagitis, and hyperplastic tissue in- or overgrowth, continues.

In order to reduce the risk of complications, several stent characteristics are important. An optimal stent design should be flexible, nontraumatic, and have an internal diameter large enough to allow normal food passage yet minimize the risks of perforation, pain, and hemorrhage. Furthermore, placement, repositioning, and removal of the stent should be easy, without risks of stent migration and nontumoral and tumoral tissue in- or overgrowth. Although the ideal stent does not exist, most currently used stents fulfill at least some of these criteria.

Since the first publication of esophageal stent placement in 1976, over 1,000 studies have been published on esophageal stents [1]. The aim of this chapter is to review data from the last decade of stent development and with corresponding outcomes of stent placement.

## Treatment Options for Malignant Dysphagia

In patients with inoperable esophageal cancer, several palliative options are available to treat malignant dysphagia [1]. These treatment options can be divided into endoscopic (stent placement, laser therapy, argon plasma coagulation (APC), dilation or nutritional support by nasogastric or nasoenteral tube, or percutaneous endoscopic gastrostomy placement) and non-endoscopic modalities (external beam radiotherapy, brachytherapy, chemotherapy, or a combination of these).

The main goal of palliation of esophageal cancer is to relieve dysphagia due to tumor obstruction. As the life expectancy of patients with inoperable esophageal cancer is often less than 6 months, palliative therapy should be rapidly

P.D. Siersema receives research support from Cook Medical Ltd., Ireland, and is an advisor of Boston Scientific Corp., USA.

P.D. Siersema, M.D., Ph.D., F.A.S.G.E., F.A.C.G. (✉)
Department of Gastroenterology and Hepatology,
University Medical Center Utrecht,
Heidelberglaan 100, Utrecht, CX 3584, The Netherlands
e-mail: p.d.siersema@umcutrecht.nl

R. Kozarek et al. (eds.), *Self-Expandable Stents in the Gastrointestinal Tract*,
DOI 10.1007/978-1-4614-3746-8_13, © Springer Science+Business Media New York 2013

effective and devoid of major complications and without adversely affecting quality of life. Homs et al. performed a large randomized controlled trial (RCT) comparing a partially covered SEMS (Ultraflex, Boston Scientific, Natick, MA) with single-dose brachytherapy and demonstrated that malignant dysphagia improved more rapidly after SEMS placement than after brachytherapy. At follow-up >3 months, recurrent dysphagia was more frequently seen in patients who underwent stent placement than in those treated with brachytherapy [2]. Complications occurred more frequently after stent placement (hemorrhage 13% vs. 5%, fistula 6% vs. 3%, perforation 2% vs. 2%, retrosternal pain 12% vs. 6%, and other complications 9% vs. 6%). In another RCT, Wenger et al. performed a health economic evaluation and confirmed that the stent-arm performed better in the first 3 months after treatment [3]. Total lifetime costs were higher in the brachytherapy arm (17,690 vs. 33,171 euro). Both studies concluded that stent placement should be reserved for patients with a short life expectancy (≤3 months) and in those with persistent or recurrent dysphagia after brachytherapy,

while brachytherapy should be used in patients with a life expectancy >3 months.

In order to determine prognosis of patients with malignant dysphagia and which patients benefit from either stent placement or brachytherapy, a prognostic model was developed based on a large cohort of patients [4]. Of several independent risk factors, such as age, male sex, tumor length, presence/absence of metastases, and the WHO score, three prognostic groups were identified. For patients with poor prognostic factors, dysphagia-adjusted survival was 23 days and favored stent placement, whereas for those with an intermediate and relatively good prognosis, dysphagia-adjusted survival was better with brachytherapy.

## Stent Designs

Results following stent placement for palliation of malignant dysphagia can be attributed to the type of stent (type of SEMS or SEPS) (Fig. 13.1). Types of SEMS are classified as partially covered and fully covered designs, with each type associated with different outcomes.

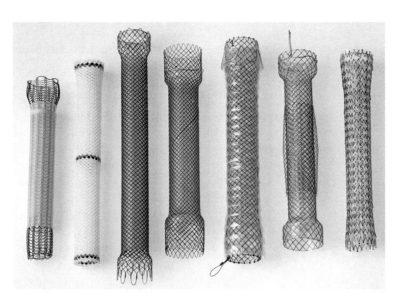

**Fig. 13.1** Currently available self-expanding metal and plastic stents (from *left* to *right*): Ultraflex (Boston Scientific, Natick, MA, USA), Polyflex (Boston Scientific), Wallflex (Boston Scientific), Evolution (Cook Medical, Limerick, Ireland), SX-Ella esophageal HV (ELLA-CS, s.r.o., Hradec Kralove, Czech Republic), double-layered Niti-S (TaeWoong Medical, Seoul, Korea), and Alimaxx-E (Merit Medical, South Jordan, UT, USA)

## Partially Covered SEMS

In general, partially covered SEMS are characterized by imbedding of the uncovered proximal and distal portions into the esophageal wall. This characteristic prevents stent migration and ensures adequate sealing of malignant and benign fistulas or perforations. A disadvantage of uncovered stent ends is the risk of recurrent dysphagia caused by granulation and/or hyperplastic tissue growth and the difficulty of stent removal, the latter especially in case of a benign disease. For benign indications, the use of partially covered SEMS is strongly discouraged, because embedment caused by this nontumoral tissue reaction may prevent easy and safe stent removal [5, 6], although stent-in-stent removal techniques placing a plastic or fully covered SEMS into the PC SEMS have allowed removal in a subset 10–14 days later because of pressure necrosis of the original hyperplastic ingrowth.

Worldwide, the Ultraflex stent is most commonly used for treatment of malignant dysphagia. This stent, made of knitted nitinol, has a central cover of polyurethane and has uncovered ends at the proximal and distal 1.5-cm stent ends. It is available in two diameters (18-mm body/23-mm proximal flare and 23-mm body/28-mm proximal flare) and lengths varying from 7 to 15 cm. After expansion, this stent foreshortens up to 30–40%. The radial force of this stent is the lowest among the currently available stents, which makes it soft and flexible. An advantage of the Ultraflex is that the distance of the upper margin of the stent to the incisors is depicted on the introducer system, which allows exact stent placement without the need for fluoroscopic guidance. The complication rate of this stent in patients with malignant strictures is 6–21%, and recurrent dysphagia occurs in 31–52% mostly due to tissue ingrowth or overgrowth (26–31%) (Fig. 13.2) and, to a lesser extent, food obstruction (2–24%) (Fig. 13.3) and migration (4–17%) [7, 8].

The Evolution (Cook Medical, Limerick, Ireland) is made from a single woven, nitinol wire with an internal and external silicone coating and uncovered distal and proximal flares. The stent is available in lengths varying from 8 to 15 cm and a

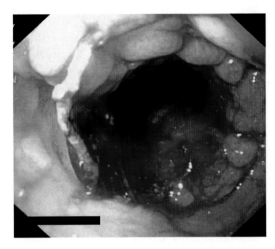

**Fig. 13.2** Nontumoral ingrowth at the uncovered *upper* end of an Ultraflex

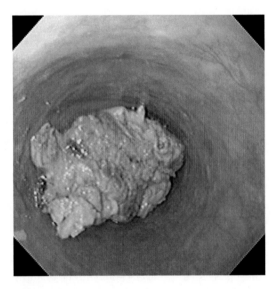

**Fig. 13.3** Food obstruction in a partially covered Ultraflex. Note the upper stent end at the 1 o'clock position

body diameter of 20 mm with flanges of 25 mm. The stent is placed with a pistol-grip delivery system which allows controlled release and recapturing, if needed. The initial results with this stent design have been promising, with a major complication rate of 9% (aspiration pneumonia and severe bleeding) and a minor complication rate of 25%. Recurrent dysphagia was observed in 25% of patients (tissue in- or overgrowth 14%, food impaction 7%, migration 4%) [9].

Controlled release and recapturing of the stent is also possible with the partially covered Wallflex (Boston Scientific). The recently introduced Wallflex stent replaces the previously available Wallstent and Flamingo Wallstent. This newly available stent design has a 1:1 stent deployment system by pulling the more distal handle toward the proximal handle which corresponds to degree of stent release. The stent is made of a multiple wire woven nitinol mesh with a silicone cover and uncovered distal and proximal flared ends. This stent is available in three lengths (10, 12, 15 cm) and two diameters (18/23 and 23/28 mm). The 18.5 Fr. (6 mm) introducer allows passage through narrow strictures. Like the Ultraflex and the Evolution, the Wallflex stent has a suture at its proximal end which allows stent repositioning or removal with a grasping forceps. The initial results in the treatment of malignant dysphagia using the Wallflex were comparable to those of the Evolution, with a major complication rate of 8% (bleeding and aspiration pneumonia); minor complications occurred in 43% (retrosternal pain and gastroesophageal reflux). Recurrent dysphagia occurred in 22% (tissue in- or overgrowth 11%, food impaction 5.5%, and migration 5.5%) [10].

## Fully Covered SEMS

When fully covered SEMS are placed, recurrent dysphagia due to hyperplastic tissue ingrowth does not occur. Because the cover prevents stent embedding, these stent designs are marketed in some countries as removable and theoretically may be more suitable for treatment of benign strictures; however, they can be used in malignant strictures as well. Unfortunately, migration rates are significantly higher with fully covered stents, which may lead to recurrent dysphagia.

The (fully covered) Evolution (Cook Medical) has succeeded the previously manufactured Z-stent which was available in two designs, with centrally placed external fixation barbs (Cook Medical Europe, Bjaeverskov, Denmark) or without these barbs (Wilson Cook Medical Inc, Winston-Salem, USA) [11]. The Evolution is available in two diameters (18/23 mm and 20/25 mm) and in 8, 10,

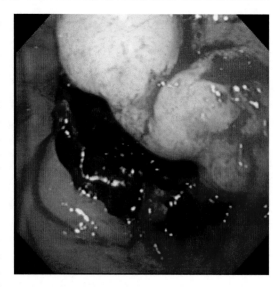

**Fig. 13.4** Tissue overgrowth at the proximal end of a double-layered Niti-S

and 12 cm lengths. So far, no results with this stent design have been reported.

The Niti-S (TaeWoong Medical, Seoul, Korea) is also available in two designs, a retrievable, fully covered, single-layer SEMS and a version with a double layer. The latter version can also be classified as partially covered SEMS, as it consists of an outer layer consisting of an uncovered nitinol mesh and a fully covered inner layer of polyurethane. This design should prevent stent migration by the combination of shouldering (flares of 26 mm wide) while allowing tissue ingrowth and embedding into the outer uncovered mesh. The inner fully covered layer, on the other hand, prevents tumoral and nontumoral tissue ingrowth. The double-layer version has been shown to reduce major complications in comparison to the single-layer version (12% vs. 58%, $p=0.006$) [12]. Another study has also suggested that this double-layer stent resulted in a low recurrent dysphagia rate (12%), due to tissue overgrowth (7%) (Fig. 13.4) and migration (5%) [13]. The Niti-S is also available with a very short (5 mm) flare, which may be useful for proximally located benign anastomotic strictures. So far, no clinical data are available with this version.

Another fully covered metal stent design, which has been suggested to function as a *removable* stent, is the Alimaxx-E (Merit Medical Endotek, South Jordan, UT, USA) [14]. This stent has a polyurethane cover over its complete length and body diameters of 18 and 22 mm and proximal flares 5 mm larger (23 and 27 mm) and distal flares 3 mm larger (21 and 25 mm), respectively. The initial design had 20 struts on the outside to prevent migration [14, 15]. Although previous studies indeed have shown that the stent is easily removable, it tended to fracture and embed due to disruption of the stent cover over time [16]. In addition, the initial stent design was associated with high migration rates (35%) [15]. For this reason, the stent design of the Alimaxx-E was adjusted to the Alimaxx-ES. This adjustment included an increase in the number of struts on the outside (to 45) in an effort to reduce migration and an inner silicone coating at the polyurethane cover to prevent chemical degradation [17]. Most published studies, however, report data on the initial stent design.

The SX-Ella esophageal HV (Ella-CS, Hradec Kralove, Czech Republic) is a new, fully covered stent. This nitinol stent has a flip-flop-type anti-migration collar at the proximal stent end. The fully covered stent design may explain the relatively low rate of recurrent dysphagia due to tissue overgrowth (5%); however, stent migration (14%) and food impaction (18%) still occur frequently. Despite the single-wire braided design of the stent which should theoretically make it less traumatic to the tissue, the stent was associated with a relatively high major complication rate (23%), particularly severe bleeding, possibly due to the anti-migration collar causing trauma to the esophageal mucosa [18].

Finally, the Wallflex (Boston Scientific) is also available in a fully covered design. While the partially covered stent has flares of similar sizes at both stent ends, the proximal diameter of the fully covered stent is 2 mm wider (25 mm) than the distal flare to prevent migration. The stent is available in two sizes, i.e., 25/18/23 and 28/23/28 mm. Results on complications and recurrent dysphagia, particularly migration, are not yet available. Due to its fully covered design, the stent may be suitable for malignant and for benign conditions; however, the application for benign disease needs further evaluation.

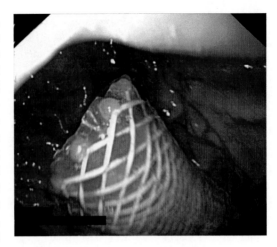

**Fig. 13.5** Migrated Polyflex in the stomach

We recently performed a prospective follow-up study with this device; however, results are pending.

## Self-Expanding Plastic Stents

The only currently available self-expanding plastic stent (SEPS) is the Polyflex (Boston Scientific), which is made of a plastic wire, fully covered with silicone and with a proximal flare. The stent has body diameters/flanges of 16/20, 18/23, and 21/25 mm and lengths of 9, 12, and 15 cm. The stent introducer has a diameter of 12–14 mm. The material of the stent has been claimed to reduce nontumoral tissue overgrowth. As a result, the stent is easily removable and therefore the only stent which is FDA approved for the treatment of benign esophageal strictures. It provides effective relief of malignant dysphagia with a major complication rate of 9% and a recurrent dysphagia rate of 37%, mostly due to stent migration (13–29%) (Fig. 13.5), tissue overgrowth (10–30%), and food impaction (5%) [7, 8].

## Comparing Different Stent Types: Randomized Controlled Trials and Pooled Data

Despite recommendations following the above-mentioned clinical trials [2, 3], stent placement is currently the most frequently used method for palliation of malignant dysphagia. Successful treatment of dysphagia with self-expanding stents can be explained by the simplicity of the procedure and the rapid effect. Almost all studies have reported that stent placement is technically successful in nearly 100% of cases and results in improvement of dysphagia score of 2 points (from 3 [liquids only] to 1 [almost all solids]) within 24–48 h. However, early enthusiasm is somewhat tempered as complications and recurrent dysphagia occur despite newer stent designs [19].

Over the last 10 years, four RCTs comparing different SEMS and SEPS for the treatment of malignant dysphagia have been performed [7, 8, 11, 20]. In 2001, 100 patients with malignant dysphagia were randomized to the three most commonly used SEMS in Europe at that time, the Ultraflex, Z-stent (without fixation barbs), and Flamingo Wallstent [11], of which only the Ultraflex is still available. Improvement of dysphagia was comparable in all three groups, but major complication rates were not significantly different and occurred in 24%, 18%, and 36% for the Ultraflex, Flamingo Wallstent, and Z-stent, respectively.

In 2003, Sabharwal et al. compared the Ultraflex and Flamingo Wallstent in 55 patients with distal esophageal cancer [20]. Improvement of dysphagia was comparable between both stent groups, as was the number of complications. Migration occurred in two patients after Ultraflex placement (6.4%) and in one patient after Flamingo Wallstent placement (4.5%). Adequate positioning was found to be more difficult with the Ultraflex, as three patients needed two Ultraflex stents because of malpositioning.

In 2007, Conio et al. performed a RCT comparing SEPS and SEMS for the treatment of malignant dysphagia [7]. In total, 100 patients were randomized to receive a Polyflex or an Ultraflex. Patients with malignancy at the esophagogastric junction were excluded. Again, there was comparable relief of dysphagia on the short term, but recurrent dysphagia occurred more often with the Polyflex, due to a higher stent migration rate (13% vs. 4%). Remarkably, tumor overgrowth and hyperplastic tissue reaction were comparable between the two stent types (30% vs. 28%).

Finally, Verschuur et al. compared the Niti-S, Ultraflex, and Polyflex in 125 patients with esophageal or gastric cardia cancer [8]. Placement of the Polyflex seemed more difficult with 83% technical success of placement versus 100% and 95% for the Ultraflex and Niti-S, respectively. As expected, improvement of dysphagia was similar for all three stent types. Complication rates were also comparable, but there was a significant difference in recurrent dysphagia (52% for Ultraflex vs. 37% for Polyflex vs. 31% for Niti-S). Particularly, stent migration was more common with the Polyflex (29%), whereas tumor in- and overgrowth and food obstruction were more frequently seen with the partially covered Ultraflex (24–31%). Migration was infrequently seen with the Niti-S (12%); however, tissue overgrowth was found in 24% of patients.

In addition to these RCTs, most new stent designs have been evaluated in single-arm, prospective, or retrospective series. After pooling these data per stent type (PCSEMS, FCSEMS, and SEPS), we compared complication rate and rate of recurrent dysphagia for the different stent types [21]. Data for partially covered SEMS showed major complications in about 18% of patients (mostly severe pain, hemorrhage, and fistula formation). These numbers seemed slightly higher for fully covered SEMS (21%). For SEPS, complication rates in individual series varied between 0% and 29%, but pooled data showed lower complication rates (10%). Pooled data show a recurrent dysphagia rate of 41% in patients treated with partially covered SEMS, 29% with fully covered SEMS, and 37% with SEPS.

In summary, partially covered and fully covered SEMS and SEPS provide similar short-term relief of dysphagia. In our experience and in others, however, the large diameter introducer of SEPS, resulting in technical difficulties during placement and high migration rates, favors SEMS for the palliation of malignant dysphagia. As only small differences between the various types of SEMS were encountered, the selection of a particular SEMS for palliation should be based on stricture type and location and on personal experience with a specific stent type. For distal esophageal and cardia tumors, which are more prone to migration, we prefer the use of partially covered stents, such as the Evolution, Wallflex, or Ultraflex, which firmly embed in the esophageal wall, or the double-layered Niti-S. In tumors located close to the upper esophageal sphincter (UES), stent placement can be associated with severe pain. In these patients, we usually place the Ultraflex, which is currently the most flexible stent, with a relatively low radial force.

## How to Minimize Re-intervention Rates

As summarized above, major complications associated with stent placement include perforation, fistula formation, bleeding, (severe) pain, and gastroesophageal reflux. Nonetheless, particularly perforation, fistula formation, and hemorrhage are now uncommon due to the use of the currently available highly flexible stent designs. The most common complication following stent placement includes recurrent dysphagia as a consequence of stent migration, tumoral or nontumoral tissue over- or ingrowth, and food obstruction of the stent. In the following, these complications will be discussed in more detail.

## Perforation, Fistula Formation, Bleeding, and Severe Pain

It is generally believed that perforation, fistula formation, bleeding, and (severe) pain can largely be prevented by using stents that have a maximum diameter of 28 mm at the flare and a diameter of 24–25 mm at the body. Another factor associated with complications, particularly pain, has been suggested to be the rigidity of the stent [10]; the more rigid the stent, the higher the risk that patients experience pain after stent placement. However, this has not been substantiated. It should be kept in mind that fistula formation and bleeding are not always the result of stent placement but can also be caused by progressive tumor growth.

These complications are difficult to treat. Perforation can be prevented avoiding dilation of the tumor prior to stent placement. If, however, perforation occurs, it can be treated by placing a covered stent that to seal the perforation. This is also true for fistula formation, which can be treated by primary or secondary stent placement. Bleeding is more difficult to treat as it is often a sign of progressive tumor growth. One may consider applying radiation therapy; however, evidence for this approach is lacking. Finally, retrosternal pain resolves after several days and can be treated by analgesics. In cases of refractory pain, stent removal may be required.

## Gastroesophageal Reflux

As the incidence of adenocarcinoma is rising, the number of patients with stents placed across the GE junction is increasing. Placement in this location not only increases the risk of stent migration but also leads to an increased risk of gastroesophageal reflux of gastric contents, as the stent bypasses the lower esophageal sphincter. Proton pump inhibitors (PPIs) reduce gastroesophageal reflux, but in some patients, symptoms persist despite PPI use. In these patients, an antireflux stent may provide a solution. A selection of antireflux stents is shown in Fig. 13.6.

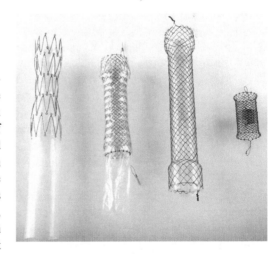

**Fig. 13.6** A selection of antireflux stents: the Z-stent with Dua valve (Cook Endoscopy Europe, Bjaeverskov Denmark), SX-Ella HV stent plus (ELLA-CS, s.r.o., Hradec Kralove, Czech Republic), Choo stent (M.I Tech, Pyeongtaek, Korea), and EndoFLUXX (Merit Medical Endotek, South Jordan, UT, USA)

Several antireflux stent designs have been evaluated in RCTs (compared to open stents) and prospective series [22–28]. In 2002, the first RCT was performed comparing open Flamingo Wallstents with Z-stents that had a windsock-type antireflux valve on the distal end in 50 patients with distal esophageal or gastric cardia cancer [25]. Reflux symptoms occurred significantly less frequently with antireflux stents (3/25) than with open stents (24/24). No objective parameters, such as pH monitoring or radiological studies, were assessed to confirm its effectiveness.

In 2004, Homs et al. performed a RCT comparing the FerX-Ella with or without an antireflux valve [22]. In total, 30 patients, blinded to stent assignment, were followed by symptom scoring and 24-h pH monitoring. Unfortunately, only one third of patients consented to pH monitoring. Surprisingly, this study showed that reflux symptoms and total acid exposure time were increased in the antireflux stent group. In addition, stent migration was common in both treatment arms (23%). Failure of this antireflux stent was thought to be due to unfavorable valve characteristics, such as a relatively short length of the windsock valve and the floppy material used for the membrane which was less stiff than the one present in the Z-stent.

Another study evaluated three different stent designs: the Do stent with a tricuspid antireflux valve (M.I. Tech, Pyeongtaek, Korea) ($n = 12$) which can be placed inside a standard stent, a newly designed antireflux stent with an S-shaped valve and long leaflets (M.I. Tech) ($n = 12$), and a standard open stent (M.I. Tech) ($n = 12$) [28]. In all patients, pH monitoring and symptom scoring were performed. This study showed that the stent with the S-shaped valve significantly reduced symptoms and total acid exposure time (3%) compared to the open stent (15%) and even more than the Do stent (29%).

In all of the above-mentioned studies, patients were included who were not routinely treated with PPIs or, in some studies, PPIs were only started when reflux symptoms occurred. A more interesting question might therefore be whether antireflux stents are superior to open stents in combination with standard PPI use. This question

was addressed by Sabharwal et al. in 2008 by comparing the outcome of open Ultraflex stent placement combined with daily omeprazole (20 mg) to placement of the antireflux FerX-Ella stent [26]. The study was terminated prematurely after 49 patients had been included, due to significant modifications that were made to the Fer X-Ella stent during the inclusion period. As expected based upon the previous study by Homs et al. [22], results with the open stent with standard PPI were not different from those of the antireflux stent (8% vs. 14%, $p = $ NS). Although the authors addressed an interesting question, the study results would have been more interesting if an antireflux stent type was used which already had shown promising results, instead of a stent which had previously been proven to be inferior to a standard open stent.

Currently, we are evaluating a newly designed antireflux valve, the EndoFLUXX, a reflux control device (Merit Medical Endotek, South Jordan, UT, USA), which can be placed inside in a previously placed "host" stent, especially in patients reflux symptoms refractory to PPI therapy. The device is a 3.5 cm long, 18 or 23 mm wide, self-expanding nitinol stent with a tricuspid valve, made of a biomimetic polymer, which opens at different pressures in each direction, allowing food passage without resistance, while reducing – if not eliminating – gastroesophageal reflux, yet still allowing vomiting and belching (Fig. 13.7a, b).

Given the conflicting results in different studies and with different antireflux stents, it can be concluded that the routine use of antireflux stents in patients with distal esophageal or gastric cardia cancer cannot be recommended [5]. If one decides not to place an antireflux stent, high-dose PPIs and antireflux precautions should be advised to prevent reflux and aspiration.

## Recurrent Dysphagia

Recurrent dysphagia, due to stent migration, reactive tissue overgrowth, or food impaction, is common and occurs in 30% of patients after stent placement for malignant dysphagia [29]. Of all patients presenting with recurrent dysphagia,

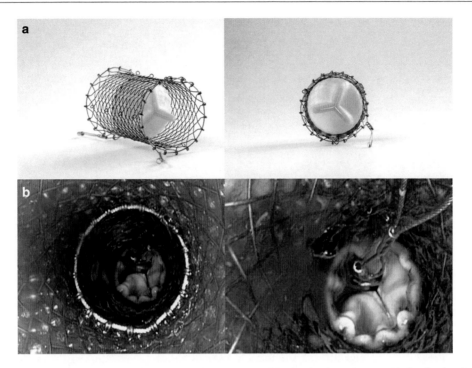

**Fig. 13.7** (**a**) The EndoFLUXX, a reflux control device (Merit Medical Endotek, South Jordan, UT, USA) (**b**) A EndoFLUXX placed within a stent that was placed in the distal esophagus with the distal end across the gastroesophageal junction

almost 90% require repeat endoscopic treatment, such as placement of a second stent, stent repositioning, or endoscopic stent cleansing.

An important aspect of preventing stent migration is to carefully consider which stent diameter should be placed. It is well known that a larger stent diameter effectively reduces both stent migration and food impaction. In less severe strictures or those in challenging locations (such as the gastroesophageal junction), a wide stent diameter is recommended. A recent retrospective review of 338 patients with malignant dysphagia showed that the risk of recurrent dysphagia was significantly reduced after placement of a large diameter stent (HR 0.35 95% CI 0.17–0.73), in particular after a large diameter (23/28 mm) Ultraflex [30].

We usually remove migrated stents endoscopically, as it has been reported that migrated stents may cause intestinal perforation or obstruction requiring abdominal surgery [31, 32].

In addition to stent diameter, the use of several stent designs specifically developed to

**Table 13.1** Stent characteristics that intend to increase or decrease the risk of recurrent dysphagia

|  | Migration | Nontumoral tissue reaction | Food impaction |
|---|---|---|---|
| Shouldering | – | +/– | +/– |
| Fully covered design | + | – | +/– |
| Large diameter | – | +/– | – |
| Covered internal mesh | +/– | +/– | – |
| Covered external mesh | + | +/– | +/– |

+ increase, +/– no effect, – decrease

reduce recurrent dysphagia can be considered (Tables 13.1 and 13.2). Such stents have increased resistance on the outside of the stent to reduce the risk of migration (double-layered Niti-S and Alimaxx-E stents). Another feature is a distinct shouldering at the upper end of the stent (Niti-S, Evolution, and Wallflex stents) to reduce migration risk. The flip-flop collar of the HV Ella stent has also been introduced in order to reduce migration.

**Table 13.2** Stent characteristics summarized per stent

| | Shouldering | Fully covered design | Covered internal mesh | Covered external mesh | Large diameter available | Other characteristics |
|---|---|---|---|---|---|---|
| Ultraflex | – | – | – | + | + | Flexible |
| Flamingo Wallstent | – | – | + | – | – | Cone shape |
| Niti-S | + | + | + | – | – | Double layered |
| Evolution (PC and FC)* | + | +/– | + | + | +/– | – |
| Wallflex (PC and FC)* | + | +/– | + | – | + | – |
| Alimaxx-E | – | + | + | – | – | 20 struts |
| SX-Ella | – | + | – | + | +/– | Anti-migration collar |
| Polyflex | – | + | + | – | +/– | Polyester material |
| SX-Ella biodegradable | – | – | – | – | + | Dissolves within 3–4 months |

– not present, +/– depending on design, + present
*PC partially covered, FC fully covered

As stated previously, the benefit of this collar is questionable, as migration still was found to occur in 6 of 44 patients (14%) [28].

Nontumoral tissue ingrowth and, to some extent, overgrowth is thought to be reduced with fully covered stents (Alimaxx-E, Wallflex, Evolution, and Niti-S stents) and non-nitinol stents (Polyflex stent). Moreover, tumoral overgrowth can also be reduced by using stents that are substantially longer (at least 2 cm) than the malignant stricture.

The risk of food obstruction can also be reduced by a larger stent diameter. An internal stent cover (as is the case with Wallflex and Evolution stents) also precludes adherence of fibrous food to the stent mesh.

## Complications Associated with Concurrent Chemotherapy and/or Radiotherapy

In a palliative setting, combination treatment of stents with chemo- and/or radiotherapy is often avoided due to concerns for an increased risk for perforation, bleeding, or stent migration. In addition, potential scatter from the metal SEMS material may complicate radiation dosimetry and increase toxicity. The initial retrospective series indeed showed that administering high-dose radiotherapy (54–64 Gy) after SEMS placement was associated with high complication rates (up to 65%) [33, 34]. These complications mostly occurred after 9–11 weeks, which was suggested to be a late effect of radiotherapy. Homs et al. compared a group of patients stented with ($n=49$) or without prior chemo- and/or radiotherapy ($n=151$) [34]. Although major complications were not different between the two groups (29% vs. 29%, respectively), prior chemoradiation therapy increased the risk of minor complications, i.e., minor retrosternal pain (41% vs. 15%).

Two recently performed RCTs showed that combination stent and chemoradiation therapy was safe and effective. In one trial, 84 patients with inoperable esophageal cancer were randomized between Ultraflex stent placement combined with external beam radiotherapy (30 Gy in ten sessions) versus Ultraflex alone [35]. The combination group showed a more sustained relief of dysphagia (7 vs. 3 months, $p=0.002$) and prolonged overall survival (180 vs. 120 days, $p=0.009$). Furthermore, combination therapy also prolonged mean dysphagia-free adjusted survival (118.$\pm$55 vs. 96$\pm$43 days, respectively; $p=0.054$). Another RCT compared conventional SEMS (MTN; Nanjing Micro Invasive Medical,

Nanjing, China) with SEMS loaded with iodine-125 seeds for brachytherapy in 53 patients [36]. This study also showed a significantly longer dysphagia-free period and longer survival in the group treated with a SEMS loaded with iodine-125 seeds. Although hemorrhage occurred in 30% of cases in both groups, patients died at an earlier stage due to severe hemorrhage in the conventional stent group.

## Conclusions

While endoscopic stent placement for relief of malignant dysphagia is widely performed, the "ideal" stent, which is effective and without complications, has not been developed. In addition, there is remarkable lack of RCTs comparing different stent designs, and only uncontrolled series focusing on various stent-related issues such as migration, nontumoral tissue in- and overgrowth, and retrosternal pain are available.

In esophageal cancer, the focus of research with stents is shifting toward a combination of stent placement with more systemic treatments, such as chemotherapy, radiation therapy, or both. The effect of these combination treatments on the occurrence of complications needs to be established. For now, it is important to realize that stent placement is associated with complications in about a third of patients. One should attempt to minimize these complications and to treat such complications in an attempt to optimize quality of life in patients with malignant dysphagia.

## References

1. Siersema PD. New developments in palliative therapy. Best Pract Res Clin Gastroenterol. 2006;20:959–78.
2. Homs MY, Steyerberg EW, Eijkenboom WM, et al. Single-dose brachytherapy versus metal stent placement for the palliation of dysphagia from oesophageal cancer: multicentre randomised trial. Lancet. 2004;364:1497–504.
3. Wenger U, Johnsson E, Bergquist H, et al. Health economic evaluation of stent or endoluminal brachytherapy as a palliative strategy in patients with incurable cancer of the oesophagus or gastro-oesophageal junction: results of a randomized clinical trial. Eur J Gastroenterol Hepatol. 2005;17:1369–77.
4. Steyerberg EW, Homs MY, Stokvis A, et al. Stent placement or brachytherapy for palliation of dysphagia from esophageal cancer: a prognostic model to guide treatment selection. Gastrointest Endosc. 2005;62:333–40.
5. Sharma P, Kozarek R, Practice Parameters Committee of American College of Gastroenterology. Role of esophageal stents in benign and malignant diseases. Am J Gastroenterol. 2010;105:258–73.
6. Hirdes MM, Vleggaar FP, Van der Linde K, et al. Esophageal perforation due to removal of partially covered self-expanding metal stents placed for a benign perforation or leak. Endoscopy. 2011;43:156–9.
7. Conio M, Repici A, Battaglia G, et al. A randomized prospective comparison of self-expandable plastic stents and partially covered self-expandable metal stents in the palliation of malignant esophageal dysphagia. Am J Gastroenterol. 2007;102:2667–77.
8. Verschuur EM, Repici A, Kuipers EJ, et al. New design esophageal stents for the palliation of dysphagia from esophageal or gastric cardia cancer: a randomized trial. Am J Gastroenterol. 2008;103:304–12.
9. van Boeckel PG, Repici A, Vleggaar FP, et al. A new metal stent with a controlled-release system for palliation of malignant dysphagia: a prospective, multicenter study. Gastrointest Endosc. 2010;71:455–60.
10. van Boeckel PG, Siersema PD, Sturgess R, et al. A new partially covered metal stent for palliation of malignant dysphagia: a prospective follow-up study. Gastrointest Endosc. 2010;72:1269–73.
11. Siersema PD, Hop WC, van Blankenstein M, et al. A comparison of 3 types of covered metal stents for the palliation of patients with dysphagia caused by esophagogastric carcinoma: a prospective, randomized study. Gastrointest Endosc. 2001;54:145–53.
12. Kim ES, Jeon SW, Park SY, et al. Comparison of double-layered and covered Niti-S stents for palliation of malignant dysphagia. J Gastroenterol Hepatol. 2009; 24:114–9.
13. Verschuur EM, Homs MY, Steyerberg EW, et al. A new esophageal stent design (Niti-S stent) for the prevention of migration: a prospective study in 42 patients. Gastrointest Endosc. 2006;63:134–40.
14. Eloubeidi MA, Lopes TL. Novel removable internally fully covered self-expanding metal esophageal stent: feasibility, technique of removal, and tissue response in humans. Am J Gastroenterol. 2009;104:1374–81.
15. Uitdehaag MJ, Hooft JE, Verschuur EM, et al. A fully-covered stent (Alimaxx-E) for the palliation of malignant dysphagia: a prospective follow-up study. Gastrointest Endosc. 2009;70:1082–9.
16. Wilson JA, DeLegge MH. Attempted removal and subsequent fragmentation of 3 self-expanding metal stents. Gastrointest Endosc. 2009;70:391–3.
17. Senousy BE, Gupte AR, Draganov PV, et al. Fully covered Alimaxx esophageal metal stents in the endoscopic treatment of benign esophageal diseases. Dig Dis Sci. 2010;55:3399–403.
18. Uitdehaag MJ, Siersema PD, Spaander MCW, et al. A new fully covered stent with antimigration properties for

the palliation of malignant dysphagia: a prospective cohort study. Gastrointest Endosc. 2010;71:600–5.

19. Ogilvie AL, Dronfield MW, Ferguson R, et al. Palliative intubation of oesophagogastric neoplasms at fibreoptic endoscopy. Gut. 1982;23:1060–7.

20. Sabharwal T, Hamady MS, Chui S, et al. A randomised prospective comparison of the Flamingo Wallstent and Ultraflex stent for palliation of dysphagia associated with lower third oesophageal carcinoma. Gut. 2003;52:922–6.

21. Hirdes MMC, Vleggaar FP, Siersema PD. Stent placement for esophageal strictures: an update review. Expert Rev Med Devices. 2011;8:733–55.

22. Homs MY, Wahab PJ, Kuipers EJ, et al. Esophageal stents with antireflux valve for tumors of the distal esophagus and gastric cardia: a randomized trial. Gastrointest Endosc. 2004;60:695–702.

23. Dua KS, Kozarek R, Kim J, et al. Self-expanding metal esophageal stent with anti-reflux mechanism. Gastrointest Endosc. 2001;53:603–13.

24. Lee S, Osugi H, Tokuhara T, et al. Self-expandable metallic stents with an anti-reflux mechanism for malignant strictures of gastroesophageal junction. Scand J Gastroenterol. 2002;37:990–1.

25. Laasch HU, Marriott A, Wilbraham L, et al. Effectiveness of open versus antireflux stents for palliation of distal esophageal carcinoma and prevention of symptomatic gastroesophageal reflux. Radiology. 2002;225:359–65.

26. Sabharwal T, Gulati MS, Fotiadis N, et al. Randomised comparison of the FerX Ella antireflux stent and the Ultraflex stent: proton pump inhibitor combination for prevention of post-stent reflux in patients with esophageal carcinoma involving the esophago-gastric junction. J Gastroenterol Hepatol. 2008;23:723–8.

27. Power C, Byrne PJ, Lim K, et al. Superiority of antireflux stent compared with conventional stents in the palliative management of patients with cancer of the lower esophagus and esophago-gastric junction:

results of a randomized clinical trial. Dis Esophagus. 2007;20:466–70.

28. Shim CS, Jung IS, Cheon YK, et al. Management of malignant stricture of the esophagogastric junction with a newly designed self-expanding metal stent with an antireflux mechanism. Endoscopy. 2005;37:335–9.

29. Homs MY, Steyerberg EW, Kuipers EJ, et al. Causes and treatment of recurrent dysphagia after self-expanding metal stent placement for palliation of esophageal carcinoma. Endoscopy. 2004;36:880–6.

30. Verschuur EM, Steyerberg EW, Kuipers EJ, et al. Effect of stent size on complications and recurrent dysphagia in patients with esophageal or gastric cardia cancer. Gastrointest Endosc. 2007;65:592–601.

31. Ko HK, Song HY, Shin JH, et al. Fate of migrated esophageal and gastroduodenal stents: experience in 70 patients. J Vasc Interv Radiol. 2007;18:725–32.

32. Zhang W, Meng WJ, Zhou ZG. Multiple perforations of the jejunum caused by a migrated esophageal stent. Endoscopy. 2011;43(Suppl 2):E145–6.

33. Nishimura Y, Nagata K, Katano S, et al. Severe complications in advanced esophageal cancer treated with radiotherapy after intubation of esophageal stents: a questionnaire survey of the Japanese Society for Esophageal Diseases. Int J Radiat Oncol Biol Phys. 2003;56:1327–32.

34. Homs MY, Hansen BE, van Blankenstein M, et al. Prior radiation and/or chemotherapy has no effect on the outcome of metal stent placement for oesophagogastric carcinoma. Eur J Gastroenterol Hepatol. 2004;16:163–70.

35. Javed A, Pal S, Dash NR, et al. Palliative stenting with or without radiotherapy for inoperable esophageal carcinoma: a randomized trial. J Gastrointest Cancer. 2012;43:63–9.

36. Guo JH, Teng GJ, Zhu GY, et al. Self-expandable esophageal stent loaded with 125I seeds: initial experience in patients with advanced esophageal cancer. Radiology. 2008;247:574–81.

Todd Baron and Richard A. Kozarek

Over the last 20–25 years, self-expandable metal stents (SEMS) have been used for palliation of malignant dysphagia and tracheoesophageal fistula. In Chap. 5, the available devices for esophageal use are described, and in Chap. 9, the indications for stent placement in benign disease are discussed. This chapter reviews the results for the use of expandable stents for the treatment of benign esophageal disease.

## Basic Principles

Partially covered SEMS (PCSEMS) and subsequently fully covered SEMS (FCSEMS) were developed to prolong the patency of uncovered SEMS. As discussed in Chap. 4, the histology and tissue responses to expandable metal stents are known from animal, autopsy, and surgical studies. Uncovered stents embed into tissue are nonremovable soon after placement and should not be used for benign disease except in extreme circumstances where other comorbidities are present and the patient otherwise has a limited life expectancy [1].

T. Baron, M.D. (✉)
Department of Medicine, Mayo Clinic,
200 First Street SW, Rochester, MN 55905, USA
e-mail: baron.todd@mayo.edu

R.A. Kozarek, M.D.
Digestive Disease Institute, Virginia Mason Medical
Center and University of Washington, 1100 9th Ave.,
C3-GAS, Seattle, WA 98111, USA

The covered portion of a SEMS prevents embedding of the metal wires into the surrounding tissue. Although temporary placement of PCSEMS has been used for treatment of benign esophageal strictures, tissue entrapment by hyperplasia occurs in the uncovered portion soon after placement and makes their removal difficult (sometimes impossible) and traumatic [2–4]. While the stent-in-stent technique of placing a FCSEMS [5] or SEPS [6] inside a PCSEMS to allow removal has been validated, PCSEMS should not be considered the first option for treatment of benign esophageal diseases. The use of PCSEMS may be considered for the management of benign diseases in patients who have experienced migration of FCSEMS [3] and/or SEPS before resolution of the underlying disease process. However, new strictures resulting from mechanical injury of the uncovered portion(s) of the stent may occur. Stent migration is more likely to occur with covered SEMS and SEPS than uncovered SEMS because of the lack of embedding into the esophageal wall.

FCSEMS are removable as long as the covering remains intact [7]. This lack of embedding has led to their temporary use for benign diseases, although most of these devices are not approved for benign disease and thus, for benign indications, are used *off-label* [8].

Self-expandable plastic stents (SEPS) do not embed, are also removable, and, although approved for malignancy, are mostly used – and approved for – treatment of benign esophageal disease (specifically refractory strictures).

R. Kozarek et al. (eds.), *Self-Expandable Stents in the Gastrointestinal Tract*,
DOI 10.1007/978-1-4614-3746-8_14, © Springer Science+Business Media New York 2013

Recently, biodegradable esophageal SEMS (BDSEMS) have been developed which are designed to preclude the need for removal. One such stent has Conformité Européenne (CE) approval for the treatment of benign strictures [9].

## Indications

There are several indications for placement of self-expandable stents for benign esophageal disease. The most common indications are treatment of benign refractory strictures, leaks, fistulas, and perforations. Less common indications include treatment of variceal bleeding, achalasia, and miscellaneous diseases. The results for these indications using the various types of stents will be discussed separately.

## Results

## Strictures

The standard therapy for esophageal strictures is dilation using either bougie or balloon dilators. In patients with refractory strictures that fail to respond or recur soon after serial dilation, with or without steroid injection, expandable stents have been used (Figs. 14.1 and 14.2).

### Uncovered SEMS

Prior to the development of CSEMS, SEPS, and biodegradable self-expandable stents (BDSES), uncovered open cell SEMS were used to treat benign strictures [10]. Unfortunately, tissue hyperplasia with resultant recurrence of strictures

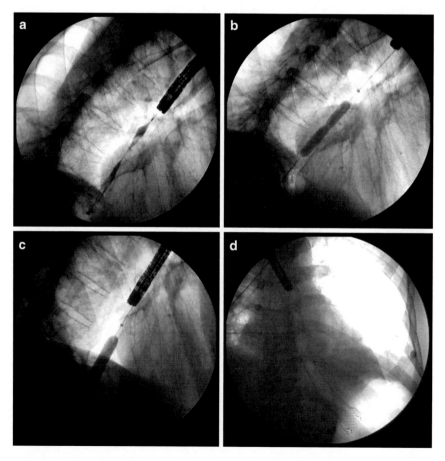

**Fig. 14.1** High-grade refractory (**a**) patient with prolapsed NG tube placement treated with balloon dilation (**b**, **c**) and fully covered self-expandable metal stent (**d**)

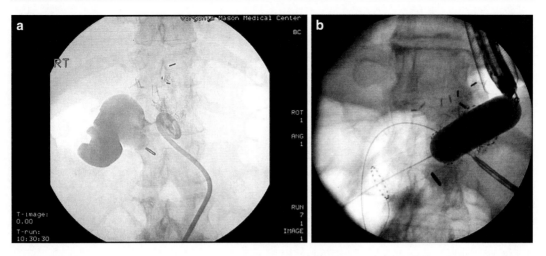

**Fig. 14.2** Chronic gastric fistula in a patient who underwent gastric stapling procedure for obesity (**a**) treated with Polyflex stent passed through overtube. Note balloon used to position Polyflex at center of the leak (**b**)

developed and these stents were nonremovable [10]. A coiled metal stent without interstices was placed in ten patients with refractory peptic, post-surgical, or postradiation esophageal strictures [11]. Although marked improvement of dysphagia was achieved, proximal and distal migration occurred in three patients and a proximal stricture occurred in another. Esophageal perforation occurred in one patient during an attempt to endoscopically remove a broken stent. Thus, for multiple reasons, uncovered SEMS are no longer used for treatment of benign strictures because of long-term complications.

### Partially Covered SEMS

There are few studies on the use of PCSEMS for the treatment of benign, refractory strictures. Early studies suggested there was potential applications and removability for benign disease [12]. In an excellent review of the available literature, which is comprised of retrospective studies, complication rates as high as 80% were reported and included new stricture formation in 41%, stent migration in 31%, pain or reflux in 21%, and fistula formation in 6%.[13].

### Fully Covered SEMS

In most countries, FCSEMS are now being used regularly *off-label* for benign strictures. There are a variety of FCSEMS available. A recent meta-analysis of studies published from January 1965 to June 2010 was performed to determine the efficacy of both FCSEMS and SEPS for treatment of refractory esophageal strictures caused by a variety of etiologies [14]. Eight studies with a total of 199 patients were included in the final analysis. Only two studies included FCSEMS [15, 16]. Overall, 46.2% of patients (95% CI 38.3–54.1%) had dysphagia improvement at an average follow-up of 74 weeks. There was a significant difference in dysphagia improvement for patients with SEPS (55.3%, 95% CI = 44.4–65.9%) versus SEMS (21.8%; 95% CI 13.7–33.7%). Factors such as patient gender, age, stricture etiology, stricture location, stricture length, time of removal, and duration of follow-up were not found to influence outcome. The overall migration rate of FCSEMS was 26.4% (95% CI 25.3–39.3%).

Other studies using FCSEMS for refractory strictures not included in the above meta-analysis have been published with mixed results [17–20]. In one study of 24 patients with refractory strictures, FCSEMS with anti-reflux valves were placed [17]. After 12 months of follow-up, 18 patients were dysphagia free. Ultimately, stricture recurrence occurred in nearly 40%. The three other studies showed long-term success rates ranging from approximately 30% to 86% and migration rates of approximately 35–40%. Thus, although it appears there is excellent short-term response to FCSEMS placement, the relapse rate is variable and dependent on the underlying disease process, and there are relatively high migration rates [13, 21].

## Self-Expandable Plastic Stents

A systematic review of studies published between 2003 and 2008 in patients who underwent SEPS placement for refractory or recurrent benign esophageal strictures included data from 10 studies (3 prospective) totaling 130 patients [22]. All patients had dysphagia at the time of SEPS insertion and had failed or recurred following one or more endoscopic dilation sessions. Stricture etiologies were postsurgical in 49 (39%), postradiation in 20 (15%), peptic in 16 (12%), and corrosive in 33 (25%) cases and other disorders in the remaining 12 (9%) patients. Stricture location was at the level of the upper esophagus in 48 (49%) cases, mid-esophagus in 36 (36%), and lower esophagus in 15 (15%) cases. In approximately half of patients, the stricture length was <2 cm. SEPS insertion was technically successful in 128 of 130 patients (98%, 95% CI = 96–100%). Median follow-up after SEPS insertion was 13 months, ranging from 6 to 23 months. At the end of this follow-up period, 68 of 130 patients were symptom free without need for further dilations, corresponding to a success rate of 52% (95% CI = 44–61%). Success was found to be significantly lower in patients with strictures in the upper esophagus than those with a mid- or lower stricture (33% vs. 54%, $P < 0.05$). Counterintuitively, the success rate was higher in patients with strictures >2 cm in length (49% vs. 28%, $P = 0.07$) (Table 14.1). Early stent migration (<4 weeks after placement) occurred in 19 (24%, 95% CI = 14–32%) cases. Post-insertion endoscopic re-intervention was needed in 25 patients (21%, 95% CI = 14–28%). Major clinical complications occurred in 12 patients (9%, 95% CI = 4–14%), including perforation, and in death in one patient.

Data from another institution, which were not included in the previously mentioned review, included 83 stent placements in 30 patients over a 5-year period [23]. Twenty-two stents were

**Table 14.1** Complications of esophageal self-expandable stents for benign disease

| Immediate |
| --- |
| Aspiration |
| Airway compromise |
| Malposition |
| Delivery system entrapment |
| Stent dislodgement |
| Perforation |
| Early |
| Bleeding |
| Chest pain |
| Nausea |
| Late |
| GERD/aspiration |
| Re-obstruction |
| Granulation tissue/tissue hyperplasia |
| Food impaction |
| Migration |
| Tracheoesophageal fistula |
| Bleeding |

placed for benign strictures, including reflux disease [4], ischemic [1], infection [1], and idiopathic or unknown [14]; 25 were placed for postsurgical anastomotic strictures, and 14 stents were placed for strictures resulting from prior radiation therapy. Stents remained in place for an average of 53 days (range 1–331 days, SD 58.2 days). Patients had initial symptomatic improvement after 77 of 83 stents placed (92.8%), but long-term relief of symptoms after stent removal was low (<10%) and stent migration was high (>50%). Overall, it does not appear that the outcome following FCSEMS is significantly different than that of SEPS, although randomized trials are lacking.

## Biodegradable Self-Expandable Stents

Biodegradable self-expandable stents (BDSES) are made from polylactic acid filaments which dissolve and absorb at variable intervals depending on the composition, but usually within 2–3 months after placement. Since the first case report in 1997, there have been multiple reports using BDSES for benign strictures showing feasibility of placement and radial force comparable to or greater than SEMS [24–28].

In one prospective study, the efficacy and safety of a biodegradable stent (Ella-BD stent, Ella-CS [Czech Republic]) in 21 patients with refractory benign esophageal strictures was assessed [29]. Stent placement was technically successful in all patients. Stent migration occurred in two patients (9.5%). After a follow-up of 6 months, 9 of 20 patients (45%) were free of dysphagia. No major complications occurred, but three patients developed severe post-stent pain requiring analgesics.

In another case series, 10 consecutive patients with symptomatic esophagogastric anastomotic strictures that occurred within 6 months after surgery and had short strictures (<3 cm), were >1.5 cm distal to the upper esophageal sphincter, and had not received previous endoscopic treatment underwent placement of a BDSES [9]. In six patients, BDSES stent placement provided a one-step treatment without the need for re-intervention during 6 months of follow-up. Re-obstruction occurred in four patients due to food impaction. Two patients had obstruction caused by hyperplasia (103–109 days after stent placement, respectively), and one patient had stricture recurrence (132 days after stent placement). Symptoms resolved after serial dilation. The mean dysphagia scores at 1 week, 3 months, and 6 months were significantly improved compared to baseline. No patient developed stent-related pain that required narcotics. At follow-up endoscopy, performed per protocol 3 months after stent placement, three stents were completely dissolved. None of the partially dissolved stents caused luminal obstruction. Tissue hyperplasia occurred in 6/10 patients, in which two were symptomatic.

Most recently, two groups of consecutively treated patients with refractory benign strictures underwent either temporary SEPS placement for 6 weeks ($n=20$) or BDSES ($n=18$); data were prospectively entered but compared retrospectively [30]. SEPS were removed in 16 (80%) patients. Stent placement was not successful in one patient, while stent removal was not performed in 3. Six (30%) patients in the SEPS group were dysphagia free after a median follow-up of 385 days (range 77–924 days). Ten (50%) developed recurrent dysphagia. Major complications occurred in two patients (1 bleeding and 1 perforation). Six patients (33%) in the BDSES group were dysphagia free after a median follow-up of 166 days (range 21–559 days). Twelve patients (67%) had recurrent dysphagia. Major complications occurred in four patients (bleeding and severe retrosternal pain in two patients each). Re-interventions were required less frequently after BDSES stent than after SEPS placement.

## Leaks, Fistulae, and Perforations

Esophageal leaks and fistulae are usually due to postoperative causes. The traditional therapy for leaks is drain placement to control the leak, surgical intervention, and avoidance of oral intake to promote leak closure. Unfortunately, if the leaks do not close with this approach, chronic fistulas develop and are much more difficult to close. Thus, early closure is more successful than closure of well-established fistula. Perforations are most often iatrogenic following dilation or transesophageal radiofrequency ablation for atrial arrhythmias but may also be spontaneous (Boerhaave's syndrome). For the purposes of this chapter, leaks, fistula, and perforations will be grouped together with the understanding that the outcomes will vary but the fundamental principle is sealing of the leak.

PCSEMS, FCSEMS, and covered BDSES have all been successfully used to close leaks, perforation, and fistulae (Figs. 14.3 and 14.4). A recent pooled analysis of available data for treatment of benign esophageal ruptures and anastomotic leaks with temporary stent placement using PCSEMS, FCSEMS, and SEPS was performed to ascertain the affect of various stent types [31]. Twenty-five studies which included 267 patients with complete follow-up on outcome were identified. Clinical success was achieved in 85% of patients and was not different between stent types (SEPS 84%, FCSEMS 85%, and PCSEMS 86%). Time of stent placement was longest for SEPS (8 weeks) followed by FCSEMS and PCSEMS (6 weeks). In total, 65 (34%) patients had a stent-related complication. Stent migration occurred more often with SEPS [$n=47$ (31%)] and FCSEMS [$n=7$ (26%)] than with PSEMS

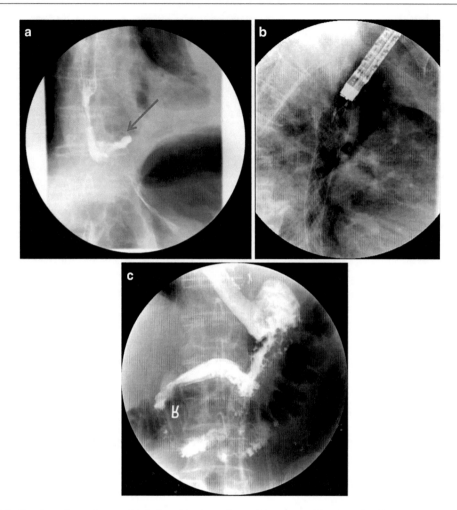

**Fig. 14.3** Boerhaave's syndrome with leak at distal esophagus (**a**) treated with covered self-expandable metal stent which is clipped x 2 to help minimize migration (**b**). UGI showing proper position, no leak (**c**)

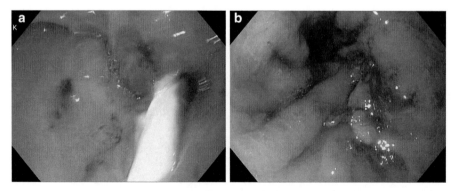

**Fig. 14.4** Esophageal fistula after second redo fundoplication. (**a**) A drain is present in the esophageal lumen causing a persistent fistula. A fully covered SEMS was placed and the drain removed. (**b**) Endoscopy 3 weeks later after stent removal shows the fistula site is closed

[$n=2$ (12%), $P \leq 0.001$], whereas there was no significant difference in tissue hyperplasia between PCSEMS [12% vs. 7% (FCSEMS) and 3% (SEPS), $P=0.68$]. Despite the absence of randomized controlled trials treating patients with surgery alone versus stent placement, the authors feel that covered stent placement for 6–8 weeks is safe and effective for closure of most benign esophageal ruptures and anastomotic leaks. Stent choice should be determined on an individual basis with factors such as stent migration when FCSEMS and SEPS are used, and risk of tissue hyperplasia and embedding when placing partially covered self-expanding metal stents.

There are scant data on the use of BDSES for closure of leaks and perforations, but in one study, five patients with anastomotic leaks or benign esophageal perforations were treated by placement of covered BDSES [32]. Postoperative anastomotic leaks were treated in four patients (1 after esophagectomy, 1 after resection of diverticulum, 2 after gastrectomy). In one patient, a perforation as a result of balloon dilatation of a benign stricture was closed. Seven covered BDSES were placed in these five patients. Clinical success (leak sealing) was achieved in four of the five patients (80%). Stent migration occurred in three patients. In two of these patients, the leak had been sealed by the time of stent migration and re-intervention was not necessary. Numerous other publications have shown benefits of CSEMS and SEPS for management of acute perforations and leaks with good results in the majority of patients [33–38].

## Variceal Bleeding

Potential indications for esophageal stent placement in the setting of varices include not only refractory variceal bleeding but also post-variceal band-induced or sclerotherapy-induced ulcer bleeding [39]. Thus far, FCSEMS have been used and been left in place for 48 h and up to 14 days [40–42]. SEMS allow patient stabilization for elective TIPS or avoidance of TIPS in patents in which it is contraindicated because of hepatic encephalopathy. In one study of 20 patients with massive, ongoing bleeding from esophageal varices in whom prior pharmacologic or endoscopic therapy failed, bleeding ceased immediately after SEMS placement in all cases. No recurrent bleeding, morbidity, or mortality occurred during SEMS placement, and all stents were extracted without complications after definitive treatment had been initiated [40]. In another study, 10 patients with variceal hemorrhage and contraindications to TIPS insertion or balloon tamponade underwent SEMS placement. Failure to control bleeding occurred in two patients (2 with gastric varices). Six patients survived the acute bleeding episode, and stents were removed endoscopically a median of 9 days after insertion. There are no cases of SEPS or BDSEMS reported for treatment of variceal bleeding.

## Achalasia

There are multiple studies showing the efficacy of temporary placement of very large diameter esophageal stents for the treatment of achalasia with comparable results to pneumatic dilation [43–47]. Long-term efficacy of these prostheses is uncertain in this setting (Fig. 14.5).

## Miscellaneous Diseases

There is only one report on using SEMS for relief of dysphagia due to extrinsic compression from benign disease. In this patient, a partially covered SEMS was placed for relief of dysphagia due to aortic compression in an elderly, nonoperative patient after a SEPS had migrated [48]. Because of the risk of long-term complications, SEMS in this setting should be reserved for patients considered to be prohibitive-risk operative candidates. To date, there are no other reports of benign extrinsic compression and none using self-expandable plastic stents SEPS or BDSES. There is one unusual report of a razor blade-induced bleeding episode successfully managed with an esophageal stent [49]. Additionally, there are reports of using a CSEMS for temporary closure of an aortoesophageal fistula as a bridge to surgery [50]. Finally, small caliber biliary CSEMS have been used to maintain patency of

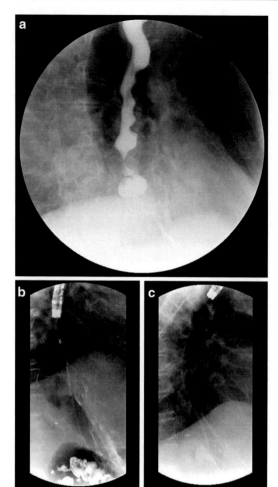

**Fig. 14.5** Barium swallow. A high-risk achalasia patient (**a**) treated with covered esophageal stent (**b, c**). Repeated stent migration into the stomach despite multiple clip placements

an esophageal neo-lumen after rendezvous reconnection of the proximal esophagus in patients who developed aphagia and esophageal obliteration after radiation for head and neck cancer [51] (Fig. 14.6).

## Complications

Complications of SEMS for benign disease are similar to that of malignant disease, and the common complications are listed in Table 14.1 and may be classified as intraprocedural and postprocedural (immediate and delayed). Procedure-related complications after SEMS placement have

remained fairly stable over the years and mainly consist of perforation, aspiration pneumonia, hemorrhage, and severe pain, the latter occurring in approximately 10% of patients. Delayed complications following stent placement include bleeding, fistula formation, GE reflux, stent migration, food bolus obstruction, and embedding of uncovered portions at either end of the stent. Repositioning or removal of a migrated stent can be achieved if tissue ingrowth has not occurred using a retrieval forceps, an inflated balloon catheter, or a polypectomy snare.

Most experts advocate the use of proton-pump inhibitors (PPIs) for patients in whom the stent crosses the lower esophageal sphincter to prevent reflux symptoms. PPIs improve reflux symptoms, but not the risk of aspiration. FCSEMS with an anti-reflux mechanism are available.

Complications associated with SEPS are similar to those associated with SEMS [52]. The need for repeat stent placement ranges from 24% to 100% in cases reported to date. Stent migration is the most common complication with frequency ranging from 7% to 75% of the cases. Overall, the rate of migration of SEPS seems to be higher than that of PCSEMS. In most instances, the stents have been removed endoscopically, and anecdotal reports on the use of endoscopic clips to secure the stent to the mucosa are disappointing. The presence of short strictures and proximal as well as distal strictures is one of the factors that may promote stent migration. In addition, the risk of fatal bleeding from SEPS placement needs to be emphasized to the patient and caregivers.

Less common complications following self-expandable stent placement include epidural abscess [53], tracheoesophageal fistula [54], and acute bronchial obstruction even in the absence of a stricture [55]. Unusual complications of BDSES include severe epithelial hyperplasia [56] and stent collapse with esophageal obstruction [57].

## Conclusions

The use of self-expandable stents seems to be safe and effective for the treatment of a variety of benign esophageal diseases, especially for closure of anastomotic leaks and perforations. However,

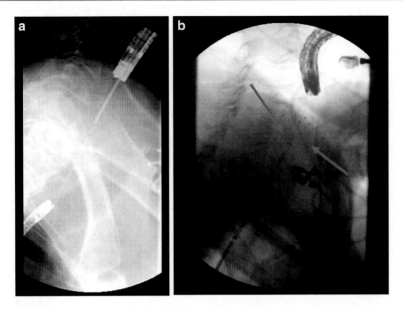

**Fig. 14.6** Rendezvous reconnection of hypopharynx and proximal esophagus working through the mouth and percutaneous endoscopic gastrostomy (PEG) tract, respectively (**a**) (*arrows*), through the PEG tract under per os direct visualization (**b**)

the data on benign esophageal strictures has been mixed. Multicenter, prospective studies are needed to evaluate the late-complication rate and long-term effectiveness in this latter, difficult-to-treat patient population.

# References

1. Kozarek RA. Expandable endoprostheses for gastrointestinal stenoses. Gastr Endosc Clin North Am. 1994;4:279–95.
2. Hirdes MM, Vleggaar FP, Van der Linde K, et al. Esophageal perforation due to removal of partially covered self-expanding metal stents placed for a benign perforation or leak. Endoscopy. 2011;43:156–9.
3. Baron TH. Esophageal avulsion following removal of a partially covered esophageal stent: lessons learned 10 year later. Clin Gastroenterol Hepatol. 2012;10:e1.
4. van Heel NC, Haringsma J, Wijnhoven BP, Kuipers EJ. Endoscopic removal of self-expandable metal stents from the esophagus (with video). Gastrointest Endosc. 2011;74:44–50.
5. Hirdes MM, Siersema PD, Houben MH, et al. Stent-in-stent technique for removal of embedded esophageal self-expanding metal stents. Am J Gastroenterol. 2011;106:286–93.
6. Evrard S, Le Moine O, Lazaraki G, et al. Self-expanding plastic stents for benign esophageal lesions. Gastrointest Endosc. 2004;60:894–900.
7. Choi EK, Song HY, Shin JH, Kim JW. Removal of a covered esophageal metallic stent 8 years after placement. J Vasc Interv Radiol. 2007;18:317–20.
8. Freeman RK, Ascioti AJ. Esophageal stent placement for the treatment of perforation, fistula, or anastomotic leak. Semin Thorac Cardiovasc Surg. 2011;23:154–8.
9. van Hooft JE, van Berge Henegouwen MI, Rauws EA, et al. Endoscopic treatment of benign anastomotic esophagogastric strictures with a biodegradable stent. Gastrointest Endosc. 2011;73:1043–7.
10. Tan BS, Kennedy C, Morgan R, et al. Using uncovered metallic endoprostheses to treat recurrent benign esophageal strictures. AJR Am J Roentgenol. 1997;169:1281–4.
11. Fiorini A, Fleischer D, Valero J, et al. Self-expandable metal coil stents in the treatment of benign esophageal strictures refractory to conventional therapy: a case series. Gastrointest Endosc. 2000;52:259–62.
12. Low DE, Kozarek RA. Removal of esophageal expandable metal stents: description of technique and review of potential applications. Surg Endosc. 2003;17:990–6.
13. Hirdes MM, Vleggaar FP, Siersema PD. Stent placement for esophageal strictures: an update. Expert Rev Med Devices. 2011;8:733–55.
14. Thomas T, Abrams KR, Subramanian V, et al. Esophageal stents for benign refractory strictures: a meta-analysis. Endoscopy. 2011;43:386–93.
15. Kim JH, Song Hy, Choi EK, et al. Temporary metallic stent placement in the treatment of refractory benign esophageal strictures: results and factors associated

with outcome in 55 patients. Eur Radiol. 2009; 19:384–90.

16. Song Ho-Y, Jung H, Park S, et al. Covered retrievable expandable nitinol stents in patients with benign esophageal strictures: initial experience. Radiology. 2000;217:551–7.

17. Liu J, Hu Y, Cui C, et al. Removable, fully covered, self-expandable metal stents for the treatment of refractory benign esophagogastric anastomotic strictures. Dysphagia. 2011 (Epub ahead of print).

18. Senousy BE, Gupte AR, Draganov PV, et al. Fully covered Alimaxx esophageal metal stents in the endoscopic treatment of benign esophageal diseases. Dig Dis Sci. 2010;55:3399–403.

19. Bakken JC, Song Kee Song LM, de Groen PC, Baron TH. Use of a fully covered self-expandable metal stent for the treatment of benign esophageal diseases. Gastrointest Endosc. 2010;72:712–20.

20. Eloubeidi MA, Talreja JP, Lopes TL, et al. Success and complications associated with placement of fully covered removable self-expandable metal stents for benign esophageal diseases (with videos). Gastrointest Endosc. 2011;73:673–81.

21. Kochman ML. Removable endoprosthetics in the management of esophageal pathology: all strictures and fistulae are not created equal.... Gastrointest Endosc. 2008;67:26–7.

22. Repici A, Hassan C, Sharma P, et al. Systematic review: the role of self-expanding plastic stents for benign oesophageal strictures. Aliment Pharmacol Ther. 2010;31:1268–75.

23. Holm AM, De La Mora Levy JG, Baron TH, Gostout CJ. Self-expanding plastic stents in treatment of benign esophageal conditions. Gastrointest Endosc. 2008;67:20–5.

24. Fry SW, Fleischer D. Management of a refractory benign esophageal stricture with a new biodegradable stent. Gastrointest Endosc. 1997;45:179–82.

25. Saito Y, Tanaka T, Andoh A, et al. Novel biodegradable stents for benign esophageal strictures following endoscopic submucosal dissection. Dig Dis Sci. 2008;53:330–3.

26. Saito Y, Tanaka T, Andoh A, et al. Usefulness of biodegradable stents constructed of poly-1-lactic acid monofilaments in patients with benign esophageal stenosis. World J Gastroenterol. 2007;13:3977–80.

27. Tanaka T, Takahashi M, Nitta N, et al. Newly developed biodegradable stents for benign gastrointestinal tract stenoses: a preliminary clinical trial. Digestion. 2006;74:199–205.

28. Stivaros SM, Williams LR, Senger C. Woven polydioxanone biodegradable stents: a new treatment option for benign and malignant oesophageal strictures. Eur Radiol. 2010;20:1069–72.

29. Repici A, Vleggaar FP, Hassan C, et al. Efficacy and safety of biodegradable stents for refractory benign esophageal strictures: the BEST (Biodegradable Esophageal Stent) study. Gastrointest Endosc. 2010; 72:927–34.

30. van Boeckel PG, Vleggaar FP, Siersema Pd. A comparison of temporary self-expanding plastic and biodegradable stents for refractory benign esophageal strictures. Clin Gastroenterol Hepatol. 2011;9:653–9.

31. van Boeckel PG, Sijbring A, Vleggaar FP, Siersema PD. Systematic review: temporary stent placement for benign rupture or anastomotic leak of the oesophagus. Aliment Pharmacol Ther. 2011;33:1292–301.

32. Cerná M, Köcher M, Válek V, et al. Covered biodegradable stent: new therapeutic option for the management of esophageal perforation or anastomotic leak. Cardiovasc Intervent Radiol. 2011;34:1267–71.

33. van Heel NC, Haringsma S, Spaander MC, et al. Short-term esophageal stenting in the management of benign perforations. Am J Gastroenterol. 2010; 105:1515–20.

34. Buscaglia JM, Ho S, Sethi A, et al. Fully covered self-expandable metal stents for benign esophageal disease: a multicenter retrospective case series of 31 patients. Gastrointest Endosc. 2011;74:207–11.

35. D'Cunha J, Rueth NM, Groth SS, et al. Esophageal stents for anastomotic leaks and perforations. J Thorac Cardiovasc Surg. 2011;142:39–46.e1.

36. Freeman RK, Vyverberg A, Ascioti AJ. Esophageal stent placement for the treatment of acute intrathoracic anastomotic leak after esophagectomy. Ann Thorac Surg. 2011;92:204–8.

37. Swinnen J, Eisendrath P, Rigaux J, et al. Self-expandable metal stents for the treatment of benign upper GI leaks and perforations. Gastrointest Endosc. 2011;73:890–9.

38. Dai Y, Chopra SS, Kneif S, H nerbein M. Management of esophageal anastomotic leaks, perforations, and fistulae with self-expanding plastic stents. J Thorac Cardiovasc Surg. 2011;141:1213–7.

39. Escorsell A, Bosch J. Self-expandable metal stents in the treatment of acute esophageal variceal bleeding. Gastr Res Pract. 2011;2011:910986.

40. Hubmann R, Bodlaj G, Czompo M, et al. The use of self-expanding metal stents to treat acute esophageal variceal bleeding. Endoscopy. 2006;38:896–901.

41. Mishin I, Ghidirim G, Dolghii A, et al. Implantation of self-expanding metal stent in the treatment of severe bleeding from esophageal ulcer and endoscopic band ligation. Dig Esophagus. 2010;23:E35–8.

42. Wright G, Lewis H, Hogan B, et al. A self-expanding metal stent for complicated variceal hemorrhage: experience at a single center. Gastrointest Endosc. 2010;71:71–8.

43. Li YD, Tang GY, Cheng YS, et al. 13-year follow-up of a prospective comparison of the long-term clinical efficacy of temporary self-expanding metallic stents and pneumatic dilatation for the treatment of achalasia in 120 patients. AJR Am J Roentgenol. 2010; 195:1429–37.

44. Cheng YS, Ma F, Li YD, et al. Temporary self-expanding metallic stents for achalasia: a prospective study with a long-term follow-up. World J Gastroenterol. 2010;16:5111–7.

45. Li YD, Cheng YS, Li MH, et al. Temporary self-expanding metallic stents and pneumatic dilation for the treatment of achalasia: a prospective study with a long-term follow-up. Dig Esophagus. 2010;23:361–7.

46. Zhu YQ, Cheng YS, Tang GY, et al. Comparison of temporary stent insertion with pneumatic dilation of the same diameter in the treatment of achalasia patients: a retrospective study. J Gastroenterol Hepatol. 2010;25:499–505.

47. Zhao JG, Li YD, Cheng YS, et al. Long-term safety and outcome of a temporary self-expanding metallic stent for achalasia: a prospective study with a 13-year single-center experience. Eur Radiol. 2009;19:1973–80.

48. Coelho-Prabhu N, Baron TH. Dysphagia and weight loss in an elderly person. Dysphagia aortica Gastroenterology. 2009;137:e1–2.

49. Kaya E, Lenz P, Lebiedq P, et al. Placement of covered self-expanding metal stent to treat razor blade-induced esophageal hemorrhage. Endoscopy. 2010;42(Suppl 2):E201–2.

50. Tsai SM, Chen YY, Chin-Yuan Y, Lai WL. Closure of an aortoesophageal fistula with an esophageal stent and hemoclip. Endoscopy. 2011;43 (Suppl2):UCTN: E302–E3.

51. Schembre D, Dever JB, Glenn M, et al. Esophageal reconstitution by simultaneous antegrade/retrograde endoscopy: re-establishing patency of the completely obstructed esophagus. Endoscopy. 2011;43:434–7.

52. Sharma P, Kozarek R. Practice parameters committee of the American college of gastroenterology. Role of esophageal stents in benign and malignant diseases. Am J Gastroen. 2010;105:258–73.

53. Boulis NM, Armstrong WS, Changler WF, Orringer MB. Epidural abscess: a delayed complication of esophageal stenting for benign stricture. Ann Thorac Surg. 1999;68:568–70.

54. Jung GE, Sauer P, Schaible A. Tracheoesophageal fistula following implantation of a biodegradable stent for a refractory benign esophageal stricture. Endoscopy. 2010;42(Suppl 2):E338–9.

55. Dechene A, Adamzik M, Gerken G, Canbay A. Acute bronchial obstruction following esophageal stent implantation for variceal bleeding. Endoscopy. 2009; 41(Suppl2):E146–7.

56. Orive-Calzada A, Alvarez-Rubio M, Romero-Izquierdo S, et al. Severe epithelial hyperplasia as a complication of a novel biodegradable stent. Endoscopy. 2009;41(Suppl 2):E137–8.

57. Nogales Rincon O, Huerta Madrigal A, Merino Rodriguez B, et al. Esophageal obstruction due to a collapsed biodegradable esophageal stent. Endoscopy. 2011;43 (Suppl 2):UCTN:E189–E190.

# Self-Expanding Metallic Stents for Malignant Hilar Biliary Obstruction

# 15

## Mustafa A. Tiewala and Martin L. Freeman

Management of malignant hilar biliary obstruction represents a major challenge for therapeutic endoscopists. There is substantial controversy regarding the optimal method for diagnosis and palliation of jaundice with respect to timing, route, method, and extent of drainage. Traditional methods of endoscopic retrograde cholangiography (ERCP) and drainage using standard opacification techniques and plastic stents have generally resulted in poor outcomes with ineffective palliation and frequent complications, especially cholangitis. Optimal results of diagnosis, staging, curative resection, and/or palliation are achieved using an advanced multidisciplinary team approach that incorporates maximal noninvasive imaging before any intervention is undertaken. It is important to decide in advance whether a patient is a candidate for surgical resection and determine further evaluation and therapy accordingly. Newly refined techniques including endoscopic ultrasound with fine needle aspiration, multidetector CT, and especially MRI and MRCP facilitate accurate diagnosis, evaluation, and staging of disease and allow optimal planning of drainage for the endoscopist or inter-

ventional radiologist if indicated. Tissue diagnosis can be made by ERCP with brush cytology, by forceps biopsy obtained under fluoroscopic guidance or under direct cholangioscopy, and by endoscopic ultrasound with fine needle aspiration, particularly of surrounding masses or lymph nodes. Intraductal ultrasound may occasionally assist with differentiation of malignant from benign obstruction, but has the disadvantage of requiring ERCP and does not provide a tissue diagnosis. Use of ERCP or percutaneous transhepatic cholangiography (PTC) should be limited primarily to palliation of jaundice in patients with unresectable tumors and to help establish a tissue diagnosis in ambiguous cases. Proof of malignancy or differentiation of malignant from benign causes of hilar obstruction such as IgG4 cholangiopathy can sometimes be challenging.

Hilar tumors can be classified into three main types based on the origin of the tumor. The first category includes tumors originating from the bile duct, including adenocarcinoma, the most common of which is cholangiocarcinoma. The second category involves local extension into the hilum by a tumor arising in an adjacent structure, such as the gallbladder, liver, or pancreas. The third category includes metastases from solid tumors, such as carcinoma of the breast, colon, or ovaries, or from lymphoma. Differentiation of metastatic lesions from primary bile duct tumors can sometimes be difficult. Patients with primary bile duct tumors may be candidates for surgical resection, whereas

M.A. Tiewala, M.D.
Division of Gastroenterology, Hennepin County Medical Center, 701 Park Avenue,
Minneapolis, MN 55415, USA

M.L. Freeman, M.D. (✉)
Division of Gastroenterology, Hepatology and Nutrition, University of Minnesota, 406 Harvard St SE, MMC36, 55455 Minneapolis, MN, USA
e-mail: freem020@umn.edu

those with extension of adjacent tumors and those with hilar metastases from distant primary sites are generally not. Attempt at curative surgical resection is appropriate for certain patients and almost always includes partial hepatectomy. Bismuth-Corlette classification alone does not determine resectability. Treatment should be governed by the clinical status of the patient and whether the patient is a surgical candidate. Liver transplantation is offered after aggressive neoadjuvant therapy at a limited number of centers for patients with locally advanced but unresectable primary tumors such as cholangiocarcinoma. Optimal therapy of hilar tumors requires a setting in which a substantial volume of patients with similar problems are seen, and advanced hepatobiliary surgery, interventional endoscopy, and interventional radiology is available.

As most patients with malignant hilar biliary obstruction are not surgical candidates, the focus of care is most often on palliation of jaundice using endoscopically or percutaneously placed stents. Additional palliative options for unresectable bile duct tumors include surgical bypass, intraluminal and external beam radiation therapy, chemotherapy, and photodynamic therapy. Even if not resectable, some hilar cancers, particularly cholangiocarcinomas and metastases from breast carcinomas, may grow slowly and allow for prolonged patient survival of up to several years with proper drainage, placing a premium on optimal stenting and palliation. Ineffective drainage, regardless of route, and associated cholangitis are major determinants of early mortality [1]. Increasing evidence suggests that metallic stents are superior to plastic stents for palliation of hilar malignant biliary obstruction in most circumstances, if optimally positioned. It remains unclear in which circumstances a single stent is sufficient for effective palliation and avoidance of cholangitis in excluded segments. With improvements in technology of guidewires, catheters, and particularly of metallic stents and their delivery systems, placement of more than one stent is technically feasible in the majority of circumstances.

## Bismuth-Corlette Classification and Liver Segmental Anatomy

Hilar tumors can be characterized by level of ductal obstruction, commonly referred to as Bismuth-Corlette classification [2] (Fig. 15.1). In type I lesions, the stenosis lies at the level of the common hepatic duct within 2 cm of the bifurcation, with intact communication between right and left hepatic ducts. In type 2, there is separate obstruction of the takeoff of the right and left hepatic ducts. Type 3A lesions involve secondary branches of the right intrahepatic duct, and type 3B secondary branches of the left intrahepatic duct with intact contralateral ducts. Type 4 lesions involve bilateral secondary or tertiary branch duct involvement or may be multifocal.

Bismuth-Corlette classification has a role in determining extent of drainage, but its importance may have been overemphasized. Understanding hepatic segmental anatomy and sectoral ductal anatomy with its many variations is a prerequisite for optimal endoscopic drainage. Both CT scan and three-dimensional MRCP, which is now routinely performed at almost all major and many smaller medical centers, greatly facilitate understanding of hepatic segmental and ductal anatomy. A number of websites have instructional materials on this topic, and endoscopists are encouraged to visit them.

Seven of the eight liver segments are usually of substantial size, excluding segment one which drains the caudate lobe. The segmental ducts typically coalesce to form three main sectoral ducts – the right anterior sectoral duct (draining segments V and VIII), the right posterior sectoral duct (draining segments VI and VII), and the left main hepatic duct (draining segments II–IV). Atrophy and variations in ductal anatomy have major implications for endoscopic stent placement. Segments may atrophy as a slowly growing tumor obstructs one sectoral duct over a prolonged period before there is obstruction of the contralateral side and thus presentation with jaundice. Drainage of such atrophic segments, even with dilated ducts, is usually ineffective at relieving jaundice and may lead to recurrent cholangitis.

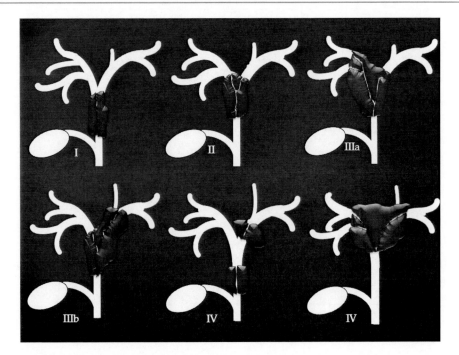

**Fig. 15.1**   Bismuth-Corlette classification of hilar tumors

In addition, there is substantial variation in segmental and sectoral anatomy (Fig. 15.2). For example, the right posterior sectoral duct (draining segments VI and VII) drains into the left hepatic duct in about one-fourth of the patients, such that a single left hepatic duct stent would drain the entire left lobe and the right posterior sectoral duct, thus draining the entire liver saved for the right anterior duct. In this situation, a *left* duct stent would actually drain a substantial portion of the right lobe. In other patients, there may be a *trifurcation* with right anterior and posterior sectoral and left ducts joining together, such that a similar bifurcation tumor might involve three equivalent sectoral ductal obstructions. In that situation, the same left hepatic duct stent as placed in the previous example would only drain one-third rather than two-thirds of the liver. In some other patients, the right posterior sectoral duct enters the common hepatic duct below the bifurcation, such that a single stent in the left hepatic duct would actually drain two-thirds of the liver. Because more than one stent may be placed in the same side of the liver (usually the right anterior and right posterior sectoral ducts),

or one stent may actually drain both sides of the liver, the concept of *unilateral* or *bilateral* drainage may be somewhat outmoded and best referred to as *single* or *multiple* stents based on sectoral anatomy.

## Single or Multiple Stents?

Whether palliative endoscopic stenting should be unilateral (perhaps best referred to as single) or bilateral (perhaps best referred to as multiple) has been debated for many years, with varying opinions based on anecdotal evidence and conflicting data. The principle governing drainage had been that only 25–50% of the liver needs to be drained for palliation, but until recently that assumption had not been formally investigated. Problems that arise from endoscopic stenting of hilar malignancy are mainly related to inadequate drainage, infection in undrained segments, or later from stent occlusion or malfunction. The prevailing point of view had been for many years that bilateral drainage was preferred; however, supporting data were mainly from retrospective case

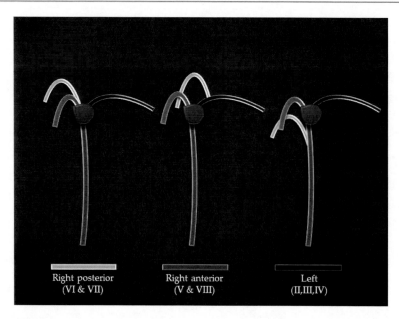

**Fig. 15.2** Anatomic variations in insertion of *right* posterior sectoral duct (shown in *white*) in three hypothetical patients with identical hilar tumors, showing implications for stenting. At *left*, trifurcation with three sectoral duct obstructions; in *middle*, insertion of *right* posterior duct into *left* duct, with two points of obstruction with one obstructing two sectors and another obstructing single sector; at *right*, *low* insertion of *right* posterior duct *below* bifurcation, with tumor separately obstructing two sectors, third below tumor

controlled series that involved the use of plastic stents and in which selective duct cannulation and opacification was not performed. In one classic retrospective study using plastic stents in 141 patients with hilar tumors, survival was significantly shorter in patients with bilateral opacification and unilateral stenting (46 days) compared with unilateral opacification and unilateral stenting (145 days) or bilateral opacification and bilateral stenting (225 days) [3]. Problems with these and other retrospective data were that multiple segmental ducts were contaminated but not drained and that many confounding variables other than drainage affect survival.

More recently, a number of authors have reported unilateral stenting to be generally satisfactory as long as selective access and opacification techniques are used. One study reported 86% efficacy and minimal complications with unilateral drainage of hilar tumors using MRCP to target endoscopic placement of single plastic stents, but the practicality of this approach was limited by the need for routine stent changes every 2 months (more than 4 per patient) [4]. A prospective

randomized trial involving plastic stents suggested that selective unilateral endoscopic drainage was superior to bilateral drainage, with significantly fewer technical failures (11.4% vs. 23.1%) and, thus, less contamination of undrained segments, resulting in fewer early complications, less early cholangitis (8.8% vs. 16.6%), and no difference in late complications [5]. Problems with these data were a relatively low technical success rate and the fact that results may not translate to metallic stents. The data do support the concept that endoscopic placement of bilateral large-bore plastic stents may be difficult or sometimes impossible, and failure to place a second stent after extensive manipulation may lead to serious complications. Unilateral targeted stenting is substantially easier to perform and allows easier endoscopic reintervention.

There are a number of prospective and retrospective case series demonstrating reasonable safety and efficacy of single metallic stents for hilar tumors [6–9]. In two prospective series involving 35 and 61 patients, respectively, approximately half of whom had Bismuth III and

IV lesions, single MRCP-targeted metallic stents resulted in resolution of jaundice in 77% and 86%, with complications occurring in 0 and 8% of cases, median stent patencies of 5.4 and 5.6 months, and repeat intervention required in 29% and 26%, respectively [7, 8]. Of note is that approximately one in five patients did not achieve palliation of jaundice with a single stent.

Most of the data comparing single versus multiple stents involve plastic endoprostheses. There are only two retrospective studies comparing outcomes of bilateral versus unilateral metallic stents. A retrospective study compared outcomes of metallic stents in 17 unilateral and 29 bilateral cases [10]. Successful drainage was achieved in nearly all patients (100% and 96%, respectively), with a trend toward fewer early complications with unilateral stents (0% vs. 10%), similar late complications (65% vs. 54%), but with substantially longer patencies for bilateral stents overall (P=0.009), especially for those patients with cholangiocarcinoma. Another retrospective study of 82 patients undergoing metallic stenting for hilar tumors found no significant difference between unilateral versus bilateral metallic stents with respect to median survival, stent patency, or complication-free survival time, but did find a significantly higher rate of liver abscess (17.6%) for bilateral versus unilateral (1.5%) stents [11]. Thus, the results of these two studies are conflicting with respect to value of dual versus single metallic stents. As with all retrospective and univariate analyses, these studies do not allow for adjustment for confounding variables such as tumor stage, functional status, Bismuth class, or other potentially important factors.

One study of palliative stenting has moved beyond the concept of *unilateral* and *bilateral* and has applied understanding of liver parenchymal volume and sectoral duct anatomy to hilar tumor drainage. In a retrospective study of 107 patients with Bismuth II–IV tumors undergoing palliative stenting with mostly plastic stents, CT scan was used to determine volume of liver in three liver sectors: the left sector (segments II–III), right posterior sector (segments VI and VII), and right anterior sector (segments V and

VIII) [12]. Segment IV could flow into the right or left duct and was accounted for based on individual biliary anatomy. On each CT slice, the relative area of each sector was calculated as a fraction of the entire liver area. Each sector was then classified as 30%, 30–50%, and >50% of the total liver volume. If the sector was less than 30%, it was considered atrophied, and if the tumor extended to greater than 75% of the total volume, then this sector also considered less than 30%. The primary outcome of this study was the effectiveness of drainage as demonstrated by a decreased bilirubin of more than 50% of the pretreatment value on day 30. In the group with more than 50% of liver volume drained, the rate of effective drainage was significantly higher with less cholangitis and longer survival than the less than 50% group. Thus, the most important take-home points from this novel study were the following: (1) More than 50% drainage of liver volume based on hepatic sectors was a strong predictor of drainage effectiveness, especially in Bismuth type three patients. (2) Intubating an atrophied sector was ineffective and was associated with increased risk of cholangitis and should thus be avoided. (3) More than 50% volume drainage is associated with a longer survival. This study involved primarily use of plastic stents. Whether or not these results can be generalized to metallic stents is unclear. An important contribution of this study is steering away from the concept of *unilateral* or *bilateral* toward single or multiple sectoral duct drainage, which sometimes involves two stents in the right hepatic duct sectors rather than a left and right hepatic duct stent.

To summarize, currently available data are conflicting for the value of bilateral versus unilateral stents, whether plastic or metallic. What is clear is that enhanced understanding of liver segment anatomy and drainage, in addition to individual tumor characteristics, and careful review of axial and reconstructed CT and MRCP images will likely lead to best outcomes (Fig. 15.3a, b). Selective access techniques, and drainage of at least 50% of the liver volume without infecting remaining segments, seem to be primary determinants of favorable results.

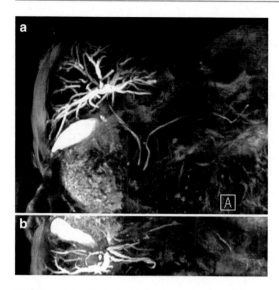

**Fig. 15.3** (**a**) MRCP showing hilar tumor with apparent communication of intrahepatic ducts (possible Bismuth I or II) and (**b**) three-dimensional rotation of MRCP showing vertical projection, revealing multiple points of obstruction (Bismuth IV)

## Plastic or Self-Expanding Metallic Stents?

It has been clearly established that for distal bile duct tumors, metal stents are superior to plastic stents with respect to patency and overall cost in patients with a minimum of 3–4 months survival [13]. For hilar tumors, there remains substantial difference of opinion and sparse data regarding choice of metal versus plastic stents [14–16]. There are many theoretical reasons why plastic stents would be less effective for hilar tumors than for distal tumors: the excessive length and lack of conformability impair bile flow, lead to early occlusion, and promote migration, and the material allows colonization of stents with biofilm, which in turn leads to infection of undrained segments and resultant cholangitis; the lack of side holes in standard stents occludes secondary branch ducts, and the relatively large insertion diameter and limited mechanical leverage render placement of multiple large-bore stents technically challenging in stenotic and complex strictures. In contrast, uncovered metallic stents have major theoretical advantages for hilar tumors, including open mesh to allow drainage of secondary branch ducts, conformability to tortuous intrahepatic ducts, and relative lack of bacterial biofilm once the stent becomes embedded in biliary mucosa.

There are, to date, only three studies comparing metallic to plastic stents in hilar tumors, of which one was a retrospective case-control study [17], one was a prospective case control with only short-term follow-up [18], and one study from two decades ago was a randomized trial [19]. In the prospective randomized trial published in 1993, bilateral large-bore plastic stents and bilateral self-expanding metal stents (8 mm) were compared in the palliative treatment of obstructive jaundice in 20 patients with Bismuth II through IV hilar malignancies [19]. Stents were placed by combined percutaneous and endoscopic route. Long-term (> 30 days) stent failure was observed in 50% of the plastic group and 18% of the metal stent group, a difference which did not quite reach statistical significance in this small study. However, even with the small sample size, the number of repeat interventions and hospitalizations for treatment of stent complications, as well as estimated overall cost of care, were significantly higher in patients treated with plastic compared with metallic stents. In a prospective multicenter case-control study, the 30-day outcomes of plastic versus self-expanding metallic stents were compared for the palliation of malignant hilar biliary obstruction [18]. Most stents were unilateral in both groups. Adverse outcomes including cholangitis, stent occlusion, migration, perforation, and/or the need for unplanned endoscopic retrograde cholangiopancreatography or percutaneous transhepatic cholangiography occurred in 11/28 (39.3%) patients with plastic versus 4/34 (11.8%) with metal stents (P=0.017). By logistic regression, factors associated with adverse outcomes included plastic stent placement (odds ratio 6.3) and higher serum bilirubin, but not study center location or Bismuth class. Finally, in a recently published retrospective case-control study of 100 patients with inoperable cholangiocarcinoma undergoing palliative stenting, the clinical effectiveness (including stent patency), complication

**Table 15.1** Complications of metal stenting for hilar tumors

| |
| --- |
| Placement in patients with benign disease |
| Placement in wrong segmental ducts |
| Precluding resection |
| Tumor ingrowth |
| Stone formation |
| Reactive hyperplasia |
| Cholangitis – early or late |
| Erosion into vessels (bleeding) |

rate, and need for salvage percutaneous transhepatic biliary drainage of SEMS and plastic stents were compared [17]. Median patencies were 1.86 months in the plastic group and 5.56 months in the SEMS group (P<0.0001). A mean of 1.53 and 4.60 reinterventions were performed in the SEMS and plastic groups, respectively (P<0.05). Median survival was not different between the two groups.

Overall, it seems from the available but limited data that metallic stents are superior to plastic stents for palliation of hilar tumors with respect to early complications, stent patencies, and need for repeat interventions. However, there are several caveats that uniquely pertain to metallic stents for hilar as opposed to distal tumors (Table 15.1). Covered stents generally are not appropriate for hilar tumors because of occlusion of secondary branch ducts. As such, hilar metallic stents are generally not removable endoscopically or even surgically. Placement of a metallic stent into intrahepatic ducts renders not only tumor staging but resection and/or liver transplantation difficult or impossible. Because there are a number of benign conditions that mimic hilar tumors, and tissue diagnosis of malignancy is often difficult to obtain, there is a further premium on accurate diagnosis and staging prior to consideration of metallic stent placement. As a result of these factors, and the theoretical and technical complexity of placement of one or more metallic stents, hilar tumor drainage is a highly specialized procedure that is best performed by expert endoscopists in the context of a specialized center dealing with all aspects of disease management.

## Technical Aspects of Metallic Stent Insertion for Hilar Tumors

Two fundamental SEMS designs that are available today include the spiral-cell type and the laser-cut open-cell type (Fig. 15.4a, b). Primary differences are that spiral stents foreshorten substantially during delivery, while open-cell stents do not, and spiral stents tend to have a tighter mesh than open-cell stents. Spiral stents include Wallflex and Wallstent (Boston Scientific, Natick MA). The Wallflex is made of Platinol, is MRI safe, and has a spiral-braided wire construction with relatively small cells. These stents probably offer the most radial force; however, they are sometimes difficult to position accurately due to foreshortening at both ends. The high axial force of these stents tends to straighten the duct and may lead to problems in hilar strictures due to tortuosity of the intrahepatic ducts. The dense mesh renders access through the stent mesh for "Y" stent placement very difficult, thus potentially locking out any undrained ducts from endoscopic access. The Niti-S (TaeWoong Medical, Goyang-Si, Korea) is made of nitinol and is a wire, flexible, fine mesh tubular prosthesis with a relatively larger cell design and substantial conformability with tortuous ducts. The D type is uniform throughout; the Y-type stent is designed with a wider mesh in the center of the stent to facilitate stent placement in a "Y" configuration.

Laser-cut nitinol stents include Zilver (Cook Endoscopy, Winston-Salem, NC), which is a self-expandable stent made of nitinol with a wide mesh open-cell design and minimal foreshortening. A major advantage of the Zilver stent is the smallest currently available outer diameter insertion diameter (6 French) and high conformability to tortuous ducts; a relative disadvantage is lower radial force. Flexxus (ConMed, Utica, NY) is quite similar to the Zilver stent, but has a gun-type deployment system, which allows easy stepwise release of the stent. The X-Suit NIR biliary stent (Olympus, Center Valley, PA) is similar to the previous two stents but has a larger diameter delivery system. The JOSTENT SelfX (Abbott

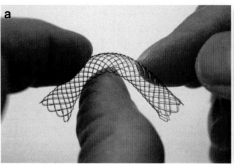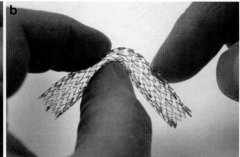

**Fig. 15.4** (**a**) Spiral configuration metallic stent (Wallflex). (**b**) Open-cell laser-cut stent (Zilver stent)

Laboratories, Abbott Park, IL) is an uncovered self-expanding nitinol stent with minimal fore-shortening. All of these open-cell stents allow placement of stent-through-stent in a "Y" configuration without special modification.

## Techniques for Single and Multiple Selective Stent Placement

Once the decision has been made to place metallic stents, whether primarily or replacing plastic stents, it is essential to carefully review imaging, including both axial and reconstructed views of the ducts. MRCP with three-dimensional reconstruction is highly recommended whenever possible, although coronal views of CT may also provide useful information. At index, ERCP contrast should only be injected to below the stricture to avoid contaminating undrained segments. Biliary sphincterotomy is recommended to reduce the otherwise elevated risk of post-ERCP pancreatitis in hilar tumor stenting and allow easy repeated access (Fig. 15.5). Sphincterotomy may not always be necessary with metallic stents positioned above the papilla. The goal should be drainage of at least 50% of the liver parenchyma, avoiding atrophic segments, and the number and position of desired stents planned in advance. The decision to place more than one metallic stent is influenced by volume of liver drained, presence of contamination of multiple sectoral ducts because of previous plastic stent placement, or cholangitis, and contamination during duct access and injection of contrast.

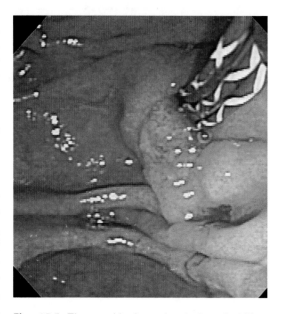

**Fig. 15.5** Three guidewires placed through biliary sphincterotomy in patient with hilar tumor

Placement of single metallic stents is straight-forward (Fig. 15.6). Enough contrast is instilled in the desired segments only to define the upper and lower extent of the intended drainage and only after selective guidewire access. The stent is then positioned with at least 2 cm above the stricture and 2 cm below the stricture, usually resulting in suprapapillary positioning. More stents can be overlapped in tandem if it is desired to extend the stents through the papilla. There is theoretical concern that transpapillary positioning of metallic stents is associated with more cholangitis due to enteric-biliary reflux [20]. In the authors' opinion, open-cell stents should be used

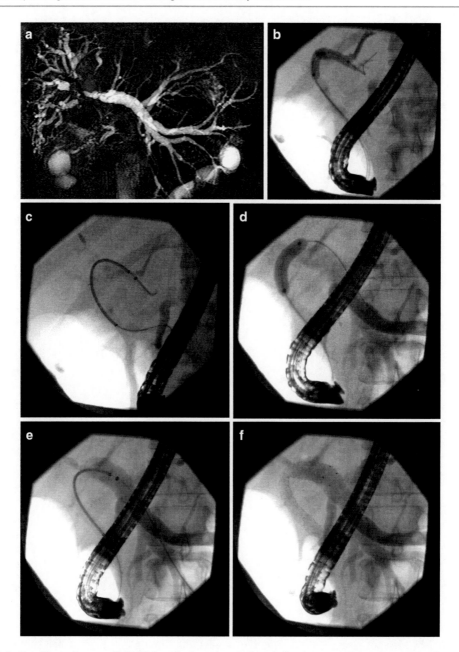

**Fig. 15.6** Case illustrating use of MRCP for selective unilateral stent placement in *left* hepatic duct of patient with hilar cholangiocarcinoma. (**a**) MRCP showing Bismuth IIIb cholangiocarcinoma arising from *right* hepatic duct with multiple points of obstruction and atrophy of the *right* lobe and hypertrophied *left* lobe. In this patient, insertion of single *left* hepatic duct stents indicated (**b**) ERCP with balloon inflated across stricture, but tip of catheter in segment IV and no access deep into segment II or III. (**c**) Stent positioned but deployment here not ideal, would not drain segments II or III adequately. (**d**) Deep-wire positioning into segment II duct with balloon reinflated. (**e**) Metallic stent positioned correctly. (**f**) Proper positioning of open-cell metallic stent into *left* hepatic duct

for single metallic stent placement in case subsequent placement of contralateral stent-through-stent is required. Access through a dense mesh stent is difficult (Fig. 15.7) and sometimes impossible endoscopically and may require percutaneous intervention (Fig. 15.8).

The original technique for placement of multiple stents typically involved endoscopic placement of

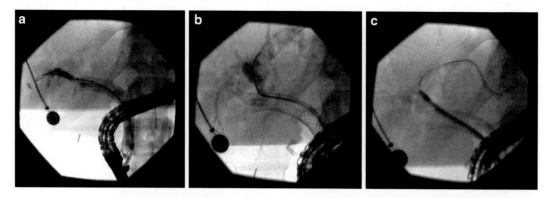

**Fig. 15.7** Sequence showing problems with dense mesh spiral stent extending beyond bifurcation; salvage using Soehendra stent extractor as dilator to rupture mesh of stent. (**a**) Wallflex stent had been placed into *right* hepatic duct across takeoff of *left* hepatic duct, with subsequent cholangitis and purulent drainage from *right* lobe.

(**b**) Steerable cannula (SwingTip, Olympus) and hydrophilic-tipped guidewire used to angle through mesh of stent into *left* hepatic duct. (**c**) 8,5-French Soehendra stent extractor (Cook Endoscopy) used to core tract through mesh of Wallflex stent to rupture mesh, with air cholangiogram visible in *left* hepatic duct

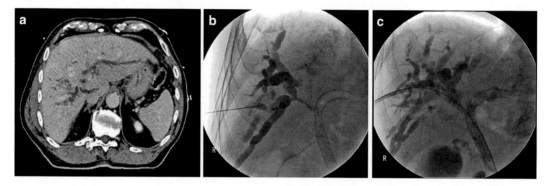

**Fig. 15.8** Demonstration of hazards of placement of dense mesh metallic Wallstent in hilar tumor: patient with unresectable hilar cholangiocarcinoma with non-atrophic *left* lobe, in whom dense mesh spiral-type single metallic stent in *left* lobe failed to relieve jaundice, could not be penetrated at repeat ERCP, requiring percutaneous access and placement of Y configuration *right* hepatic duct stent. (**a**) CT scan showing hilar tumor with mildly hypertrophied *left*

lobe, subsequently single *left* stent placed as predicted to be adequate for drainage. (**b**) Percutaneous access to obstructed *right* hepatic duct because of persistent jaundice; after repeat ERCP showed patent *left* hepatic duct stent, but unable to traverse dense mesh to access *right* hepatic duct. (**c**) After percutaneous placement of second stent-through-mesh of endoscopically placed *left* hepatic duct stent in Y configuration, with successful relief of jaundice

one stent and percutaneous placement of the contralateral stent via a percutaneous or combined endoscopic-percutaneous *rendezvous* technique [21]. Subsequently, improvements in endoscopic techniques for accessing multiple sectoral ducts and improved stent characteristics with smaller insertion diameters have facilitated stent placement such that success rates for multiple endoscopic stents now approach 100%. Dual metallic stent placement by the endoscopic route is generally done using the side-by-side configuration or stent-through-stent (Y) configuration. The earliest

reports of multiple stent placement mostly included side-by-side placement with the stents protruding through the papilla (Fig. 15.9) [21]. In this method, dual wires are placed, the strictures balloon dilated, and first one stent is deployed, then the second stent passed beyond the first stent and into the contralateral duct. Using Wallstents as originally reported, the 30–40% foreshortening requires a stent of 10 cm or longer length or overlapping stents to span the distance from the intrahepatic ducts across the papilla. Despite optimal positioning during ERCP, foreshortening of the

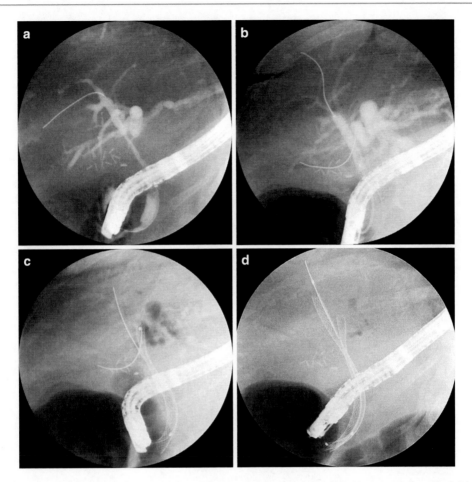

**Fig. 15.9** Placement of bilateral Wallstents using side-by-side technique and extending across the papilla. (**a**) Cholangiogram showing Bismuth II cholangiocarcinoma. (**b**) Balloon dilation of *right* (and *left* not shown) duct strictures. (**c**) First stent has been deployed in *left* hepatic duct and extending across papilla, with second guidewire *left* in place beside first stent. (**d**) Second stent has been passed beside *left* stent and deployed in *right* hepatic duct

stents may result in eventual contraction of the stents upward across the papilla. During placement of dual side-by-side metallic stents positioned above the papilla, the second stent may not pass the opened bottom of the first stent, rendering second stent placement impossible and creating a potential hazard for undrained segmental cholangitis. Although complex modifications of techniques have been reported to overcome this obstacle, including placement of large-bore plastic stent as a conduit, the sequential side-by-side technique is limited [22].

Simultaneous deployment of side-by-side stents was first described using a prototype large caliber ERCP duodenoscope [23]. Subsequently, the availability of very small caliber (6 French)

delivery systems has rendered the technique of simultaneous positioning of two side-by-side stents prior to deployment feasible and quite easy using standard therapeutic duodenoscopes with a 4.2-mm working channel. Technical success rates approach 100% with these prostheses (Figs. 15.10, 15.11, and 15.12). The stents can be released sequentially or simultaneously. Challenges with side-by-side simultaneous stent deployment include lining up the distal ends of the stents exactly. Due to the fact that the distal bile duct is often small caliber (6–8 mm) in patients with hilar obstruction, presence of dual 8-mm stent results in overcrowding of the distal duct and nearly inevitable compression of one stent by the other even if exactly aligned.

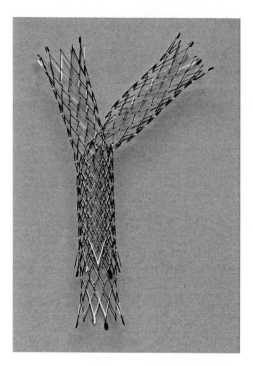

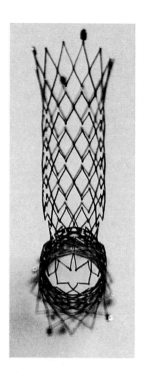

**Fig. 15.10** Two standard metallic stents in Y configuration with one inserted through the other without special modification (Flexxus, ConMed)

**Fig. 15.11** Different view of Y configuration Flexxus stents showing minimal *caging* effect with large lumen

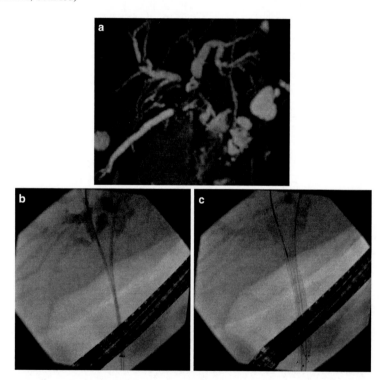

**Fig. 15.12** Sequence showing simultaneous side-by-side deployment of 6-French Zilver stents in patient with Bismuth IIIa tumor. (**a**) MRCP showing Bismuth IIIa cholangiocarcinoma with mild atrophy of *left* lobe. Plan is to drain *left* sector (segments II–IV) and *right* anterior sectoral duct (segments V and VIII). (**b**) Dual 6-French 8-mm diameter, 8-cm length Zilver stents have been positioned simultaneously with *bottom* ends exactly even inside distal bile duct above papilla. (**c**) After simultaneous deployment, there is compression of distal end of one stent by the other, a common problem with this technique especially in patients with small caliber bile duct

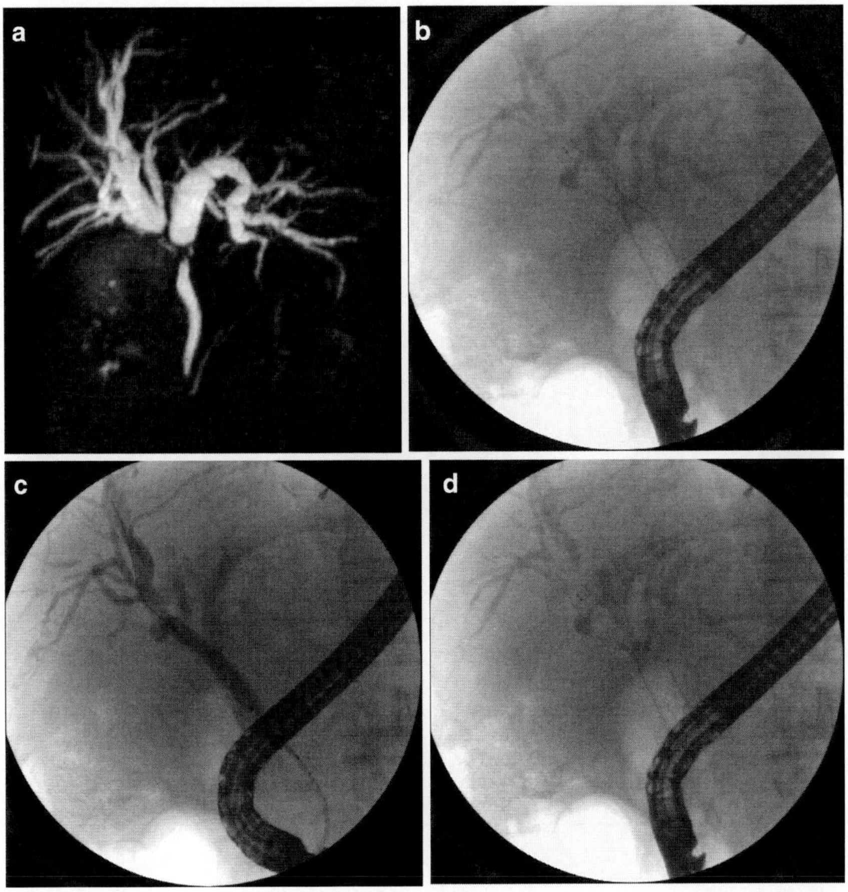

**Fig. 15.13** Sequence showing MRCP-targeted placement of bilateral metallic Zilver stents in Y configuration in a patient with Bismuth II tumor. (**a**) MRCP showing Bismuth II tumor 1. (**b**) After wires placed in *left* and *right* anterior sectoral ducts, first metallic stent positioned in *left* hepatic duct. (**c**) After deployment of *left* hepatic duct stent, additional guidewire passed through lumen of *left* stent into *right* hepatic duct paralleling other *right* hepatic duct wire, followed by balloon dilation of tract through open-mesh stent into *right* hepatic duct. (**d**) After deployment of bilateral Zilver stents in Y configuration

As a result, later selective access for cleaning or re-stenting can be difficult.

A stent-through-stent technique (Y configuration) was initially described using spiral stents such as the Wallstent, but was very challenging due to the tight mesh of such stents. Subsequent proliferation of open-cell stents with small caliber delivery systems has greatly facilitated placement of Y stents (Fig. 15.13) [24–27]. The Niti-S Y-type stent was specifically designed stent to have a more open mesh in the central portion to theoretically facilitate bilateral stent placement. However, conventional stents including Zilver, Flexxus, X-Suit, and JOSTENT SelfX are easily placed using the stent-through-stent technique. Not only can this be done at initial placement, but if a single stent fails to relieve jaundice, or results in cholangitis such that a second stent-through-stent is later necessary, salvage access through the mesh can be done at a later date in contrast to tight mesh spiral stents. The availability of steerable catheters (SwingTip, Olympus Endoscopy) greatly facilitates selective access through the open mesh for placement of a second stent by angling the catheter tip perpendicularly into the side of the initial stent. Hydrophilic wires and hybrid wires, both straight and angled tip, can be used in combination with steerable catheters to allow access to virtually any intrahepatic duct. Correlation with MRCP allows assurance that the desired duct is accessed before the stent is deployed. Revision of Y stents is fairly straightforward as access can generally be obtained through the side of the mesh using steerable catheters and guidewires (Figs. 15.14 and 15.15).

Complications of metal stenting occur in approximately 8–15% of patients within the first

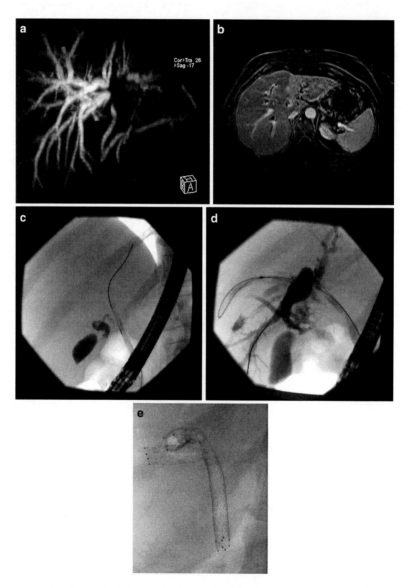

**Fig. 15.14** Sequence showing dual *right* hepatic duct metallic stent in Y configuration in patient with Bismuth IV cholangiocarcinoma with atrophied *left* hepatic duct, separately obstructed *right* anterior and posterior sectoral ducts. (**a**) MRCP showing Bismuth IV cholangiocarcinoma with atrophied *left* hepatic duct, separately obstructed *right* anterior and posterior sectoral ducts. (**b**) Axial image from MRCP showing atrophied *left* lobe. (**c**) Initial ERCP showing wire access into *left* hepatic duct, no contrast injected, wire withdrawn and redirected toward *right* lobe. (**d**) Selective access into *right* anterior and posterior sectoral ducts, which were separately obstructed. (**e**) Open-mesh stents placed into *right* anterior and posterior ducts in Y configuration

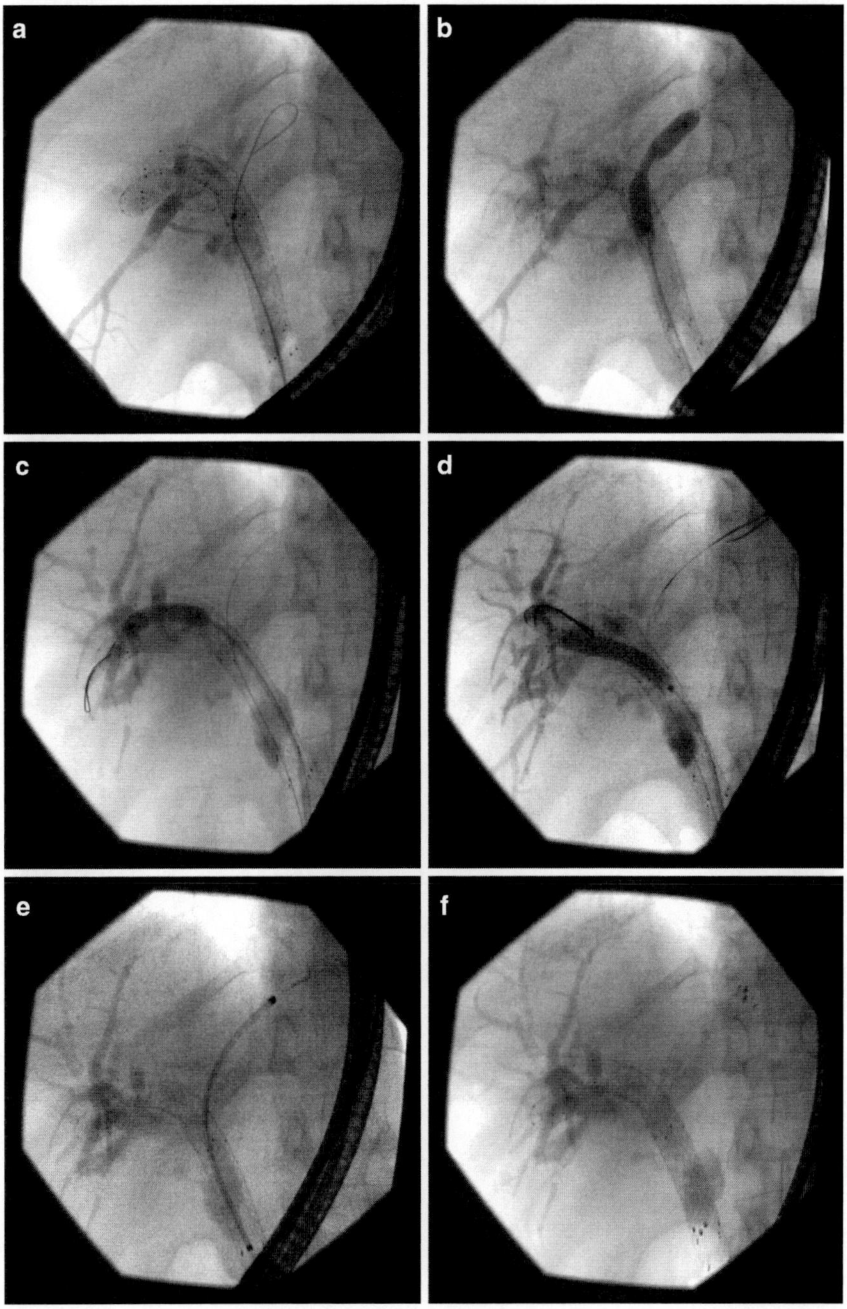

**Fig. 15.15** (**a**) After 4 months, ERCP is repeated because patient developed cholangitis with purulent drainage from atrophied *left* lobe duct; steerable catheter (SwingTip, Olympus) is used to access through dual layer of mesh into *left* hepatic duct. (**b**) Balloon dilation of tract through mesh of stent into *left* hepatic duct. (**c**) Selective access using steerable catheter into *right* anterior hepatic duct stent for balloon dilation and clearance of debris. (**d**) Similar access into *right* posterior sectoral duct. (**e**) Zilver stent positioned in *left* hepatic duct through mesh of initial stents. (**f**) Final deployment of salvage *left* hepatic duct metal stent through dual *right* hepatic duct stents, for total of three endoscopically placed Y configuration stents in *right* anterior, *right* posterior, and *left* hepatic ducts

30 days and in approximately 30% of patients at some point during palliation (6–8). Early cholangitis is relatively rare (0–8%) using selective wire-access techniques and avoidance of opacification of undrainable segments. Major complications include strategic errors, i.e., inappropriate placement in a benign stricture or a resectable lesion. Placement in wrong segmental ducts can lead to cholangitis and substantial difficulty with revision, sometimes requiring percutaneous salvage. Tumor ingrowth and reactive hyperplasia and stone formation may lead to late cholangitis. Occasionally, erosion of the stent into vessels may result in bleeding.

## Special Challenges with Metallic Stents: Revision of Stents and Photodynamic Therapy

Revision of single metallic stent is easy and generally involves insertion of a new metallic stent inside the previous stent. In general, a second SEMS insertion in occluded SEMS provides significantly longer patency time than secondary plastic stents, but such data regarding hilar tumors are limited [28]. Revision of multiple hilar metallic stents can be challenging. As previously mentioned, endoscopic access to both stents for side-by-side intraductal stents can be impossible and requires percutaneous access and drainage with at least one of the stents. Endoscopic access to Y stents using open-cell stents is relatively easy, using steerable catheters and hydrophilic-tipped guidewires. The lumens can be cleaned of stone debris, balloon dilated, and/or new stents placed within the old stents.

Photodynamic therapy (PDT) has been shown to add survival advantage compared with plastic stents alone in retrospective case-control studies and in the one prospective randomized trial of patients with inoperable cholangiocarcinoma [29, 30]. There are limited reports demonstrating the feasibility of combining PDT with metallic stents for cholangiocarcinoma, with PDT performed before or after metallic stent insertion [31, 32]. In a retrospective case-control study of 21 patients with hilar cholangiocarcinoma receiving bilateral JOSTENT SelfX stents, the 8 patients who underwent additional PDT had significantly longer survival (16.5 months vs. 12.3 months), without adding to cumulative hospital time [32]. As of the current time, if PDT is intended in conjunction with multiple metallic stents, side-by-side metallic stent placement with transpapillary extension is probably ideal to allow easy access to both stent lumens.

## References

1. Paik WH, Park YS, Hwang JH, et al. Palliative treatment with self-expandable metallic stents in patients with advanced type III or IV hilar cholangiocarcinoma: a percutaneous versus endoscopic approach. Gastrointest Endosc. 2009;69:55–62.
2. Bismuth H, Castaing D, Traynor O. Resection or palliation: priority of surgery in the treatment of hilar cancer. World J Surg. 1988;12:39–47.
3. Chang WH, Kortan P, Haber GB. Outcome in patients with bifurcation tumors who undergo unilateral versus bilateral hepatic duct drainage. Gastrointest Endosc. 1998;47:354–62.
4. Hintze RE, Abou-Rebyeh H, Adler A, et al. Magnetic resonance cholangiopancreatography-guided unilateral endoscopic stent placement for Klatskin tumors. Gastrointest Endosc. 2001;53:40–6.
5. De Palma GD, Galloro G, Siciliano S, et al. Unilateral versus bilateral endoscopic hepatic duct drainage in patients with malignant hilar biliary obstruction: results of a prospective, randomized, and controlled study. Gastrointest Endosc. 2001;53:547–53.
6. Cheng JL, Bruno MJ, Bergman JJ, et al. Endoscopic palliation of patients with biliary obstruction caused by nonresectable hilar cholangiocarcinoma: efficacy of self-expandable metallic wall stents. Gastrointest Endosc. 2002;56:33–9.
7. De Palma GD, Pezzullo A, Rega M, et al. Unilateral placement of metallic stents for malignant hilar obstruction: a prospective study. Gastrointest Endosc. 2003;58:50–3.
8. Freeman ML, Overby C. Selective MRCP and CT-targeted drainage of malignant hilar biliary obstruction with self-expanding metallic stents. Gastrointest Endosc. 2003;58:41–9.
9. Peters RA, Williams SG, Lombard M, Karani J, Westaby D. The management of high-grade hilar strictures by endoscopic insertion of self-expanding metal endoprostheses. Endoscopy. 1997;29:10–6.
10. Naitoh I, Ohara H, Nakazawa T, et al. Unilateral versus bilateral endoscopic metal stenting for malignant hilar biliary obstruction. J Gastroenterol Hepatol. 2009;24:552–7.
11. Iwano H, Ryozawa S, Ishigaki N, et al. Unilateral versus bilateral drainage using self-expandable metallic stent for unresectable hilar biliary obstruction. Dig Endosc. 2011;23:43–8.

12. Vienne A, Hobeika E, Gouya H, et al. Prediction of drainage effectiveness during endoscopic stenting of malignant hilar strictures: the role of liver volume assessment. Gastrointest Endosc. 2010;72:728–35.

13. Levy MJ, Baron TH, Gostout CJ, et al. Palliation of malignant extrahepatic biliary obstruction with plastic versus expandable metal stents: an evidence-based approach. Clin Gastroenterol Hepatol. 2004;2:273–85.

14. Coelho-Prabhu N, Baron TH. Endoscopic retrograde cholangiopancreatography in the diagnosis and management of cholangiocarcinoma. Clin Liver Dis. 2010;14:333–48.

15. Kozarek RA. Malignant hilar strictures: one stent or two? Plastic versus self-expanding metal stents? The role of liver atrophy and volume assessment as a predictor of survival in patients undergoing endoscopic stent placement. Gastrointest Endosc. 2010;72:736–8.

16. Freeman ML, Sielaff TD. A modern approach to malignant hilar biliary obstruction. Rev Gastroenterol Disord. 2003;3:187–201.

17. Raju RP, Jaganmohan SR, Ross WA, et al. Optimum palliation of inoperable hilar cholangiocarcinoma: comparative assessment of the efficacy of plastic and self-expanding metal stents. Dig Dis Sci. 2011;56:1557–64.

18. Perdue DG, Freeman ML, Disario JA, et al. Plastic versus self-expanding metallic stents for malignant hilar biliary obstruction: a prospective multicenter observational cohort study. J Clin Gastroenterol. 2008;42:1040–6.

19. Wagner HJ, Knyrim K, Vakil N, et al. Plastic endoprostheses versus metal stents in the palliative treatment of malignant hilar biliary obstruction. A prospective and randomized trial. Endoscopy. 1993;25:213–8.

20. Okamoto T, Fujioka S, Yanagisawa S, et al. Placement of a metallic stent across the main duodenal papilla may predispose to cholangitis. Gastrointest Endosc. 2006;63:792–6.

21. Neal CP, Thomasset SC, Bools D, et al. Combined percutaneous-endoscopic stenting of malignant biliary obstruction: results from 106 consecutive procedures and identification of factors associated with adverse outcome. Surg Endosc. 2010;24:423–31.

22. Dumas R, Demuth R, Buckley M, et al. Endoscopic bilateral metal stent placement for malignant hilar stenoses: identification of optimal technique. Gastrointest Endosc. 2000;51:334–8.

23. Saleem A, Baron TH, Gostout CJ. Large-diameter therapeutic channel duodenoscope to facilitate simultaneous deployment of side-by-side self-expandable metal stents in hilar cholangiocarcinoma. Gastrointest Endosc. 2010;72:628–31.

24. Kawamoto H, Tsutsumi K, Harada R, et al. Endoscopic deployment of multiple JOSTENT SelfX is effective and safe in treatment of malignant hilar biliary strictures. Clin Gastroenterol Hepatol. 2008;6:401–8.

25. Kim JY, Kang DH, Kim HW, et al. Usefulness of slimmer and open-cell-design stents for endoscopic bilateral stenting and endoscopic revision in patients with hilar cholangiocarcinoma (with video). Gastrointest Endosc. 2009;70:1109–15.

26. Lee JH, Kang DH, Kim JY, et al. Endoscopic bilateral metal stent placement for advanced hilar cholangiocarcinoma: a pilot study of a newly designed Y stent. Gastrointest Endosc. 2007;66:364–9.

27. Chahal P, Baron TH. Expandable metal stents for endoscopic bilateral stent-within-stent placement for malignant hilar biliary obstruction. Gastrointest Endosc. 2010;72:628–31.

28. Ridtitid W, Rerknimitr R, Janchai A, et al. Outcome of second interventions for occluded metallic stents in patients with malignant biliary obstruction. Surg Endosc. 2010;24:2216–20.

29. Kahaleh M, Mishra R, Shami VM, et al. Unresectable cholangiocarcinoma: comparison of survival in biliary stenting alone versus stenting with photodynamic therapy. Clin Gastroenterol Hepatol. 2008;6:290–7.

30. Ortner ME, Caca K, Berr F, et al. Successful photodynamic therapy for nonresectable cholangiocarcinoma: a randomized prospective study. Gastroenterology. 2003;125:1355–63.

31. Dumoulin FL, Gerhardt T, Fuchs S, et al. Phase II study of photodynamic therapy and metal stent as palliative treatment for nonresectable hilar cholangiocarcinoma. Gastrointest Endosc. 2003;57:860–7.

32. Gerhardt T, Rings D, Höblinger A, et al. Combination of bilateral metal stenting and trans-stent photodynamic therapy for palliative treatment of hilar cholangiocarcinoma. Gastroenterol. 2010;48:28–32.

Dong Ki Lee

An unresectable distal malignant bile-duct lesion is the best indication for a self-expanding metal stent (SEMS). The emergence of SEMS was a turning point in endoscopic biliary drainage because most clinical trials failed to demonstrate improvement in the patency using plastic stents (PS). Considering that effective biliary drainage is the most important factor determining quality of life, developing and improving the performance of SEMS affects treatment outcome because patients with malignant biliary obstruction generally have a shorter life expectancy.

Although SEMS have a more prolonged patency than that of PS and are considered to be the first choice for unresectable malignant biliary obstruction, they still have problems and limitations, requiring further improvement. Treatment outcomes, complications, and ongoing trials of SEMS have been described for distal malignant duct lesions. Many clinical trials on SEMS extend over a span of 20 years, and improvements in techniques over time may influence differences between studies. Thus, studies mostly published after the year 2000 will be discussed.

D.K. Lee, M.D., Ph.D. (✉)
Department of Internal Medicine, Gangnam Severance Hospital, Yonsei University, 712 Eonjuro, Gangnam-gu, Seoul 135-720, Republic of Korea
e-mail: gidept@chollian.net

## Outcomes

Although design and material modifications, as well as many other efforts to prolong stent patency, have not greatly affected the patency of PSs, efforts are currently underway to improve the performance of SEMS.

## Plastic Versus SEMS

When SEMS were first introduced, even prototypes demonstrated more prolonged patency than PS. Although PS have been used in clinical practice since 1979 [1], the only strategy found to reliably prolong stent patency was the use of larger caliber stents. This finding led to the use of SEMS technology. Newer SEMS had fewer complications with prolonged patency due to improvements in the delivery system, fewer deployment problems, and the addition of various designs. The larger internal caliber of SEMS lead to a prolonged median stent patency of 9 months, as confirmed in several prospective studies [2, 3].

According to a meta-analysis of seven studies that compared PS to the Wallstent® (Boston Scientific, Natick, MA, USA), from the 1990s until the early 2000s, no difference was observed between metal and PS in terms of technical success, therapeutic success, or complications [4]. However, metal stents had a significantly reduced relative risk (RR) of recurrent biliary obstruction prior to death/end of study (RR, 0.52; 95%

confidence interval [CI], 0.39–0.69). Importantly, a significantly reduced risk of recurrent biliary obstruction was observed at the early time point of 4 months (RR, 0.44; 95% CI, 0.3–0.63; $p < 0.01$) with metal stents. Two studies reported a higher number of endoscopic retrograde cholangiopancreatographies (ERCPs) per patient in the PS group (mean 1.6 vs. 1.0 per patient).

In a multicenter randomized study [5] comparing SEMS and a 10-Fr PS, the probability of stent occlusion was 2.8-fold greater for PSs than for SEMS and the overall complication rate was significantly lower in the SEMS group versus the PS group (20 vs. 31%; $p < 0.05$).

Most studies have confirmed that SEMS patency is twice as long as that of PSs, with a decreased need for hospital readmission and endoscopic re-intervention for recurrent biliary obstruction. The prolonged patency offered by SEMS often avoids the need for repeated ERCP in patients with relatively prolonged survival and who outlive the patency of their PS. However, PS are preferred in patients with short predicted survival (< 6 months). In a randomized study from Sweden [6], the median survival of patients was 4.5 months; 65% of patients in the SEMS group and 49% in the polyethylene group died before stent failure.

A review of randomized controlled trials suggests that SEMS are associated with improved patency over PS, as early as 4 months after insertion. The additional initial cost of metal stents is offset by the reduction in re-intervention rates in patients who have prolonged survival [7]. Thus, metal stents appear to be more cost effective than PS if the patient survives beyond 4–6 months. This is applicable in countries where the cost of ERCP is low compared with that of a metal stent [8]. To conclude, a SEMS is the best choice for treating patients with unresectable distal malignant biliary obstruction, except those whose remaining life expectancy is very short.

## Bare Versus Covered SEMS

Covered self-expandable metal stents (CSEMS) are used for middle and distal bile-duct lesions, because the covered membrane does not block the opening of the intrahepatic duct and the stent must overlap with the lesion by approximately 2 cm. Theoretically, because CSEMS block tumor ingrowth, they were thought to offer more prolonged patency than bare SEMS. However, actual clinical data do not confirm this. Reasons include the higher migration rate and more frequent impaction of sludge or food material within CSEMS versus that of the bare type. After insertion of a bare SEMS, the metal mesh becomes embedded into the bile-duct tissue, lining the bile duct with tissue, causing far less attachment and formation of sludge. SEMS are more prone to the formation of sludge than the bare type when food materials are impacted at the distal tip of the stent and are a nidus for sludge formation. Additionally, the tight stricture occasionally restricts full expansion of a CSEMS because of the covered membrane. Thus, the stent lumen may remain restricted, making it more prone to obstruction from biliary sludge [3].

Clinical trials have been numerous, but there is likely a trade-off, for the cause of stent occlusion, from tissue ingrowth and hyperplasia to sludge formation resulting from the covering. For these reasons, as shown in Table 16.1 [9–14], although there is a trend favoring covered SEMS, overall stent patency rates between covered and bare SEMS have not differed significantly to date.

Two recent multicenter randomized trials [12, 13], comparing uncovered and partially covered SEMS in the palliation of distal malignant biliary obstruction, showed no difference in time to recurrent biliary obstruction or patient survival between the two groups. In one study [12], partially covered SEMS were more commonly associated with more serious adverse events, particularly migration. However, that study included patients between 2002 and 2008 and used the Wallstent, which has stronger axial force. Another randomized study [13], which divided 400 patients from 2006 to 2008 into two groups, found no significant difference in stent patency, patient survival time, or complication rate between covered and uncovered nitinol metal stents for the palliative treatment of

**Table 16.1** Studies comparing covered and uncovered self-expanding metal stents (SEMSs) for malignant distal biliary obstruction

| Citation | Study design | Comparison | Stent patency (days) | Stent obstruction (%) (p value) |
|---|---|---|---|---|
| Isayama et al. 2004 [9] | RCT | PU Diamond (n=57) | 255 (11–1,155) | 8 (14%) |
| | | Diamond (n=55) | 193 (12–810) | 21 (38%) |
| | | | NS | (<0.001) |
| Yoon et al. 2006 [10] | Retrospective cohort | PU Wallstent (n=36) | 245±48 | 9 (25.0%) |
| | | Wallstent (n=41) | 202±29 | 15 (36.6%) |
| Park et al. 2006 [11] | Retrospective + prospective cohort | PU Wallstent (n=98) | 148.9 (3–667) | 21 (21.4%) |
| | | Wallstent (n=108) | 143.5 (3–910) | 20 (18.5%) |
| Telford et al. 2010 [12] | RCT | PU Wallstent (n=68) | 357 (264–1,302)[a] | 20 (29%) |
| | | Wallstent (n=61) | 711 (283 – unknown[b]) | 11 (18%) |
| Kullman et al. 2010 [13] | RCT | PC-PU nitinol (n=200) | 154 | 47 (23.5%) |
| | | Nitinol (n=200) | 199 | 45 (22.5%) |
| Gwon et al. 2010 [14] | Retrospective cohort (percutaneous insertion) | PTFE nitinol (n=58) | 98/91/76/76[c] | 7 (12.1) |
| | | Zilver (n=58) + Sentinel | 83/72/57/57 | 19 (32.8) |
| | | | | (0.013) |

*PU*, polyurethane; *PC-PU*, polycarbonate-polyurethane; *PTFE*, polytetrafluoroethylene
[a]Medium days to biliary obstruction
[b]Largest value was censored
[c]Cumulative stent patency rate at 3, 6, 9, and 12 months of the stent insertion

malignant distal biliary obstructions. Clinical data comparing SEMS patency according to covering material is not available. However, polyurethane is readily dissolved by bile acids and tumor ingrowth.

## SEMS Design

SEMS can be classified into three structural types according to the manufacturing methods: braided, specially braided, and laser-cut types. The metal mesh of SEMS is classified as closed-cell and open-cell types, based on the manufacturing method. Furthermore, there are two types of metal (nitinol, stainless steel) and three types of covering membrane (silicone, polyurethane, e-PTFE). According to these characteristics, SEMSs have different mechanical properties, including radial force, chronic outward force, force to recover to a straight position after bending (axial force), and flexibility. All of these factors can affect clinical performance, such as patency and complications [15].

To date, there are few clinical data to compare the efficacy of SEMS based on design. Yang et al. [16] compared double-woven SEMS (Niti-D biliary uncovered stent, n=41) with single-woven SEMS (Wallstent, n=60). The former SEMS is manufactured from nitinol and has both a "hook-and-cross"-type wire structure to create a D-shaped cavity at deployment and a wide stent mesh. These characteristics were intended to maximize flexibility and conformability of the stent and to minimize stent shortening without loss of radial force. In contrast, the Wallstent has a cross-type wire structure and a tight stent mesh, which increases radial force. The Wallstent has high axial force and low conformability. This study, however, showed no significant difference in patency or complication rates between the two groups. The Niti-D only showed a significantly prolonged median duration of stent patency compared with the Wallstent (249 days vs. 76 days; p=006) in a hilar obstruction subgroup. Due to the small sample size and nonrandomized, retrospective nature of the study, it was not possible to explore the efficacy and complication rates between the two groups. Loew et al. [17] compared 10-mm Zilver and 10-mm Wallstents. Zilver is representative of the open-cell type of SEMS, and Wallstents are closed-cell-type SEMS. The mean number of days of stent patency was 185.8 and 186.7, respectively, and the occlusion rates were similar (23.9% vs. 21.4%). Earlier clinical trials [18, 19] comparing the spiral Z-stent and the Wallstent and the Zilver and Wallstent found no difference between the stents in terms of technical success, stent occlusion, median patency rates, or complications.

Isayama et al. [15] proposed that ComVi stents were ideal because they maintained appropriately high values of radial force with less migration, but exhibited extremely low axial force because of their unique doubly overlapped structure. Ingrowth is prevented by a thin e-PTFE membrane sandwiched between the two metal mesh layers without being fixed to the wires. However, their clinical trial [20] failed to document the superiority of this stent for managing distal malignant biliary obstructions. ComVi stents (n=47) were compared with the same number of covered Wallstents, but no significant difference in stent patency (208.1+173.3 vs. 151.1+130 days) or stent occlusion (27.7% vs. 21.3%) was found. However, there was a difference for the cause of stent occlusion between the two groups. In the ComVi group, the incidence of food impaction was higher (14.9% vs. 2.1%; p=0.0588) and that of bile-duct kinking was lower than those in the covered Wallstent group (0% vs. 8.4%; p=0.1170). The high incidence of food impaction was presumed to be due to the inner surface roughness of the exposed wire. However, diet composition, such as fiber, may be a factor affecting stent occlusion.

These studies showed that stent design is not an important factor determining SEMS occlusion rates. However, unlike the PS, in which the diameter of the stent is the only factor determining stent patency, newly designed SEMSs promising longer patency are awaiting clinical trials.

## SEMS Diameter

Most commercially available SEMSs are 10 mm in diameter; thus, only a few studies have compared patency based on stent diameter. Loew et al. [17] compared the outcomes of 6-mm

Zilver, 10-mm Zilver, and 10-mm Wallstents. At the interim analysis, a significant increase in occlusions was noted in the 6-mm Zilver group at the P=0.04 level, resulting in arm closure, but continued follow-up. The final study arms included 64, 88, and 89 patients receiving 6-mm Zilver, 10-mm Zilver, and 10-mm Wallstents, respectively. Stent occlusion occurred in 39.1, 23.9, and 21.4% of the cases, respectively. The mean number of days of stent patency was 142.9, 185.8, and 186.7, respectively. SEMS occlusion was much less frequent, but equivalent, in the two 10-mm SEMS, despite major differences in stent design and material, suggesting that diameter was a critical feature, as found for PSs.

## Peroral Versus Percutaneous Application

No reported study has directly compared percutaneous and peroral methods of SEMS insertion. Nevertheless, treatment outcomes between percutaneous and peroral methods are not significantly different. Prolonged duration of treatment and an increased rate of early complications due to formation of a percutaneous tract have been reported. Numerous noncomparative studies assessing percutaneous biliary drainage and stenting (PTBD) and ERCP for treating distal bile-duct obstruction suggest no significant difference in technical success rates between percutaneous and endoscopic treatments [21–23]. Furthermore, complication rates and mortality are comparable, although the type of complication differs. Pancreatitis is more often seen after ERCP, whereas bile leakage is more frequently seen after PTBD. An advantage of ERCP over PTBD is the absence of a percutaneous drainage tube, which can be uncomfortable for patients.

In clinical practice, the peroral method is preferred when the ampulla is endoscopically approachable. However, if the peroral method fails for any reason, the percutaneous method should be attempted. Subsequent percutaneous stent placement is successful in the majority of patients in whom endoscopic stent placement fails [22].

**Table 16.2** Causes of stent obstruction and complications: comparison of covered and uncovered self-expanding metal stents (SEMSs) for malignant distal biliary obstruction

| Citation | Comparison | Tumor ingrowth ($p$ value) | Tumor overgrowth | Sludge/food ($p$ value) | Cholecystitis | Pancreatitis | Migration ($p$ value) |
|---|---|---|---|---|---|---|---|
| Isayama | CSEMS | 0 | 4 | 2 | 2 | 5 | 1 |
| et al. 2004 [9] | UCSEMS | 16 (<0.001) | 2 | 2 | 0 | 1 | 0 |
| Yoon et al. | CSEMS | 0 | 5 | 2 | 1 | 0 | 1 |
| 2006 [10] | UC-SEMS | 5 | 8 | 1 | 0 | 0 | 0 |
| Park et al. | CSEMS | 0 | 1 | 20 | 5 | 6 | 6 |
| 2006 [11] | UC-SEMS | 17 (.000) | 0 | 3 (.000) | 1 | 2 | 0 (.011) |
| Telford et al. | CSEMS | 6 | 3 | 4 | 3 (7%)[a] | 0 | 6 |
| 2010 [12] | UC-SEMS | 8 | 0 | 1 | 3 (7%) | 1 | 0 |
| Kullman et al. | CSEMS | 9 | 18 | 12 | 2 | 3 | 6 |
| 2010 [13] | UC-SEMS | 21 | 10 | 4 | 2 | 4 | 0 (0.03) |
| Gwon et al. | CSEMS | 0 | 1 | 4 | 1 | 0 | 2 |
| 2010 [14] | UC-SEMS | 14 | 1 | 4 | 0 | 0 | 0 |

[a]% patients with gallbladder

## Surgery Versus SEMS

Only one reported study [24] has compared clinical outcomes between surgical bypass (n=40) and endoscopic SEMS placement (n=46) for the palliation of patients with malignant distal common bile-duct obstruction. The SEMS group had a lower rate of procedure-related mortality (2 vs. 7.5%; p=0.01), a lower frequency of early complications (8.7 vs. 45%; p=0.02), and a shorter hospital stay (median 6 versus 12 days; p=0.01). Recurrent jaundice occurred in three patients in the surgical bypass group (7.5%) and in eight patients in the SEMS group (17.3%; p=0.198). Despite the early benefits of stenting, no significant difference in median overall survival was found between the two groups.

## Complications

Immediate, early, and late complications may occur as a result of attempting to place SEMS [25]. Inadequate positioning of the stent, incomplete removal of the covering membrane, failure of the stent to expand, and the inability to remove the introducing catheter after stent release are examples of problems that may occur during the procedure. Malpositioning of SEMS is generally attributed to operator error and may occur during deployment of SEMS with a higher axial force.

Early complications, defined as those occurring within the first week after stent placement, include stent migration, perforation, cholangitis, and hemobilia. The most common late complication related to SEMS is stent occlusion. However, these complications can occur at any time during follow-up after SEMS placement, according to the clinical situation. Table 16.2 [9–14] details the causes of obstruction and complications between covered and uncovered metal stents.

## SEMS Occlusion

The occlusion rate of SEMS during follow-up appears to vary greatly among investigators and stent types. Although SEMS have a lower occlusion rate and prolonged patency, and patients with pancreas and biliary malignancies currently survive longer than historical controls, stent occlusion does occur while patients are alive. Several studies [10, 11, 13, 16, 26–28] have shown that the stent occlusion rate for both covered and uncovered SEMS is between 20% and 38%.

The causes of early occlusion within 7 days after SEMS insertion are incomplete deployment, food impaction, or a blood clot due to bleeding.

Tumor ingrowth is the most common cause of late occlusion in bare SEMS, whereas sludge is the most common cause in CSEMS. In a postmortem examination of ten patients with malignant biliary obstruction who received polyurethane-covered stents, only one case showed a small quantity of protruding tumor tissue through a pinhole in the polyurethane membrane [29]. However, tumor ingrowth is possible, due to membrane degradation by bile acids or the tumor itself, if CSEMS are in place for longer than 6 months. No reported study has been conducted on differences between membrane materials.

Ingrowth is the most common cause of uncovered SEMS failure, particularly for smaller diameter SEMS. However, whether failures are, in fact, caused by true tumor ingrowth is debated. According to biopsies of ingrowth tissue performed by Loew et al. [17], of the 40% of ingrowth cases, half were caused by epithelial hyperplasia. To date, most studies of ingrowth were dependent on cholangiographic findings. Thus, misclassification may have occurred, causing a substantial underrepresentation of benign tissue hyperplasia. SEMS occlusion caused by tissue ingrowth is more likely to be benign epithelial hyperplasia in a narrower 6-mm stent than with a 10-mm stent. However, the small number of biopsy results in that study did not allow for definite conclusions concerning the exact tissue characteristics causing ingrowth.

Tumor overgrowth can be the cause of occlusion in both types of SEMS. Thus, it is recommended that the stent be placed to overlap the tumor-involved segment by approximately 2 cm and no less than 1 cm.

It remains unclear which stricture-related or stent-related factor(s) influences stent patency. In one multicenter study [30], early stent expansion (70% within 24 h) and easy passage of large-caliber instruments through the stricture were favorable for the long-term patency of Wallstents. However, no significant difference in patency rates according to patient age, initial serum bilirubin level, primary tumor type, length and morphological type of stricture, or length and location of the distal end of the stent was found. Theoretically, if tumor tissue is soft, the metallic

stent mesh can rapidly penetrate the tumor and lead to early occlusion. However, this result could be interpreted as indicating that the consistency of most malignant biliary strictures is hard rather than soft. A tight stricture may resist full expansion of a covered SEMS because of the covering membrane. Thus, the covered stent lumen may remain restricted and is, therefore, more prone to obstruction by biliary sludge, similar to smaller PSs, with a corresponding reduction in the overall covered SEMS stent patency [3].

## Management of Occluded SEMS

Therapeutic options for managing SEMS occlusion include mechanical cleansing using a basket or balloons, insertion of a PS, or deployment of another SEMS within the occluded metal stent. Among these methods, regardless of the cause of obstruction, re-occlusion is faster with mechanical cleansing than with re-stenting [31]. Comparative studies [31–34] between PSs and SEMS revealed that SEMS generally have longer patency than plastic stents. However, Yoon et al. [35] reported that subsequent biliary drainage with PSs offers similar patency and number of additional biliary drainage procedures compared with SEMS for managing occluded SEMS. Tumor ingrowth, as with initial SEMS occlusion, was the only factor associated with a shorter time to the second stent occlusion, regardless of the material used for the second stent. The initial SEMS embedded in the tumor tissue and the tumor itself may serve as a rigid framework, adding more resistance to the expanding force of a subsequent SEMS. If this is the case, a PS with its fixed diameter may not be inferior to SEMS for subsequent biliary stenting. Covered SEMS with sufficient radial force may be useful in this setting.

Several studies have confirmed that covered SEMS are superior to uncovered SEMS for re-intervention. The first extensive data from Ornellas et al. [26] were presented, directly comparing covered SEMS placement as a primary procedure versus re-intervention in malignant biliary obstruction. The duration of stent patency in the re-intervention group tended to be shorter than that of the primary stent placement group, although the difference was not statistically significant. For the re-intervention group, patency rates at 3, 6, and 12 months were 90, 78, and 48%, respectively (100, 93, and 82%, respectively, in the primary placement group), which were at or below the low end of the previously reported ranges for primary stent placement. The observed patency rates indicated that substantial clinical benefit can be gained by re-intervention with covered SEMS, as judged by the comparatively high patency rate through 6 months. Cho et al. [33] retrospectively evaluated patients who underwent secondary biliary stent insertion for prior biliary stent occlusion. The use of covered SEMS at revision showed a significantly longer patency than that of a PS, but not compared with bare metal stents. A multivariate analysis showed that bare SEMS had a worse cumulative stent patency and survival time than the use of covered SEMS. With regard to patient age, causative disease, and antitumor treatment, bare SEMS had 2.0 times the risk of occlusion of CSEMS and 2.4 times the risk of death during follow-up compared with covered SEMS. They suggested that SEMS placement using at least one covered SEMS (in the primary and/or secondary procedure) might provide longer cumulative stent patency and survival than using uncovered SEMS during both procedures.

## Dislocation

Stent migration can occur both as a short-term and as a long-term complication. SEMS migration rate has been reported to range from 0% to 12%, based on stent design and the presence of covering material [11, 13, 16, 26, 27, 36]. Migration after placement of uncovered SEMS seems very rare. However, partially covered SEMSs show a higher migration, of 4–12%. Migration does not appear to be related to prior PS placement or sphincterotomy [37]. Isayama et al. [15] suggested that SEMS migration may be related to increased axial force, which is high in Wallstents. The axial force is the straightening force exerted by high axial force, which may be

associated with stent kinking and biliary wall injury, as well as migration. Thus, a combination of the covering and high axial force may lead to stent migration. Currently, introducing SEMS with low axial force and high conformability results in very low migration rates, regardless of the covering.

## Cholecystitis

Acute cholecystitis is a rare complication in patients managed with a PS, with an incidence of 0-1.6% [38–42]. However, the incidence of cholecystitis in patients treated with covered SEMS varies from 0% to 11.5% [9, 26, 27, 29, 36, 43–48]. In one report [49], the most serious complication of covered biliary stent placement was acute cholecystitis, which occurred in 10% of the cases and was responsible for one death. The development of acute cholecystitis appears to have been independent of cystic duct invasion by the tumor and was observed only a few days after stent insertion. Thus, the author believed that the biliary stent was responsible, due to overlapping of the cystic duct orifice.

However, no difference in cholecystitis occurred between the covered and uncovered SEMS insertion group (5.8% vs. 4.0% and 9.1% and 10.4%, respectively) in two comparative clinical studies [50, 51]. These studies suggested that an obstruction by a tumor across the cystic duct is the major determinant of cholecystitis after SEMS insertion, regardless of stent type. The onset of cholecystitis was 4.6 (range, 1–26) days [50]. However, late-onset cholecystitis (99 and 123 days after SEMS insertion) was noted in one study [49].

For a further explanation of these results, Isayama et al. [51] suggested an interesting hypothesis. According to this, even if the cystic duct orifice is involved, bile flow is not obstructed completely, but the orifice may narrow and lose elasticity. However, even a small amount of compression caused by stent expansion or a displaced tumor may lead to impaired efflux of gallbladder bile. Cholecystitis can develop when gallbladder bile is infected with gut bacteria intruding at

ERCP. In contrast, an intact cystic duct orifice may be elastic and allow space for bile from the gallbladder to pass through.

A percutaneous cholecystostomy is the treatment of choice for cholecystitis. Suk et al. [50] reported that a percutaneous cholecystostomy should be performed as soon as cholecystitis is diagnosed and that the clinical outcome was good, with 87% (13/15) of patients recovering. The remaining two patients underwent subsequent cholecystectomies.

## Pancreatitis

In the majority of prior Wallstent studies, pancreatitis has ranged from 0% to 9% [9, 10, 16, 36, 49, 52]. These data are limited by small sample size, and thus, they were unable to control for known and potential confounding predictors of post-ERCP pancreatitis. Pancreatitis is rare in patients with pancreatic cancer because the pancreatic duct is usually already obstructed. However, pancreatitis is possible by the following mechanisms: a larger diameter SEMS, in conjunction with radial expansion after deployment, may cause obstruction of the pancreatic orifice or distortion of the common channel, increasing the risk for post-ERCP pancreatitis. This risk may be further exacerbated by CSEMS through pancreatic orifice occlusion.

Cote et al. [52] compared post-ERCP pancreatitis between 248 SEMS (102 covered) and 296 PS groups. The frequency of post-ERCP pancreatitis was significantly higher in the SEMS group (7.3%) than that in the PS group (1.3%; OR, 5.7; 95% CI, 1.9–17.1). In a univariate analysis, patient age of <40 years, a history of post-ERCP pancreatitis, and at least one pancreatic duct injection were significant predictors of pancreatitis, whereas female gender and the presence of pancreatic duct cancer were not. However, the frequency of post-ERCP pancreatitis was similar between covered (6.9%) and uncovered (7.5%) SEMS (OR, 0.9; 95% CI, 0.3–2.4). Purported SEMS-specific risk factors, including the use of CSEMS, overlapping SEMS, or undergoing a

biliary sphincterotomy, did not significantly contribute to a higher risk. Percutaneous insertion of SEMS also does not increase pancreatitis [21, 53]. However, fully covered SEMS have been reported to cause a higher rate (47%) of pancreatitis, and some cases (11.8%) lead to severe pancreatitis [54]. Prompt removal of a SEMS can avoid progression to severe pancreatitis when post-ERCP pancreatitis occurs after SEMS placement, and symptoms persist or intensify.

## Cholangitis

The frequency of cholangitis after SEMS placement ranges from 6.5% to 22% in reported series [55–60]. Restenosis and placement across the main duodenal papilla are undoubtedly associated with the occurrence of cholangitis. In a recent study [61] using barium, free reflux occurred through the SEMS in all patients (Fig. 16.1). However, reflux itself does not imply clinical cholangitis. The presence of food material in the bile-duct and stent blockage as a result of impacted food can, nevertheless, be a cause of cholangitis. In a study reported by Okamoto et al. [60],

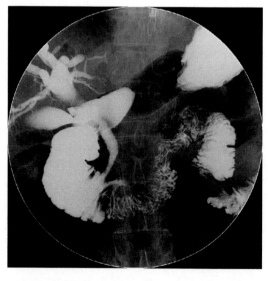

**Fig. 16.1** Reflux of contrast media into common bile duct through the SEMS in a patient with pancreatic cancer during hypotonic duodenography

cholangitis occurred in 12 of 108 patients (11.1%), but more frequently in a subgroup with transpapillary stent placement (21.6%). Cholangitis can also occur unrelated to stent occlusion [26, 49]. Cholangitis, in this case, was treated successfully with antibiotic therapy alone.

SEMS may be placed above the level of the papilla, allowing the biliary sphincter to remain intact. This avoids duodenal content reflux into the bile duct and, consequently, may decrease the incidence of cholangitis. However, this procedure can only be undertaken with strictures when the distal end is more than 2 cm above the papilla. However, to date, there are no reported clinical trials examining SEMS patency with regard to stent position.

## Unusual Complications

Distal SEMS migration rarely causes duodenal perforation [62]. When an excessive length of SEMS is placed into the duodenum with resulting ulceration of the contralateral duodenal wall or bleeding, argon beam plasma coagulation can be used to trim the excess length [63, 64]. Hemobilia can occur during SEMS placement through a friable tumor. Such bleeding may produce clots and early stent obstruction requiring endoscopic treatment [25]. The high expansive force of SEMS has also been purported to cause choledocho-duodenal fistulas [65].

SEMS fracture is another rare late complication associated with periampullary malignant biliary obstructions, which can also contribute to recurrent biliary obstruction. In a retrospective study [66], stent fractures were detected in 8% of patients, most of them between 9 and 21 months after stent placement, and all patients had a nitinol stent [67]. Stent fracture was probably related to metal fatigue, due to the constant and repetitive bending and stress at the site of maximum leverage of the prosthesis. Nitinol stents may be stiffer than other bile-duct non-nitinol stents and, therefore, less resistant to bending. However, the paucity of stent fracture data may suggest the possibility of manufacturer failure of specific stents.

## SEMS in Special Clinical Situations

### SEMS Applications Based on Resectability

The practice of placing SEMS in potentially resectable patients is still evolving and is currently restricted to highly select patients. In light of poor results with PS, preoperative biliary drainage during the period of neoadjuvant treatment may be best achieved with metal stents, which have a higher patency rate than PS and do not affect surgical outcome, in contrast to malignant hilar lesions [68–70]. Furthermore, shorter periods of drainage do not benefit outcomes [71], and longer periods of drainage raise the risk of stent occlusion, as well as the very real possibility of closing the window of opportunity for cure in a patient with a potentially resectable tumor. The prolonged patency and removability of CSEMS makes them an attractive option for biliary decompression, regardless of resectability. A strategy of initial covered SEMS placement has been purported to be the most cost-effective strategy for pancreatic malignancy regardless of resectability [72]. Covered SEMS placement may be the best option for cases of delayed surgery or if neoadjuvant therapy is being considered.

### SEMS Insertion in a Duodenal Obstruction

Endoscopic palliation can be achieved in patients who require relief from both biliary and duodenal obstruction, although this can be technically difficult to achieve, depending on the level of duodenal obstruction in relation to the major papilla [73]. Endoscopic ultrasound-guided biliary drainage (EUSBD) with one-step placement of a fully covered SEMS can be applied in patients for whom endoscopic stent placement is not possible because of tumor infiltration that limits transpapillary access [74–79]. This method can substitute for percutaneous transhepatic biliary drainage. A fully covered SEMS with both ends flared has been designed to prevent stent migration. EUSBD can be conducted using either an intra- or extrahepatic approach. The overall rate of procedure-related complications, such as bile leakage or pneumoperitoneum, for extrahepatic approaches with PS is 19% [74–79]. In contrast, Park et al. [80] reported no such procedural complications with fully covered SEMS in 14 patients with malignant biliary obstruction who had duodenal strictures or periampullary tumor infiltration, making transpapillary cannulation impossible.

Another EUS-guided drainage method is the antegrade advancement of a SEMS after EUS-guided wire placement across malignant strictures in patients with an endoscopically inaccessible biliary orifice [81]. Rather than transluminal (transgastric or transduodenal) stent placement, stents are deployed traversing the stricture and crossing the ampulla. Transgastric access is the preferred method for this procedure. Transgastric access to the intrahepatic bile ducts is not limited by morbid obesity or ascites, which may prevent external access in comparison with EUS-guided transmural drainage (hepaticogastrostomy or choledochoduodenostomy). Placing a SEMS across a stricture and entirely within the duct preserves the intended use of tubular stents for lumen recanalization and should eliminate reported complications associated with transmural drainage, including bile leaks and stent dislodgement.

The use of a dedicated duodenal stent with a central portion designed to facilitate passage of a biliary stent through the interstices has been reported in a small number of patients [82] to manage simultaneous biliary and duodenal obstruction. However, two-thirds of patients with tumor infiltration of the major papilla failed bile-duct cannulation and required a rendezvous procedure. These methods can be successfully applied in patients with combined duodenal and biliary malignant obstruction. However, these methods require comparative clinical trials with percutaneous placement of SEMS to determine efficacy, complications, and long-term results.

# Future of Biliary SEMS

## Modification of SEMS Design

The ideal SEMS provides very low axial force to prevent kinking and other adverse effects, such as biliary wall damage and migration, yet has a medium level of radial force that is strong enough to keep the domain open for a smooth flow of bile but not too high as to cause damage to the biliary duct wall [15]. Although new types of SEMS are currently commercially available, well-designed randomized prospective clinical trials with sufficient sample size should be conducted to assess whether their use is associated with superior clinical results.

The most common cause of obstruction in CSEMS is impaction of biliary sludge or food impaction. Although the diameter of SEMS is far wider than that of PSs, it is not free of luminal sludge formation caused by duodenal reflux. To minimize this effect, the friction coefficient of the covering membrane should be low and the metal mesh should not be exposed to the lumen. Thus, the concept of a sandwich-design SEMS, recently introduced commercially, is disadvantageous and modification is necessary.

SEMS covered with polyurethane, silicone, or Gore-Tex membranes are now commercially available. Clinical trials are still insufficient to conclude which covering membrane is most beneficial. According to an in vitro study, silicone was more refractory to membrane degradation by bile acids than polyurethane. However, further clinical trials are needed.

Several studies have reported the presence of plant fibers in bile ducts and blocked PSs as a result of food material reflux. This situation is similar to that observed for SEMS. To prevent reflux of duodenal contents, Hu et al. [83] developed a new anti-reflux metal stent. A hemispheric silicone valve with a cross-shaped outlet was attached to the distal end of a nitinol-wire SEMS. This modification allowed for one-way flow of bile as a check valve. A pilot study showed that the median duration of patency for this stent was 14 months, with cumulative patency rates at 3, 6, and 12 months of 95%, 74%, and 56%, respectively. The impact of anti-reflux SEMS to prolong stent patency deserves further randomized evaluation.

## Drug-Eluting Stent

No drug-eluting stent (DES) for nonvascular use has been developed commercially to date. Recently, however, an animal experiment and a human pilot study on the use of a DES in bile ducts have been conducted, and a comparative study between the use of conventional nondrug-coated stents and DES is in progress. Lee et al. [84] developed a metallic stent covered with a membrane incorporating paclitaxel. Paclitaxel, an antineoplastic agent that binds to β-tubulin and stabilizes polymerized microtubules, is currently used to treat several types of cancer. Paclitaxel enhances the assembly of extraordinarily stable microtubules, interrupts cell proliferation, and triggers molecular signaling of the mitochondrial pathway for apoptosis. Paclitaxel dose-dependently inhibits the proliferation of human gallbladder epithelial cells, fibroblasts, and pancreatic adenocarcinoma cells, suggesting that local delivery of paclitaxel may reduce tumor cell proliferation. In animal experiments and an in vitro study, the nature of histological changes and the effectiveness of drug release associated with 10% paclitaxel were superior to the results of treatment with 20% paclitaxel-coated stents. The same group conducted a pilot study [85] in 21 human patients diagnosed with an unresectable malignant biliary obstruction. The mean patency of a 10% paclitaxel-coated covered SEMS was 429 days (median, 270 days; range, 68–810 days), and the cumulative patency rates at 3, 6, and 12 months were 100%, 71%, and 36%, respectively. A human pilot comparative study [86] conducted by another group failed to demonstrate the superiority of DES over conventionally covered SEMS. Furthermore, that study did not clearly validate the drug incorporation method and in vitro release profile of paclitaxel.

It is important to develop a technique that would allow chemotherapeutic agents to remain effectively incorporated in the membrane and, thus, maintain steady release of the drug over an extended period. To achieve this, a polyurethane/pluronic F-127 mixture as a surfactant was incorporated into the drug-containing membrane material, which resulted in more effective drug release from the membrane [87]. Pluronic block copolymers are an efficient drug delivery system with multiple effects. Further clinical studies using effective local drug delivery systems are expected.

Despite a negative or unconfirmed, single-center clinical study, other drugs could potentially have a significant effect on biliary stent patency when used for malignant obstruction, although it is expected that such stents would be significantly more costly and unlikely to result in prolonged survival [88]. It is expected that DES may be another turning point in the palliative treatment of malignant biliary obstruction.

## Conclusions

The introduction of SEMS for the palliative treatment of unresectable distal malignant bile-duct obstruction is a highlight in terms of prolonging stent patency and improving the quality of patient life. SEMS, however, are foreign bodies and bile drainage conduits that can cause complications. This is the driving force for the continuous evolution and improvement of SEMS.

Significant advances in the development of SEMS have occurred over the years. Manufacturers can now adjust the axial and radial forces of SEMS and even their conformability. Various coverings for SEMS are also commercially available. Additionally, functioning SEMS with anti-tumor effects, such as the DES, are awaiting clinical trials. However, as many clinical trials have shown, there is unfortunately still no ideal SEMS that can fulfill all needs. Although improvements have been gradual, an ideal SEMS may eventually be available in the future.

## References

1. Soehendra N, Reynders-Frederix V. Palliative biliary duct drainage. A new method for endoscopic introduction of a new drain. Dtsch Med Wochenscher. 1979;104:206–7.

2. Levy MJ, Baron TH, Gostout CJ, et al. Palliation of malignant extrahepatic biliary obstruction with plastic versus expandable metal stent: an evidence-based approach. Clin Gastroenterol Hepatol. 2004;2:273–85.

3. Cipolletta L, Rotondano G, Marmo R, et al. Endoscopic palliation of malignant obstructive jaundice: an evidence-based review. Dig Liver Dis. 2007;39:375–88.

4. Moss AC, Morris E, Leyden J, MacMathuna P. Malignant distal biliary obstruction: a systemic review and meta-analysis of endoscopic and surgical bypass results. Cancer Treat Rev. 2007;33:213–21.

5. Carr-Locke DL, Ball TJ, Connors PJ, et al. Multicenter, randomized, trial of Wallstent biliary endoprosthesis versus plastic stents. Gastrointest Endosc. 1993; 39:A310.

6. Soderlund C, Linder S. Covered metal versus plastic stents for malignant common bile duct stenosis: a prospective, randomized, controlled trial. Gastrointest Endosc. 2006;63:986–95.

7. Moss AC, Morris E, Leyden J, MacMathuna P. Do the benefits of metal stents justify the costs? A systematic review and meta-analysis of trials comparing endoscopic stents for malignant biliary obstruction. Eur J Gastroenterol Hepatol. 2007;19:1119–24.

8. Yon WJ, Ryu JK, Yang KY, et al. A comparison of metal and plastic stents for the relief of jaundice in unresectable malignant biliary obstruction in Korea: and emphasis on cost-effectiveness in a country with a low ERCP cost. Gastrointest Endosc. 2009;70:284–9.

9. Isayama H, Komatsu Y, Tsujino T, et al. A prospective randomized study of "covered" versus "uncovered" diamond stents for the management of distal malignant biliary obstruction. Gut. 2004;53:729–34.

10. Yoon WJ, Lee JK, Lee KH, et al. A comparison of covered and uncovered Wallstents for the management of distal malignant biliary obstruction. Gastrointest Endosc. 2006;63:996–1000.

11. Park DH, Kim M-H, Choi JS, et al. Covered versus uncovered Wallstent for malignant extrahepatic biliary obstruction: a cohort comparative analysis. Clin Gastroenterol Hepatol. 2006;4:790–6.

12. Telford JJ, Carr-Locke DL, Baron TH, et al. A randomized trial comparing uncovered and partially covered self-expandable metal stents in the palliation of distal malignant biliary obstruction. Gastrointest Endosc. 2010;72:907–14.

13. Kullman E, Frozanpor F, Soderlund C, et al. Covered versus uncovered self-expandable nitinol stents in the palliative treatment of malignant distal biliary obstruction: results from a randomized, multicenter study. Gastrointest Endosc. 2010;72:915–23.

14. Gwon DI, Ko G-Y, Kim JH, et al. A comparative analysis of PTFE-covered and uncovered stents for palliative treatment of malignant extrahepatic biliary obstruction. AJR Am J Roentgenol. 2010;195:W463–9.

15. Isayama H, Nakai Y, Toyokawa Y, et al. Measurement of radial and axial forces of biliary self-expandable metallic stents. Gastrointest Endosc. 2009;70:37–44.

16. Yang KY, Ryu JK, Seo JK, et al. A comparison of the Niti-D biliary uncovered stent and the uncovered Wallstent in malignant biliary obstruction. Gastrointest Endosc. 2009;70:45–51.

17. Loew BJ, Jowell DA, Sandeers MK, et al. Comparative performance of uncoated, self-expanding metal biliary stents of different design in 2 diameters: final results of an international multicenter, randomized, controlled trial. Gastrointest Endosc. 2009;70:445–53.

18. Shah RJ, Howell DA, Desilets DJ, et al. Multicenter randomized trial of the spiral Z-stent compared with the Wallstent for malignant biliary obstruction. Gastrointest Endosc. 2003;57:729–34.

19. Howell DA, Sanders MK, Bernadino KP, et al. Randomized controlled trial of a new nitinol non-foreshortening self-expanding metal stent for malignant biliary obstruction: an international multi-center comparison to Wallstent. Gastroenterology. 2006;130(Suppl. 2).

20. Isayama H, Kawabe T, Nakai Y, et al. Management of distal malignant biliary obstruction with the ComVi stent, a new covered metallic stent. Surg Endosc. 2010;24:131–137.

21. Pinol V, Castells A, Bordas JM. Percutaneous self-expanding metal stents versus endoscopic polyethylene endoprostheses for treating malignant biliary obstruction: randomized clinical trial. Radiology. 2002;225:27–34.

22. van Delden OM, Lameris JS. Percutaneous drainage and stenting for palliation of malignant bile duct obstruction. Eur Radiol. 2008;18:448–56.

23. Dahlstrand U, Sandblom G, Eriksson L-G, et al. Primary patency of percutaneously inserted self-expanding metallic stents in patients with malignant biliary obstruction. HPB (Oxford). 2009;11:358–63.

24. Castano R, Lopes TL, Alvarez O, et al. Nitinol biliary stent versus surgery for palliation of distal malignant biliary obstruction. Surg Endosc. 2010;24:2092–8.

25. Ferreira LEC, Baron TH. Endoscopic stenting for palliation of a malignant biliary obstruction. Expert Rev Med Devices. 2010;7:681–91.

26. Ornellas LC, Stefanidis G, Chuttani R, et al. Covered Wallstents for palliation of malignant biliary obstruction: primary stent placement versus reintervention. Gastrointest Endosc. 2009;70:676–83.

27. Kahaleh M, Tokar J, Conaway MR, et al. Efficacy and complications of covered Wallstents in malignant distal biliary obstruction. Gastrointest Endosc. 2005;61: 528–33.

28. Kubota Y, Mukai H, Nakaizumi A, et al. Covered Wallstent for palliation of malignant common bile duct stricture: prospective multicenter evaluation. Dig Endosc. 2005;17:218–23.

29. Isayama H, Komatsu Y, Tsujino T, et al. Polyurethane-covered metal stent for management of distal malignant biliary obstruction. Gastrointest Endosc. 2002;55:366–70.

30. Kim HS, Lee DK, Kim HG, et al. Features of malignant biliary obstruction affecting the patency

of metallic stents: a multicenter study. Gastrointest Endosc. 2002;55:359–65.

31. Bueno JT, Gerdes H, Kurtz RC. Endoscopic management of occluded biliary Wallstents: a cancer center experience. Gastrointest Endosc. 2003;58:879–84.

32. Ridtitid W, Rerknimitr R, Janchai A, et al. Outcome of second interventions for occluded metallic stents in patients with malignant biliary obstruction. Surg Endosc. 2010;24:2216–20.

33. Cho JH, Jeon TJ, Park JY, et al. Comparison of outcomes among secondary covered metallic, uncovered metallic, and plastic biliary stents in treating occluded primary metallic stents in malignant distal biliary obstruction. Surg Endosc. 2011;25:475–82.

34. Katsinelos P, Beltsis A, Chatzimavroudis G, et al. Endoscopic management of occluded biliary uncovered metal stents: a multicenter experience. World J Gastroenterol. 2011;7:98–104.

35. Yoon WJ, Ryu JK, Lee JW, et al. Endoscopic management of occluded metal biliary stents: Metal versus 10F plastic stents. World J Gastroenterol. 2010;14: 5347–52.

36. Nakai Y, Isayama H, Komatsu Y, et al. Efficacy and safety of the covered Wallstent in patients with distal malignant biliary obstruction. Gastrointest Endosc. 2005;62:742–8.

37. Artifon EL, Sakai P, Ishioka S, et al. Endoscopic sphincterotomy before deployment of covered metal stent is associated with greater complication rate; a prospective randomized control trial. J Clin Gastroenterol. 2008;42:815–9.

38. Smith AG, Dowset JF, Rassell RCG, et al. Randomized trial of endoscopic stenting versus surgical bypass in malignant low bile duct obstruction. Lancet. 1994; 344:1655–60.

39. Anderson JR, Sonsen SM, Kruse A, et al. Randomized trial of endoscopic endoprosthesis versus operative bypass in malignant obstructive jaundice. Gut. 1989;30:1132–5.

40. Davids PHP, Groen AK, Rauws EAJ, et al. Randomized trial of self-expanding metal stents versus polyethylene stents for distal malignant biliary obstruction. Lancet. 1992;340:1488–92.

41. Knyrim K, Wagner HJ, Pausch J, et al. A prospective, randomized, controlled trial of metal stents for malignant obstruction of the common bile duct. Endoscopy. 1993;25:207–12.

42. Ainley CC, Williams SJ, Smith AC, et al. Gallbladder sepsis after stent insertion for bile duct obstruction: management by percutaneous cholecystectomy. Br J Surg. 1991;78:961–3.

43. Saito H, Sakurai Y, Takamura A, et al. Biliary endoprosthesis using Gore-Tex covered expandable metallic stents: preliminary clinical evaluation [in Japanese with English abstract]. Nippon Acta Radiologica. 1994;54:180–2.

44. Kawase Y, Motoyama A, Kawanishi M, et al. Experience with Strecker stent covered with polyurethane membrane for malignant biliary strictures [in Japanese with English abstract]. Gastroenterol Endosc. 1995;37:1229–35.

45. Miyayama S, Matsui O, Terayama N, et al. Covered Gianturco Stent for malignant biliary obstruction: preliminary clinical evaluation. J Vasc Interv Radiol. 1997;8:641–8.

46. Shim CS, Lee YH, Cho YD, et al. Preliminary results of a new covered biliary metal stent for malignant biliary obstruction. Endoscopy. 1998;30:345–50.

47. Bezzi M, Zolovkins A, Cantisani V, et al. New ePTFE/FEP-covered stent in the palliative treatment of malignant biliary obstruction. J Vasc Interv Radiol. 2002; 13:581–9.

48. Schoder M, Rossi P, Uflacker R, et al. Malignant biliary obstruction: treatment with ePTFE-FEP-covered endoprostheses initial technical and clinical experiences in a multicenter trial. Radiology. 2002;225:35–42.

49. Fumex F, Coumaro D, Napoleon B, et al. Similar performance but higher cholecystitis rate with covered biliary stents: results from a prospective multicenter evaluation. Endoscopy. 2006;38:787–92.

50. Suk KT, Kim HS, Baik SK, et al. Risk factors for cholecystitis after metal stent placement in malignant biliary obstruction. Gastrointest Endosc. 2006;64:522–9.

51. Isayama H, Kawabe T, Nakai Y, et al. Cholecystitis after metallic stent placement in patients with malignant distal biliary obstruction. Clin Gastroenterol Hepatol. 2006;4:1148–53.

52. Cote GA, Kumar N, Ansstas M, et al. Risk of post-ERCP pancreatitis with placement of self-expandable metallic stents. Gastrointest Endosc. 2010;72:748–54.

53. Han YH, Kim M-Y, Kim SY, et al. Percutaneous insertion of Zilver stent in malignant biliary obstruction. Abdom Imaging. 2006;31:433–8.

54. Bakhru M, Ho HC, Wang AY, et al. Fully covered self expandable metal stents in malignant biliary strictures: mid-term evaluation. J Gastroenterol Hepatol. 2011;26:1022–7.

55. Nicholson AA, Royston CMS. Palliation of inoperable biliary obstruction with self-expanding metallic endoprostheses: a review of 77 patients. Clin Radiol. 1993;47:245–50.

56. Stoker J, Lameris JS, Jeekel J. Percutaneously placed Wallstent endoprosthesis in patients with malignant distal biliary obstruction. Br J Surg. 1993;80:1185–7.

57. Boguth L, Tatalovic S, Antonucci F, et al. Malignant biliary obstruction: clinical and histopathologic correlation after treatment with self-expanding metallic prostheses. Radiology. 1994;192:669–74.

58. Stocker J, Lameris JS. Complications of percutaneously inserted biliary Wallstent. J Vasc Interv Radiol. 1993;4:767–72.

59. Hatzidakis AA, Tsetis D, Chrysou E, et al. Nitinol stents for palliative treatment of malignant obstructive jaundice: should we stent the sphincter of Oddi in every case? Cardiovasc Intervent Radiol. 2001;24:245–8.

60. Okamoto T, Fujioka S, Yanagisawa S, et al. Placement of a metallic stent across the main duodenal papilla

may predispose to cholangitis. Gastrointest Endosc. 2006;63:792–6.

61. Misra SP, Dwivedi M. Reflux of duodenal contents and cholangitis in patients undergoing self-expanding metal stent placement. Gastrointest Endosc. 2009;70:317–21.

62. Thumbe VK, Houghton AD, Smith MS. Duodenal perforation by a Wallstent. Endoscopy. 2000;32:512–5.

63. Vanbiervliet G, Piche T, Caroli-Bosc FX, et al. Endoscopic argon plasma trimming of biliary and gastrointestinal metallic stents. Endoscopy. 2005;37: 434–8.

64. Chen YK, Jakribettuu V, Springer EW, et al. Safety and efficacy of argon plasma coagulation trimming of malpositioned and migrated biliary metal stents: a controlled study in the porcine model. Am J Gastroenterol. 2006;101:1–6.

65. Moon SK, Cheung DY, Kim JH, et al. A case of choledochoduodenal fistula as a delayed complication after biliary metallic stent placement in distal cholangiocarcinoma. Korean J Gastroenterol. 2008;51:314–8.

66. Rasmussen IC, Dahlstrand U, Sandblom G, et al. Fractures of self-expanding metallic stents in periampullary malignant biliary obstruction. Acta Radiol. 2009;23:730–7.

67. Peck R, Wattam J. Fracture of Memotherm metallic stents in the biliary tract. Cardiovasc Intervent Radiol. 2000;23:55–6.

68. van der Gaag NA, Rauws EAJ, van Eijck CHJ, et al. Preoperative biliary drainage for cancer of the head of the pancreas. N Engl J Med. 2010;362:129–37.

69. Mullen JT, Lee JH, Gomez HF, et al. Pancreaticoduodenectomy after placement of endobiliary metal stents. J Gastrointest Surg. 2005;9: 1094–104.

70. Decker C, Christein JD, Phadnis MA, et al. Biliary metal stents are superior to plastic stents for preoperative biliary decompression in pancreatic cancer. Surg Endosc. 2011;25:2364–7.

71. Wang Q, Gurusamy KS, Lin H, et al. Preoperative biliary drainage for obstructive jaundice. Cochrane Database Syst Rev. 2008;3:CD005444.

72. Kahaleh M, Brock A, Conaway MR, et al. Covered self-expandable metal stents in pancreatic malignancy regardless of resectability; a new concept validated by a decision analysis. Endoscopy. 2007;39:319–24.

73. Baron TH. Management of simultaneous biliary and duodenal obstruction: the endoscopic perspective. Gut Liver. 2010;4(Suppl. 1):S50–6.

74. Burmester E, Niehaus J, Leineweber T, et al. EUS-cholangio-drainage of the bile duct: report of 4 cases. Gastrointest Endosc. 2003;57:246–51.

75. Kahaleh M, Hernandez AJ, Tokar J, et al. Interventional EUS-guided cholangiography: evaluation of a technique in evolution. Gastrointest Endosc. 2006;64:52–9.

76. Itoi T, Itokawa F, Sofuni A, et al. Endoscopic ultrasound-guided choledochoduodenostomy in patients with failed endoscopic retrograde cholangiopancreatography. World J Gastroenterol. 2008;14:6078–82.

77. Yamao K, Bhatia V, Mizuno N, et al. EUS-guided choledochoduodenostomy for palliative biliary drainage in patients with malignant biliary obstruction: results of long-term follow-up. Endoscopy. 2008;40:340–2.

78. Itoi T, Yamao K. EUS 2008 Working Group document: evaluation of EUS-guided choledochoduodenostomy (with video). Gastrointest Endosc. 2009;69:S8–12.

79. Siddiqui AA, Sreenarasimhaiah J, Lara LF, et al. Endoscopic ultrasound-guided transduodenal placement of a fully covered metal stent for palliative biliary drainage in patients with malignant biliary obstruction. Surg Endosc. 2011;25:549–55.

80. Park DH, Koo JE, Oh J, et al. EUS-guided biliary drainage with one-step placement of a fully covered metal stent for malignant biliary obstruction: a prospective feasibility study. Am J Gastroenterol. 2009;104:2168–74.

81. Nguyen-Tang T, Binmoeller KF, Shah JN. Endoscopic ultrasound-guided transhepatic antegrade self-expandable metal stent placement across malignant biliary obstruction. Endoscopy. 2010;42:232–6.

82. Moon JH, Choi HJ, Ko BM, et al. Combined endoscopic stent-in-stent placement for malignant and duodenal obstruction by using a new duodenal metal stent (with video). Gastrointest Endosc. 2009;70:772–7.

83. Hu B, Wang T-T, Shi Z-M, et al. A novel antireflux metal stent for the palliation of biliary malignancies: a pilot feasibility study (with video). Gastrointest Endosc. 2011;73:143–148.

84. Lee DK, Kim HS, Kim K-S, et al. The effect on porcine bile duct of a metallic stent covered with a paclitaxel-incorporated membrane. Gastrointest Endosc. 2005;61:296–301.

85. Suk KT, Kim JW, Kim HS, et al. Human application of a metallic stent covered with a paclitaxel-incorporated membrane for malignant biliary obstruction: multicenter pilot study. Gastrointest Endosc. 2007;66:798–803.

86. Song TJ, Lee SS, Yun SC, et al. Paclitaxel-eluting covered metal stents versus covered metal stents for distal malignant biliary obstruction: a prospective competitive pilot study. Gastrointest Endosc. 2011;73:727–33.

87. Lee DK. Drug-eluting stent in malignant biliary obstruction. J Hepatobiliary Pancreat Surg. 2009;16: 628–32.

88. Baron TH. Endoscopic retrograde cholangiopancreatography (DDW highlight). Endoscopy. 2010;42: 938–43.

## Further Reading

89. Kaasis M, Boyer J, Dumas R, et al. Plastic or metal stents for malignant stricture of the common bile duct? Results of a randomized prospective study. Gastrointest Endosc. 2003;57:178–82.

90. Schmassmann A, von Gunten E, Knuchel J, et al. Wallstents versus plastic stents in malignant biliary obstruction: effects of stent patency of the first and second stent on patient compliance and survival. Am J Gastroenterol. 1996;91:654–9.

# Benign Biliary Diseases

17

## John T. Cunningham

In the context of assessing the use of self-expanding metal stents (SEMS) for benign biliary disease, several aspects need to be addressed prior to their use. What is the expected survival of the patient? What is the natural course of the disease being treated and are there any advantages over conventional therapy? Stent design will also play an important role when dealing with benign disease, with significant differences between uncovered stents (uSEMS), partially covered stents (pcSEMS), and fully covered stents (fcSEMS). The standard endoscopic treatment has been some form of therapy with plastic stents, and to date, there are no prospective controlled trials comparing plastic to metal stents for benign disease. The outcome and potential complications could also be influenced by the mechanical characteristics of the stents. The two principles involved are radial force (RF) and axial force (AF). RF is the expanding force of the stent, and the higher the force, the greater its ability to reach its manufactured size. The AF is the property of the device to resist remaining in a nonmanufactured configuration, i.e., curvature of the bile duct, and the force created to return to its manufactured straight shape. Isayama [1] reported the AF and RF of 14 covered and uncovered stents and discusses how the understanding of both principles in an individual device could have an effect on one's selection. One of the theoretical advantages of metal stents over conventional stenting with multiple stents is the long duration of stenting requiring multiple stents on a scheduled exchange interval; however, several recent studies saw no difference in the rate of clinical occlusion in patients in whom three or more stents were left in place for greater than 6 months versus those with a scheduled every-3-month change [2, 3].

## Initial Experience with Uncovered Metal Stents

Early use of uSEMS in benign disease has demonstrated that, over time, there is a significant risk of mucosal hyperplasia or stone/debris formation within the stent, leading to recurrent occlusion and cholangitis [4–6]. This led one author to advise against their use in a review article on metal stents for benign disease unless extenuating circumstances existed [7]. Most of the problems addressed in this chapter have the potential to be treated over a finite period of time, and to have a device which is removable is a definite advantage. Silvis et al. were the first to demonstrate in a dog model the advantage of a membrane covering on a metal stent in preventing stent occlusion by inhibiting the formation of mucosal hyperplasia [8].

J.T. Cunningham, M.D. (✉)
Department of Internal Medicine,
Section of Gastroenterology and Hepatology,
University of Arizona, 1501 N. Campbell Ave.,
Room 6402, Tucson, AZ 85724, USA
e-mail: cunning1@u.arizona.edu

R. Kozarek et al. (eds.), *Self-Expandable Stents in the Gastrointestinal Tract*,
DOI 10.1007/978-1-4614-3746-8_17, © Springer Science+Business Media New York 2013

## Benign Biliary Strictures

### Chronic Pancreatitis

The conventional treatment of benign strictures, like in malignancy, is plastic stents. Initial series on the use of single plastic stents in chronic pancreatitis (CP) reported high failure rates of 62% and 69% [9, 10]. This led multiple authors to report series that have shown the advantage of multiple plastic stents over single stents for biliary strictures secondary to CP [11, 12]. The theoretical advantage is a larger luminal diameter conferred by multiple stents to fully ablate the stricture which will delay or prevent restenosis. The disadvantage is that the current protocol is serial endoscopic retrograde cholangiopancreatographies (ERCPs) with the addition of more stents at each procedure [11–13]. The mean number of endoscopic procedures is variable, depending on the protocol used, with most adding one stent every 3 months [13]. The potential advantage of metal stents in this context is that fewer procedures will be necessary and the increased cost of metal stents will be outweighed by the decreased procedural costs. An initial report by Deviere [14] demonstrated a 90% patency in 20 patients with CP who had uSEMS at 3 years follow-up. But additional series have demonstrated a significant occlusion rate secondary to mucosal hyperplasia and a low success rate in stent extraction, requiring either repeat metal stents, insertion of plastic stents, or surgery [4, 5, 15]. The longer the follow-up, the higher the frequency of stent malfunction [4]. Two studies with a pcSEMS (Wallstent, Boston Scientific, Natick, Mass) in CP report success comparable to multiple plastic stents [16, 17]. However, the design of these studies was quite different. The study by Cantu placed 10-mm stents with no scheduled removal and had 100%

patency at 18 months. Thereafter, there was a decrement in function to 50% at 24 months and 35% at 30 months [16]. There is no mention of long-term follow-up. The study by Kahaleh placed pcSEMS in 32 CP patients and reported a 77% success rate [17]. The duration of stent placement was highly variable, and the criteria for removal were vague. Follow-up was relatively short, with a median of 12 months (range 1–28 months). One small series of 19 patients with fcSEMS (Viabil, Conmed, Utica, NY) reported a 65% success in CP, but with only a brief follow-up of 3.9 months [18]. To date, there are no controlled comparative trials of metal versus plastic prostheses, and because of the variability of the number of plastic stents used, it is difficult to get valid comparability. The theoretical goal is to dilate the stricture to the point of full ablation relative to native duct size. Table 17.1 demonstrates the relative degree of stricture dilation achieved by various stent regimens.

One of the major predictors of failure of stenting in CP is the presence of pancreatic calcifications [10, 12]. However, in these two series, there were either a single stent or only two or three used. Catalano, using four or five 10F stents, had 100% success in noncalcific disease and 83% in calcific pancreatitis in a small case series of 12 patients with mean follow-up of 3.9 years [13]. They used historical controls from their own institution with serial single 10F stents with a success rate of only 24%. None of the pcSEMS or fcSEMS series mention the presence or absence of calcific disease.

### Postoperative Strictures

Conventional management of biliary strictures was surgery, but with the introduction of biliary stenting, there has been a gradual change to

**Table 17.1** Comparison of the amount of stricture dilation that can be achieved by two conventional metal stent sizes in comparison with three 10F plastic stent configurations

| Maximum circumference of various stent configurations | | | | | |
| --- | --- | --- | --- | --- | --- |
| Stent | 8-mm metal | 10-mm metal | 3–10F | 4–10F | 5–10F |
| Circumference (mm) | 25.3 mm | 31.6 mm | 23 mm | 27 mm | 31 mm |

endoscopic therapy and the suggestion that surgery be reserved for complete transections, prior failed repairs, and failed endoscopic therapy [19]. A more recent nonrandomized study of surgery versus stenting for postcholecystectomy strictures suggested a comparable outcome in the two groups, although most of the stented patients had only one or two plastic stents [20].

Stenting for postoperative and particularly posttransplant strictures has been undertaken with plastic stents with the best success being reported for multiple stents [3, 11, 21–26]. Success in these reports ranges from 82% to 100%. Most of the plastic stent series have used a 3-month or shorter procedure interval based on the expected stent occlusion within 3–4 months. Two series have suggested that if three or more stents are in place, the incidence of cholangitis with longer dwell times is extremely low, and this would allow for longer stent placement intervals and fewer ERCPs [2, 3]. The variables involved are the number of stents to be used and the duration of stenting required. A multicenter, prospective study of a 10-mm pcSEMS (Wallstent, Boston Scientific, Natick, NY) reported the use in 22 posttransplant patients with anastomotic strictures [27]. The stents were left in place for 2 months, and three had outward migration with residual stricture formation. In the remaining 19 patients after 12 months of follow-up, there was a 47% stricture recurrence. A single center reported with the same 10-mm stent in 16 orthotopic liver transplantation (OLTX) patients, and a 4-month dwell time for the device demonstrated 15/16 (94%) resolution of the stricture, but median follow-up was only 4 months [17]. They also reported 100% success for other benign biliary strictures (non-OLTX and nonpancreatic). Fully covered SEMS have been placed by several centers in small case series after failure of plastic stents to resolve strictures or stricture with leaks. The first used 10-mm fcSEMS (Niti-S ComVi, Taewoong Medical, Korea) in 16 patients (11 stenosis alone and 5 leaks and stenosis). All had failed multiple ERCPs with two 10F or 11.5F stents [28]. All stents were deployed successfully and left in place for 2 months. At retrieval ERCP, six stents had migrated out, but the cholangiogram showed stricture resolution in all six. Two patients had persistent stricturing at stent removal, and one recurred at 6 months follow-up, giving an overall success of 81%. The second series had eight patients in whom the authors used a 10-mm WallFlex (Boston Scientific, Natick, Mass) after failure of one or two 10F plastic stents for at least three endoscopic sessions [29]. Stent migration occurred in four out of the eight, and successful management was reported in 75%. There were two failures, one in the migrated stent group and one in the full stent interval group.

## Stents for Leaks

Conventional treatment of postcholecystectomy leaks has been either biliary sphincterotomy [30, 31] or endoscopic stent with or without sphincterotomy [31–34]. One series reported a 95% success with endoscopic therapy if the leak is seen on ERCP, but a 33% failure if the treatment was sphincterotomy alone [31]. This is supported in a dog model reported by Marks where biliary stenting was more effective than sphincterotomy alone [35]. A prospective randomized, controlled trial (RCT) looked at 10F versus 7F plastic stents in postcholecystectomy leaks, with resolution in 93% for the 7F group and 97% in the 10F group. The two failures in the 7F group resolved with an additional endoscopic treatment with a 10F stent [34]. This success has led one author to state that bridging the papilla with short 10F stents without sphincterotomy should be the standard for postcholecystectomy leaks, thus avoiding the potential complication of sphincterotomy [33]. Similar success has been reported in biliary fistulas after complex liver resection with an overall success of 96% using a variety of stents (5F to 10F), but using longer stents, most of which bridged the leak [36]. There are three small case series of metal stents for biliary leaks not associated with liver transplant, some for failed prior plastic stenting (Fig. 17.1) or the presence of a significant comorbidity on first stent placement [37–39]. The first series included three cases of persistent leak after attempted cholecystectomy, two were pcSEMS (Wallstent, Boston Scientific, Natick,

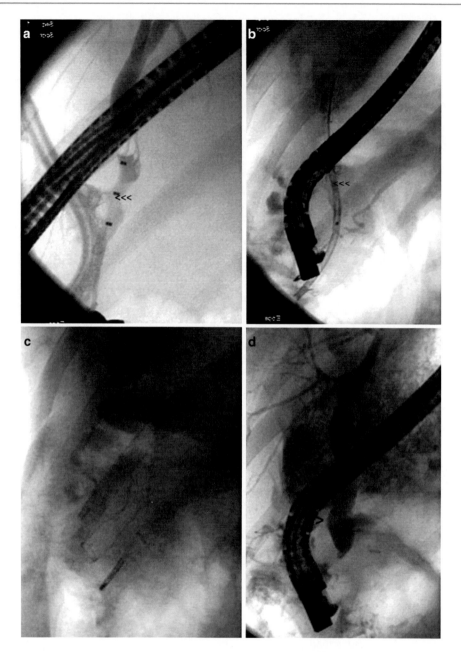

**Fig. 17.1** Patient with pancreatic trauma and (**a**) a high volume distal biliary leak (*arrow*) into a JP drain. (**b**) Continued leak (*arrow*) despite a 10F stent placed 6 weeks earlier. (**c**) Transpapillary placement of a 10 mm × 8 cm Viabil® fcSEMS. (**d**) Poststent removal cholangiogram done 1-month poststent extraction showing leak resolution and no residual effects from stent placement

Mass), one crossing the leak and one crossing the ampulla but not the cystic duct, and the third was a fcSEMS (Viabil, Conmed, Utica, NY) also just bridging the ampulla. All three leaks resolved with successful stent removal after 3–9 weeks [37]. The second series reported 15 patients, eight cystic duct leaks, five duct of Luschka leaks, and two with partial cholecystectomy [38]. The stent used was a 10-mm Wallstent (Boston Scientific, Natick, Mass) and seven had failed prior plastic stents. The stent crossed the cystic duct for cystic leaks and partial resections, but only the ampulla for duct of Luschka leaks. The duration of stenting was a median of 3 months (range 1–17 months). The authors reported 94% resolution of the leaks. There were three outward migrations, but only one was associated with failure of leak closure. The final series from the same institution used fcSEMS (Viabil, Conmed, Utica, NY) in eight patients with successful resolution of the leaks in all the cases, and no migrations were reported [39].

## Leaks in Orthotopic Liver Transplantation Patients

Endoscopic therapy for choledochocholedocal from T-tube tracts or choledochocholedostomy anastomoses soon became a preferred method of treatment and included the use of nasobiliary catheters [40, 41] or indwelling stents [42, 43]. One series reported their 9-year experience in 219 patients with duct-to-duct anastomosis [43]. There were 26 leaks identified at ERCP, and 24/26 had stents bridging the anastomosis. In the other two either a transpapillary or nasobiliary drain was placed. Eleven patients had an anastomotic leak, and the remainder, a leak from the cystic duct or T-tube tract. Initial stent placement resolved the leaks in 23/26 (88%) of cases, including all from the anastomosis. Two of the initial failures responded to a second stent and one went to surgery, resulting in an overall success of 96% [43]. For anastomotic leaks, the preferred method of stent placement has been long stents which bridge the surgical anastomosis. The success with plastic stents was high for T-tube leaks in both series, but Pfau reported less success with anastomotic leaks in three of seven (43%) despite all having had prostheses placement across the surgical anastomosis [42]. Metal stents have been used in several series [28, 29, 39, 44, 45]. A single case report of resolution with a partially covered Wallstent (Boston Scientific, Natick, Mass) has been reported [44]. Fully covered SEMS have also been reported in four series [28, 29, 39, 45]. Two reports with the

Viabil fcSEMS (Conmed, Utica, NY) from the same institution report 22 patients, 20/22 anastomotic, with leak resolution in 21 [39, 45]. The deployment bridged the anastomosis in all but one case. Another center used the Niti-S ComVi (Taewoong Medical, Korea) in five patients with stricture and leaks, with resolution in all [28]. Finally, a smaller series of three patients treated with the covered WallFlex (Boston Scientific, Natick, Mass) reported two successes and one failure secondary to stent migration [29]. The latter patient underwent surgical bypass.

## Covered Stents for Postsphincterotomy Bleeding

An interesting use of fcSEMS has been reported by two authors [46, 47]. The first series had five patients, three had bleeding recognized at the time of the sphincterotomy and two were delayed. Four had failed some form of endoscopic control including endoclips, thermal coagulation, and epinephrine injection, and one failed interventional radiologic embolization [46]. One patient had immediate placement of a 10-mm stent for a pulsatile bleed. All patients had either 10-mm or 8-mm biliary WallFlex stents (Boston Scientific, Natick, Mass). All had control of the bleeding. Stents had scheduled removal at 4–6 weeks. Two had migrated without rebleeding in either case. The second series included 11 patients, 10 with delayed bleeding, all of whom failed some form of endoscopic therapy [47]. Eight patients had placement of pcSEMS (Wallstent, Boston Scientific, Natick, Mass) and three with fcSEMS (two WallFlex, Boston Scientific, Natick, Mass, and one Combi, Taewoong, Soul, Korea). Ten resolved with a single stent, and one required a second fcSEMS [47].

## Complications

### Uncovered Stents

Many of the complications of SEMS can be related to the stent design or the anatomic conditions when the stents are placed. The first metal stents available were uncovered metal stents being placed in patients for diseases which have a potential long-term survival. The 3-year follow-up in patients with benign strictures revealed a patency rate of 55% for a variety of uncovered metal stents, stent occlusion in 28%, and 17% non-stent-related mortality [6]. A 68% occlusion rate in another study [4] resulted in two reviews arguing that alternative therapies are preferable [7, 48]. Removal of uncovered stents has been reported [49–53], but in the largest reported series of 39 uSEMS patients, the success is only 13% or 38% [52]. The removal technique is usually cumbersome and entails removing the wires of the Wallstent one at a time.

## Partially Covered Stents

To resolve the problem of ingrowth, either by tumor or mucosal hyperplasia, a stent has been marketed with a Permalume ® (Wallstent, Boston Scientific, Natick, Mass) membrane. The proximal end has a 3-mm open mesh flare to try to prevent migration, and the distal end also has 5 mm of open mesh [54]. A large series of 396 biliary patients treated with this pcSEMS (247 malignant and 149 benign stenoses) had an overall complication rate of 18% [54]. Duodenal migration occurred in 6.8%, proximal migration in 2.3%, cholecystitis in 3.3%, and debris stent occlusion in 1.6%. Three patients with benign biliary disease developed mucosal hyperplasia with stricture at the proximal margin of the stent noted at the time of stent removal which was managed with plastic stents. When either a complication occurs or upon reaching the therapeutic endpoint, removal of a pcSEMS is advised. There was 93% removability in 13 of 14 instances of Wallstent (Boston Scientific, Natick, Mass) in one reported series [51] and 24 of 26 (92%) in another using a variety of pcSEMS [52]. The reason for failure was ingrowth or duodenal tumor extension in these three patients, and there is no mention if any had benign disease. Distal migration occurs in a significant portion of patients in whom pcSEMS are used for benign disease, but in many instances, the therapeutic goal has already been reached, such as stricture or leak

resolution [16, 38]. Failed therapy can be managed by repeat stenting. Proximal migration is more difficult to manage due to tissue hyperplasia and stricture formation in the distal uncovered mesh, and many have been managed by a second SEMS or insertion of plastic stents [17, 54]. Partial migration with impaction in the duodenal wall has been reported to preclude stent extraction in 2/65 cases, and a bile duct perforation during balloon-assisted stent extraction for a pcSEMS has also been reported [17].

## Fully Covered SEMS

Stent migration of fcSEMS has also been noted in benign disease. Two series of migration in patients with post-OLTX strictures or leaks have been reported [28, 29]. In the first, migration of a Niti-S ComVi (Taewoong Medical, Korea) was noted in 6/16 patients [28], but there was total resolution of the treatment indication. The second used the WallFlex (Boston Scientific, Natick, Mass) for the same indication and reported migration in 5/11 patients. In three of the five, migrations were association with failure of therapy [29]. Both stents have a flared proximal margin as an anchoring mechanism. To address the migration issue, Park et al. have reported a prospective RCT from two centers using two different design fcSEMS in 43 patients with benign biliary disease [55]. More than 90% of the patients had failed prior treatment with plastic stents. Twenty-one patients received conventional stents which were flared proximally and distally (FS) (Standard Sci Tech, Seoul, Korea) or a newly designed 10-mm stent with distal flared end and single row of four proximal anchoring flaps (AF) (M.I. Tech, Seoul, Korea) in 22 patients. They scheduled stent removal at 4–6 months postplacement. There were no proximal or distal migrations in the AF group and 33% migration (6/21 distal and 1/21 proximal) in the FS group. All remaining stents were extracted successfully with no complications and no stent-related strictures on postextraction cholangiography. There are several reports on the use of another fcSEMS which is covered with a Teflon®-based membrane (Viabil, W.L.

Gore, Flagstaff, AZ, and distributed by Conmed, Utica, NY) in a variety of benign conditions [39, 45, 56]. The first series of 13 patients with biliary leaks reported no distal migrations and a single proximal migration, and all of the stents were successfully removed. On cholangioscopy, 4/6 were noted to have "ulcerations" presumably at the anchoring fins site. A single long-term complication of stricture in one posttransplant patient may have been ischemic or stent related [39]. Ductal damage has also been reported with plastic stents in a series of 30 patients, 17 of whom were stented for 4 weeks preoperatively prior to surgical resection [57]. The obstructed, but nonstented ducts showed mild inflammation and fibrosis when compared to the stent group which showed "severe inflammation, fibrosis and ulcerative lesions" [57]. A second series used the Viabil® fcSEMS as first-line treatment in 16/17 patients with posttransplant biliary leaks, and one patient with failed plastic stents for 2 months, has been reported [45]. The authors placed 10-mm stents in 15/17 and 8 mm in 2/17 cases. There was one full outward migration, one proximal migration, and six significant strictures which required endoscopic therapy. It is difficult to discern from the study, but of the six patients

requiring further stenting for stricture, at least two had strictures at different locations than pretreatment. Stricture formation in OLTX patients with transanastomotic plastic stents for anastomotic leaks has also been reported in 7/11 patients (64%) after the stents were removed but in none of the other 15 patients with leaks from other sites [43]. This raises the question of whether the presence of leak from an anastomosis engenders an additional risk of complications itself. One multicenter study looked at the complications associated with Viabil® stent removal in 37 patients with both benign and malignant disease [56]. All stents were removed successfully with no complications associated with the extraction. In the 17 patients with benign disease, there were three stent-related strictures reported, one proximal stricture, and two distal strictures in patients who had intraductal stent placement (Fig. 17.2). All three were retreated with the same fcSEMS with stricture resolution. In each instance, the authors felt that the original stent was oversized in relation to the native duct diameter and the high radial force of this device was thought to contribute to ischemic damage. They advised better sizing of the stent to duct caliber.

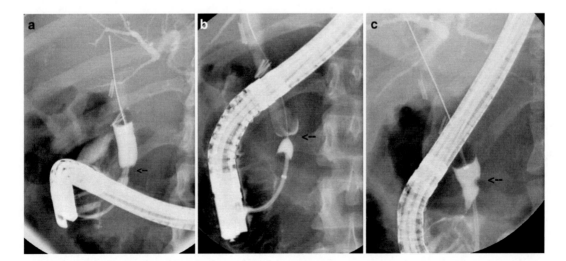

**Fig. 17.2** Poststent extraction of a 10-mm Viabil® which had been placed intraductally for a postoperative CHD stricture. (**a**) Note the waist (*arrow*) at the deployment site of the distal margin of the stent and resolution of the upper stricture. (**b**) Patient returns 18 weeks later with pain and elevated liver tests, and on an occlusion cholangiogram, a tight distal stricture (*arrow*) in the CBD at the site of the distal stent margin is noted. A transpapillary 10-mm Viabil® was placed through the stricture. (**c**) Stent extraction 3 months later with stricture resolution (Courtesy of Paul Tarnasky, MD, Dallas, TX)

## Pancreatitis and Cholecystitis

Post-ERCP pancreatitis (PEP) as a complication of metal stent insertion is a subject of some controversy, and whether a biliary sphincterotomy prior to the stent insertion will alter it is also debated [58–60]. A retrospective study from Indiana University reported an incidence of post-ERCP pancreatitis of 7.5% for uSEMS and 6.9% for cSEMS versus 1.3% for plastic stents with the performance of a sphincterotomy not being a variable [59]. All of these placements were for malignant biliary obstruction. Another retrospective study of 104 patients with both benign and malignant indications had only one case of PEP, and that was in a patient with a sphincterotomy [58]. A prospective study of 83 patients randomized to sphincterotomy versus no sphincterotomy prior to covered metal stent insertion found an increased incidence of complications in the sphincterotomy group, but no pancreatitis in either group [61]. The majority of the patients in these studies had malignancy, and pancreatic cancer made up a significant proportion of the malignancy. How this translates to benign indications is unknown. Review of patients with metal stents for benign disease is difficult to interpret as many of the series have had prior plastic stents and sphincterotomy. However, one series with fcSEMS and no sphincterotomy at stent deployment reported PEP in 14%; however, almost all had some form of plastic stenting prior to entry in the study [55]. Another study with sphincterotomy in 17 with post-OLTX leaks had no pancreatitis [45]. The same institution reported PEP in 4% of 79 patients with benign disease in whom a pcSEMS was placed; two were mild and one severe with development of an infected pseudocyst [17]. Whether sphincterotomy is necessary will await the results of prospective studies, as none exists at this time.

Cholecystitis has been reported as a complication of placing a covered metal stent across the cystic duct orifice. However, the main reports have been in patients with malignant biliary obstruction [62, 63]. In the largest series looking for risk factors for development of gallbladder infection, the two major factors were the tumor crossing the cystic duct orifice (67%) and the presence of stones in the gallbladder (40%) [63]. They also found that the incidence for uSEMS versus cSEMS was 33% and 27%, respectively [63]. Many conditions for stenting in benign disease, to include post-OLTX and postsurgical leaks, already have a gallbladder resection. Patients who may have a gallbladder in situ would be patients with chronic pancreatitis. To date, there is a single report of cholecystitis, and in that case the stent did not cross the cystic duct [16]. Another series reported no cholecystitis in 20 patients with chronic pancreatitis, but a low cystic duct insertion was an exclusion criterion for cSEMS placement [64]. Additional reports using cSEMS in patients with an intact gallbladder would be welcomed.

## References

1. Isayama H, Nakai Y, Toyokawa Y, et al. Measurement of radial and axial forces of biliary self-expandable metallic stents. Gastrointest Endosc. 2009;70:37–44.
2. Lawrence C, Romagnuolo J, Payne KM, et al. Low symptomatic premature stent occlusion of multiple plastic stents for benign biliary strictures: comparing standard and prolonged stent change intervals. Gastrointest Endosc. 2010;72:558–63.
3. Tabibian JH, Asham EH, Han S, et al. Endoscopic treatment of postorthotopic liver transplantation anastomotic biliary strictures with maximal stent therapy (with video). Gastrointest Endosc. 2010;71:505–12.
4. O'Brien SM, Hatfield ARW, Craig PI, et al. A 5-year follow-up of self-expanding metal stents in the endoscopic management of patients with benign bile duct strictures. Eur J Gastroenterol Hepatol. 1998;10: 141–5.
5. Van Berkel AM, Cahen DL, van Westerloo DJ, et al. Self-expanding metal stents in benign biliary strictures due to chronic pancreatitis. Endoscopy. 2004;36: 381–4.
6. Maccioni F, Rossi M, Salvatori FM, et al. Metallic stents in benign biliary strictures: three-year follow-up. Cardiovasc Intervent Radiol. 1992;15:360–6.
7. Rosch T. Metal stents for benign and malignant bile duct strictures stents for benign and malignant bile duct strictures. Endoscopy. 1998;30:A247–52.
8. Silvis SE, Sievert CE, Vennes JA, et al. Comparison of covered versus uncovered wire mesh stents in the canine biliary tract. Gastrointest Endosc. 1994;40: 17–21.
9. Cahen DL, van Berkel AM, Oskam D, et al. Long-term results of endoscopic drainage of common bile duct strictures in chronic pancreatitis. Eur J Gastroenterol Hepatol. 2005;17:103–8.

10. Kahl S, Zimmermann S, Genz I, et al. Risk factors for failure of endoscopic stenting of biliary strictures in chronic pancreatitis: a prospective follow-up study. Am J Gastroenterol. 2003;98:2448–53.

11. Draganov P, Hoffman B, Marsh W, et al. Long-term outcome of in patients with benign biliary strictures treated endoscopically with multiple stents. Gastrointest Endosc. 2002;55:680–6.

12. Pozsar J, Sahin P, Laszlo F, et al. Medium-term results of endoscopic treatment of common bile duct strictures in chronic calcifying pancreatitis with increasing numbers of stents. J Clin Gastroenterol. 2004;38:118–23.

13. Catalano MF, Linder JD, George S, et al. Treatment of symptomatic distal common bile duct stenosis secondary to chronic pancreatitis: comparison single vs. multiple simultaneous stents. Gastrointest Endosc. 2004;60:945–52.

14. Deviere J, Cremer M, Baize M, et al. Management of common bile duct stricture caused by chronic pancreatitis with metal mesh self expandable stents. Gut. 1994;35:122–6.

15. Yamaguchi T, Ishihara T, Seza K, et al. Long-term outcome of endoscopic metallic stenting for biliary stenosis associated with chronic pancreatitis. World J Gastroenterol. 2006;12:426–30.

16. Cantu P, Hookey LC, Morales A, et al. The treatment of patients with symptomatic common bile duct stenosis secondary to chronic pancreatitis using partially covered metal stents: a pilot study. Endoscopy. 2005;37:735–9.

17. Kahaleh M, Behm B, Clarke BW, et al. Temporary placement of covered self-expandable metal stents in benign biliary strictures: a new paradigm? (with video). Gastrointest Endosc. 2008;67:446–54.

18. Mahajan A, Ho H, Sauer B, et al. Temporary placement of fully covered self-expandable metal stents in benign biliary strictures: midterm evaluation (with video). Gastrointest Endosc. 2009;70:303–9.

19. Davids PHP, Tanka AKF, Rauws EAJ, et al. Benign biliary strictures surgery or endoscopy? Ann Surg. 1993;217:237–43.

20. Tocchi A, Mazzoni G, Liotta G, et al. Management of benign biliary strictures: biliary enteric anastomosis vs. endoscopic stenting. Arch Surg. 2000;135:153–7.

21. Tuvignon N, Liguory C, Ponchon T, et al. Long-term follow-up after biliary stent placement for postcholecystectomy bile duct strictures: a multicenter study. Endoscopy. 2011;43:208–16.

22. Costamagna G, Pandolfi M, Mutignani M, et al. Long-term results of endoscopic management of post operative bile duct strictures with increasing numbers of stents. Gastrointest Endosc. 2001;54:162–8.

23. Costamagna G, Tringali A, Mutignani M, et al. Endotherapy of postoperative biliary strictures with multiple stents: results after more than 10 years of follow-up. Gastrointest Endosc. 2010;72:551–7.

24. Morelli G, Fazel A, Judah J, et al. Rapid-sequence endoscopic management of posttransplant anastomotic biliary strictures. Gastrointest Endosc. 2008;67:879–85.

25. Kuzela L, Oltman M, Sutka J, et al. Prospective follow-up of patients with bile duct strictures secondary to laparoscopic cholecystectomy, treated endoscopically with multiple stents. Hepatogastroenterology. 2005;52:1357–61.

26. Morelli J, Mulcahy HE, Willner IR, et al. Long-term outcomes for patients with post-liver transplant anastomotic biliary strictures treated by endoscopic stent placement. Gastrointest Endosc. 2003;58:374–9.

27. Chaput U, Scatton O, Bichard P, et al. Temporary placement of partially covered self-expandable metal stents for anastomotic biliary strictures after liver transplantation: a prospective, multicenter study. Gastrointest Endosc. 2010;72:1167–74.

28. Triana M, Tarantino I, Barresi L, et al. Efficacy and safety of fully covered self-expandable metallic stents in biliary complications after liver transplantation: a preliminary study. Liver Transpl. 2009;15:1493–8.

29. Marin-Gomez LM, Sobrino-Rodriguez S, Alamo-Martinez JM, et al. Use of fully covered self-expandable stent in biliary complications after liver transplantation: a case series. Transplant Proc. 2010;42:2975–7.

30. Liguory C, Vitale GC, Lefebre JF, et al. Endoscopic treatment of post-operative biliary fistulae. Surgery. 1991;100:779–84.

31. Kaffes AJ, Hourigan L, De Luca N, et al. Impact of endoscopic intervention in 100 patients with suspected postcholecystectomy bile leak. Gastrointest Endosc. 2005;61:269–75.

32. Wootton FT, Hoffman BJ, Marsh WH, et al. Biliary complications following laparoscopic cholecystectomy. Gastrointest Endosc. 1992;38:183–5.

33. Bjorkman DJ, Carr-Locke DL, Lichtenstein DR, et al. Post surgical bile leaks: endoscopic obliteration of the transpapillary pressure gradient is enough. Am J Gastroenterol. 1995;90:2128–33.

34. Katsinelos P, Kountouras J, Paroutoglou G, et al. A comparative study of 10-Fr vs. 7-Fr straight plastic stents in the treatment of postcholecystectomy bile leak. Surg Endosc. 2008;22:101–6.

35. Marks JM, Ponsky JL, Shillingstad RB, et al. Biliary stenting is more effective than sphincterotomy in the resolution of biliary leaks. Surg Endosc. 1998;12:327–30.

36. Farhat S, Bourrier A, Gaudric M, et al. Endoscopic treatment of biliary fistulas after complex liver resection. Ann Surg. 2011;253:88–93.

37. Baron TH, Poterucha JJ. Insertion and removal of covered expandable metal stents for closure of complex biliary leaks. Clin Gastroenterol Hepatol. 2006;4:381–6.

38. Kahaleh M, Sundaram V, Condron SL, et al. Temporary placement of covered self-expandable metallic stents in patients with biliary leak: midterm evaluation of a pilot study. Gastrointest Endosc. 2007;66:52–9.

39. Wang AY, Ellen K, Berg CL, et al. Fully covered self-expandable metallic stents in the management of complex biliary leaks: preliminary data-a case series. Endoscopy. 2009;41:781–6.

40. Ostroff JW, Roberts JP, Gordon R, et al. The management of T-tube leaks in orthotopic liver transplant recipients with endoscopically placed nasobiliary catheters. Transplantation. 1990;49:922–4.

41. Bourgeois F, Deviere J, Yeaton P, et al. Diagnostic and therapeutic endoscopic retrograde cholangiography after liver transplantation. Gastrointest Endosc. 1995;42:527–34.

42. Pfau PR, Kochman M, Lewis JD, et al. Endoscopic management of postoperative biliary complications in orthotopic liver transplantation. Gastrointest Endosc. 2000;52:55–63.

43. Morelli J, Mulcahy HE, Willner IR, et al. Endoscopic treatment of post-liver transplantation biliary leaks with stent placement across the leak site. Gastrointest Endosc. 2001;54:471–5.

44. Di Pisa M, Traina M, Miraglia R, et al. Use of self-expandable metallic stent for large bile leakage following orthotopic liver transplant. Endoscopy. 2009;41:E4–5.

45. Phillips MS, Bonatti H, Sauer BG, et al. Elevated stricture rate following the use of fully covered self-expandable metal biliary stents for biliary leaks following liver transplantation. Endoscopy. 2011;43:512–7.

46. Shah JN, Marson F, Binmoeller KF. Temporary self-expandable metal stent placement for treatment of post-sphincterotomy bleeding. Gastrointest Endosc. 2010;72:1274–8.

47. Itoi T, Yasuda I, Doi S, et al. Endoscopic hemostasis using covered metallic stent placement for uncontrolled post-endoscopic sphincterotomy bleeding. Endoscopy. 2011;43:369–72.

48. Van Boeckel PGA, Vleggaar FP, Siersema PD. Plastic or Metal Stents for benign extrahepatic biliary strictures: a systematic review. BMC Gastroenterol. 2009;17:9–96.

49. Ahmed A, Keefe EB, Imperial JC. A novel technique for endoscopic removal of expandable biliary Wallstent. Gastrointest Endosc. 1999;50:279–81.

50. Egan LJ, Baron TH. Endoscopic removal of an embedded biliary Wallstent by piecemeal extraction. Endoscopy. 2000;32:492–4.

51. Kahaleh M, Tokar J, Le T, et al. Removal of self-expandable metallic Wallstents. Gastrointest Endosc. 2004;60:640–4.

52. Familiari P, Bulajic M, Mutignani M, et al. Endoscopic removal of malfunctioning biliary self-expandable metallic stents. Gastrointest Endosc. 2005;62:903–10.

53. Lahlal M, Gigot JF, Annet L, et al. Successful endoscopic extraction of a double uncovered expandable metal stent. Endoscopy. 2009;41:E98–9.

54. Ho H, Mahajan A, Gosain S, et al. Management of complications associated with partially covered biliary metal stents. Dig Dis Sci. 2010;55:516–22.

55. Park DH, Lee SS, Lee TH, et al. Anchoring flap versus flared end, fully covered self-expandable metal stents to prevent migration in patients with benign biliary stricture: a multicenter, prospective comparative pilot study (with videos). Gastrointest Endosc. 2011;73:64–70.

56. Kasher JA, Corasanti JG, Tarnasky PR, et al. A multicenter analysis of safety and outcome of removal of a fully covered self-expandable metal stent during ERCP. Gastrointest Endosc. 2011;73:1292–7.

57. Karsten TM, Coene P-PLO, van Gulik TM, et al. Morphologic changes of extrahepatic bile ducts during obstruction and subsequent decompression by endoprosthesis. Surgery. 1992;111:562–8.

58. Banerjee N, Hilden K, Baron T, et al. Endoscopic biliary sphincterotomy is not required for transpapillary SEMS placement for biliary obstruction. Dig Dis Sci. 2011;56:591–5.

59. Cote GA, Kumar N, Ansstas M, et al. Risk of post-ERCP pancreatitis with placement of self-expandable metallic stents. Gastrointest Endosc. 2010;72:748–54.

60. Adler DG, Baron TH. Biliary self-expandable metal stents and the risk of post-ERCP pancreatitis: the jury is still out. Gastrointest Endosc. 2011;73:1070.

61. Artifon ELA, Sakai P, Ishioka S, et al. Endoscopic sphincterotomy before deployment of covered metal stent is associated with greater complication rate. J Clin Gastroenterol. 2008;42:815–9.

62. Kahaleh M, Tokar J, Conaway MR, et al. Efficacy and complications of covered Wallstents in malignant distal biliary obstruction. Gastrointest Endosc. 2005;61:528–33.

63. Suk KT, Kim HA, Kim JW, et al. Risk factors of cholecystitis after metal stent placement in malignant biliary obstruction. Gastrointest Endosc. 2006;64:522–9.

64. Behm B, Brock A, Clarke BW, et al. Partially covered self-expandable metallic stents for benign biliary strictures due to chronic pancreatitis. Endoscopy. 2009;41:547–51.

## Maarten W. van den Berg and Jeanin E. van Hooft

Enteral stent placement was first reported in the early 1990s and since then has gained popularity, especially for the treatment of symptomatic malignant gastric outlet obstruction (GOO) [1]. It has been suggested that stent placement for GOO is less invasive with a faster relief of symptoms compared to conventional open or laparoscopic gastrojejunostomy [2–4]. In this chapter, we will mainly focus on the results including complications of enteral stenting as a treatment for malignant GOO. After a brief elaboration on definitions, several outcome parameters and complications will be discussed point by point, and, if applicable, influences for different indications and material will be taken into consideration. We will round up with some miscellaneous indications and a summary.

## Defining Results and Complications

There is no clear definition of results regarding enteral stenting. A composite of several outcome parameters is often described as results. Reviewing the literature, the following outcome measures are stated in the majority of articles: technical success (adequate positioning and deployment of

M.W. van den Berg • J.E. van Hooft (✉)
Department of Gastroenterology and Hepatology,
Academic Medical Center, University of Amsterdam,
Meibergdreef 9, Amsterdam, AZ 1105, The Netherlands
e-mail: m.w.vandenberg@amc.nl; J.E.vanHooft@amc.nl

the stent) and clinical success (relief of symptoms and/or improvement of oral intake predominantly defined by improvement of the GOO Scoring System (GOOSS) score, Table 18.1).

A great number of publications also report on median survival and procedure-related hospitalization time, where only some articles elaborate on cost and quality of life. Complications related to enteral stenting are often divided into major and minor complications [6–10] and/or into early and late complications [6, 7, 11–14] in an attempt to render the severity and determine which complications might be procedure-related. Unfortunately, the definitions used to classify complications differ between the main publications [6–9, 11, 12]. In this chapter, it was therefore decided to just mention the type of complication, e.g., perforation or migration, and refrain from judging the severity and the possible relation to the procedure.

## Results

To obtain an up-to-date insight in the results of enteral stenting as a treatment for malignant GOO, a critical review of the literature has been performed. All studies published between October 2003 and May 2011 that met the following criteria were reviewed: information on technical and clinical success, publication in English, and a study population of more than ten patients were included and are summarized in Table 18.2.

R. Kozarek et al. (eds.), *Self-Expandable Stents in the Gastrointestinal Tract*,
DOI 10.1007/978-1-4614-3746-8_18, © Springer Science+Business Media New York 2013

**Table 18.1** The gastric outlet obstruction scoring system (GOOSS)

| Level of oral intake | GOOSS score |
|---|---|
| No oral intake | 0 |
| Liquids only | 1 |
| Soft solids | 2 |
| Low-residue or full diet | 3 |

Adapted from Adler and Baron [5], with permission

## Technical Success

### Overall Technical Success

In the vast majority of the patients with malignant GOO, adequate positioning and deployment of the enteral stent is achieved. The overall technical success ranges from 77% to 100% with a mean of 97% (2175/2,243) in our pooled population (Table 18.2). The technical failures occurring in 3% of the patients, are mainly caused by either the inability to cannulate the stricture with the guide wire or unsuccessful deployment of the enteral stent. Adequate positioning of the guide wire might be hampered by the tightness of the stenosis or looping in the distended stomach of either the endoscope or guide wire [6, 17, 30, 34, 40]. Deployment failures are mostly related to a tortuous anatomy, causing too many or too sharp bends on the delivery device impeding the deployment force [22].

### Type of Procedure and Technical Success

There are two types of procedures for enteral stent placement: either endofluoroscopic (combination of endoscopic and fluoroscopic guidance performed by endoscopist) or fluoroscopic (performed by radiologist). There are, however, no studies published that compare these techniques. Pooled analysis of the larger studies (n > 50) in which either an endofluoroscopic [8, 15, 17, 19, 26] or fluoroscopic technique [22, 34, 38] was combined with one type of stent reveals technical success rates of, respectively,

97% (280/288) and 96% (372/387). Based on these data, no conclusions can be drawn about the preferred type of procedure. To answer the question, very large randomized controlled trials would be needed as the success rates appear to be rather similar. Regarding the current data, one could also argue that both success rates are high and that the choice for either one should be determined by local expertise.

### Tumor Characteristics and Technical Success

As mentioned before, the tightness of the stenosis and the anatomic position may well influence the technical success rate of enteral stent placement in patients with malignant GOO. Studies specifically assessing a relationship between tumor characteristics like type of malignancy or site of the lesion are, however, sparse [22, 37, 41]. A study by Kim et al., in which stents were placed under fluoroscopic guidance by radiologists, showed a statistically significant difference for technical success rates depending on the site of the lesion: peripyloric region 98%, duodenum 93%, and anastomosis (gastroduodenostomy and gastrojejunostomy) 82% [22]. The authors state that severe loop formation of the catheter-guide wire system in the distended stomach and curved configuration of the duodenal C-loop are the main causes of the lower success rate in the latter two groups. Another study of Kim et al. found that the technical success rate was not statistically different, depending on the type of malignancy: primary gastric carcinoma 100% versus pancreatic carcinoma 100% [41]. Although stent placement was technically successful in all patients, the radiologists found stent placement more challenging in the pancreatic carcinoma group for the same reasons as mentioned in their previous study.

Lindsay et al. performed a retrospective study in which stents were placed under endofluoroscopic guidance in groups of patients with GOO, caused by either pancreaticobiliary or gastric carcinoma, and found technical success rates of 100% in both groups [37].

**Table 18.2** Overview of literature regarding results of enteral stenting as a treatment for gastric outlet obstruction after September 2003 until May 2011 meeting the following criteria: information on technical and clinical success, publication in English, and a study population of more than ten patients

| Publication | Study design | Procedure | Stent type | N | Technical success (%) | Clinical success (%) | Hospital stay (days) | Survival (days) |
|---|---|---|---|---|---|---|---|---|
| Van Hooft et al. 2011 [15] | Prospective multicenter | EF | D-Weave Niti-S duodenal stent (Taewoon Medical, Seoul, Korea) | 52 | 96 | 77 | 2 | 82 |
| Jeurnink et al. 2010 [7] | Randomized prospective (GJJ vs. stent) multicenter | EF | WallFlex (Boston Scientific, Matick, MA, USA) | 21[a] | 95 | 86 | 7 | 56 |
| Shi et al. 2010 [16] | Prospective single center | EF | Big Cup Nitinol stent | 13 | 92 | 84 | ns | 195[b] |
| Kim et al. 2010 [9] | Randomized prospective (covered vs. uncovered) single center | EF | Covered (Niti-S Pyloric, Niti-S Comvi Pyloric(Taewoon Medical, Seoul, Korea)) | 80 | 100(c) | 95(c) | ns | 182(c) |
| | | | Uncovered (Wallstent, WallFlex) | | 100(u) | 90(u) | | 133(u) |
| Shaw et al. 2010 [17] | Prospective single center | EF | WallFlex | 70 | 93 | 89 | 2 | 54 |
| Kim et al. 2010 [18] | Prospective single center | EF | Niti-S Comvi Pyloric | 25 | 100 | 88 | ns | 112 |
| Lee et al. 2009 [11] | Nonrandomized prospective (covered vs. uncovered) single center | EF | Niti-S Pyloric (covered and uncovered) | 154 | 100(c) 100(u) | 99(c) 96(u) | ns | 115(c) 108(u) |
| van Hooft et al. 2009 [19] | Prospective multicenter | EF | WallFlex | 51 | 98 | 84 | 3 | 62 |
| Havemann et al. 2009 [20] | Prospective single center | EF | Hanaro (M.I. Tech, Ltd., Seoul, Korea) | 45 | 91 | 63 | 13[b] | 121[b] |
| Gutzeit et al. 2009 [21] | Retrospective single center | EF | Wallstent | 29 | 97 | 86 | ns | 52 |
| Phillips et al. 2008 [13] | Prospective (n = 43) & retrospective (n = 3) single center | EF | Wallstent Alimaxx (Alveolus, Charlotte, NC, USA) | 46 | 100 | 91 | ns | 152[b] |
| Jeurnink et al. 2007 [6] | Comparative retrospective (GJJ vs. stent) single center | EF | Wallstent WallFlex Choo stent (M.I. Tech, Ltd., Seoul, Korea) | 53[a] | 93 | 75 | 6 | 70 |

(continued)

**Table 18.2** (continued)

| Publication | Study design | Procedure | Stent type | N | Technical success (%) | Clinical success (%) | Hospital stay (days) | Survival (days) |
|---|---|---|---|---|---|---|---|---|
| Kim et al. 2007 [22] | Prospective single center | F | Niti-S Pyloric | 213 | 94 | 92 | ns | 99 |
| Lee et al. 2007 [23] | Prospective preliminary single center | EF | Niti-S Comvi Pyloric | 11 | 100 | 91 | ns | 122 |
| Maetani et al. 2007 [24] | Prospective multicenter | EF | Niti-S enteral colonic (Taewoon Medical, Seoul, Korea) | 37 | 97 | 94 | 10 | 118 |
| Huang et al. 2007 [25] | Prospective single center | F | Wallstent | 15 | 100 | 86 | ns | 69[b] |
| Lowe et al. 2007 [12] | Prospective and retrospective single center | EF | Wallstent Hanaro stent Choo stent Flamingo | 87 | 97 | 87 | ns | 86 |
| Kim et al. 2007 [8] | Retrospective single center | EF | Niti-S Pyloric | 53 | 100 | 81 | ns | 145[b] |
| van Hooft et al. 2007 [26] | Retrospective multicenter | EF | WallFlex | 62 | 100 | 85 | 6 | ns |
| Mehta et al. 2006 [27] | Randomized prospective (GJJ vs. stent) single center | F | Wallstent | 13[a] | 77 | 77 | 5 | ns |
| Espinel et al. 2006 [28] | Nonrandomized prospective (GJJ vs. stent) single center | EF | Wallstent | 24[a] | 100 | 100 | 7 | 140 |
| Kazi et al. 2006 [29] | Retrospective single center | EF | Wallstent | 23 | 91 | 91 | 4 | 58 |
| Maire et al. 2006 [30] | Retrospective single center | EF | Hanaro | 25 | 96 | 88 | ns | ns |
| Del Piano et al. 2005 [31] | Comparative retrospective (GJJ vs. stent) single center | EF | Wallstent Ultraflex (Boston Scientific, Matick, MA, USA) | 24[a] | 96 | 92 | 3[b] | 96[b] |
| Maetani et al. 2005 [32] | Comparative retrospective (GJJ vs. stent) single center | EF | Ultraflex | 22[a] | 100 | 77 | Unclear | 65 |
| Mosler et al. 2005 [33] | Retrospective single center | EF | Gianturco Z-stent (Wilson-Cook Inc, Winston-Salem, NC, USA) Endocoil (InStent Inc, Eden Prairie, MN, USA) Ultraflex Wallstent | 36 | 92 | 81 | ns | 105[b] |

| Study | Technique | Stent | N | | | | |
|---|---|---|---|---|---|---|---|
| Bessoud et al. 2005 [34] Retrospective single center | F | Wallstent | 72 | 97 | 90 | ns | 120[b] |
| Johnsson et al. 2004 [35] Nonrandomized prospective (GJJ vs. stent) single center | EF | Wallstent | 21[a] | 100 | 76 | 7 | 56 |
| Maetani et al. 2004 [36] Comparative retrospective (GJJ EF vs. stent) single center | EF | Ultraflex Z-stent (Cook, Bloomington, IN, USA) | 20[a] | 100 | 80 | 15 | 55 |
| Holt et al. 2004 [5] Prospective single center | EF | Wallstent Flamingo (microvasive) | 28 | 93 | 93 | 7 | 51 |
| Kim et al. 2004 [10] Retrospective single center | EF | Niti-S Pyloric (covered and uncovered type) | 49 | 100 | 92 | 7 | 70 |
| Lindsay et al. 2004 [37] Retrospective single center | EF | Wallstent | 40 | 100 | 80 | ns | 49 |
| Song et al. 2004 [38] Prospective single center | F | Dual stent (S&G Biotech, Seoul, Korea) | 102 | 99 | 83 | ns | 73 |
| Dormann et al. 2004 [39][c] | EF & F | Wallstent Ultraflex Choo stent InStent (InStent Inc, Eden Prairie, MN, USA) | 606 | 97 | 87 | ns | 85[b] |

*N* study population, *ns* not specified, *GJJ* gastrojejunostomy, *EF* endofluoroscopy, *F* fluoroscopic, *c* covered, *u* uncovered

[a]Patients who received stent

[b]Mean instead of median

[c]Included all relevant studies published between January 1992 and September 2003

In conclusion, data suggest that sec fluoroscopic enteral stent placement might be more challenging in distally located obstructions. Data with regard to endofluoroscopic stent placement are too sparse for any conclusion.

## Type of Stent and Technical Success

There are no data directly comparing the different kinds of enteral stents. Looking at Table 18.2, only one study reveals a deviating finding with regard to technical success. In this study by Mehta et al., a technical success rate of 77% was found in a small study population (n = 13) using the Wallstent enteral stent (Boston Scientific, Natick, MA, USA) [27]. Other studies using the Wallstent enteral stent report technical success rates ranging from 91% to 100% [12, 21, 25, 28, 29, 34, 35, 37]. Therefore, it seems reasonable to assume that the Wallstent enteral stent has similar outcomes regarding technical success compared to other stent types.

In contrast to the different types of stents, clusters of stents have been compared. A prospective randomized trial comparing endoscopic placement of covered stents (Niti-S Pyloric and Niti-S Comvi Pyloric (TaeWoong Medical, Seoul, Korea)) (n = 40) with uncovered stents (Wallstent and WallFlex (Boston Scientific, Natick, MA, USA)) (n = 40) as a treatment for malignant pyloric obstruction in gastric cancer showed no difference concerning technical success rate (both 100%) [9]. This result is consistent with another prospective, nonrandomized comparative study which compared endoscopic placement of covered (Niti-S Pyloric) (n = 70) stents with uncovered stents (Niti-S Pyloric) (n = 84) as a treatment for malignant GOO, also revealing technical success rates of 100% in both groups [11]. In the guidelines for fluoroscopic placement of gastroduodenal stents by Sabharwal et al., it is however stated that the delivery systems of covered stents are less flexible and larger and therefore more difficult to deploy at distant locations through tortuous anatomy [42]. Notwithstanding there are no data in the current literature which can objectively support this statement.

The technical success rate of enteral stent placement for GOO is really high. Neither the type of procedure nor the type of stent seems to make any distinctive difference. On the contrary, tumor characteristics might have their influence, especially when the obstruction is more distally located.

## Clinical Success

### Overall Clinical Success

Clinical success defined as relief of symptoms and/or improvement of oral intake is achieved on mean in 87% of the patients (1979/2,271), ranging from 63% to 100% (Table 18.2). The difference might be caused by a variety in definitions of clinical success. The studies with lower clinical success rates (<80%) did define clinical success as an improvement of the GOOSS score instead of "relief of symptoms and/or an improvement of the GOOSS-score" [15, 20, 27, 32]. Furthermore, some patients do not improve even after successful stent placement because of unidentified sites of malignant obstruction, diffuse peritoneal carcinomatosis with bowel encasement [22, 34, 38], or functional gastric outlet obstruction either from neural (celiac axis) tumor involvement or as side effect of narcotic pain medication [15, 19, 40].

### Type of Procedure and Clinical Success

There are no studies comparing the two types of enteral stent placement with regard to clinical success. Pooled analysis of the larger studies (n > 50) in which either an endofluoroscopic [8, 15, 17, 19, 26] or fluoroscopic technique [22, 34, 38] was combined with one type of stent reveals almost similar clinical success rates of, respectively, 84% (241/288) and 89% (346/387). Based on these results, one could suggest that it is unlikely that the type of procedure does influence the clinical success rate.

## Tumor Characteristics and Clinical Success

At present there are two studies which specify clinical outcomes of enteral stent placement in relationship to the type of malignancy [37, 41]. The study of Kim et al., specifically set up to compare outcomes of enteral stent placement in the palliative treatment of GOO caused by either gastric carcinoma or pancreatic carcinoma, did not show a significant difference with regard to the clinical success. The study of Lindsay et al. found clinical success rates of both 80% in a group of patients with gastric carcinoma and a group with pancreaticobiliary cancer [37]. Currently, there are no data that show any influence of tumor characteristics on the clinical success.

## Type of Stent and Clinical Success

Though there is a rather large spreading of clinical success rates between studies, there are no data, whether randomized or comparative, that support a relation with a specific type of enteral stents. Clusters of stents, e.g., covered and uncovered, have been compared in prospective studies [9, 11]. These studies did not reveal a significant difference; the clinical success rates were, respectively, 95% and 90% (covered vs. uncovered) in the study of Kim et al. and 98.6% and 96.4% in the study of Lee et al. [9, 11]. At the moment, there is no scientific basis to prefer a specific type or cluster of enteral stents with regard to clinical success.

Though the overall clinical success rate is high, there is a wide range in reported values, which could be explained by a difference in used definitions for clinical success. From the current data, it is not possible to draw any firm conclusions regarding the influence on clinical success of the type of procedure, the tumor characteristics, or the type of stent.

## Procedure-Related Hospital Stay, Survival, and Stent Patency

Procedure-related hospital stay is an essential outcome parameter because the majority of patients with malignant GOO have a poor life expectancy, and therefore, a short hospital stay is desirable. Pooled analysis of all studies reporting on medians (Table 18.2) revealed an overall median hospital stay after stent placement of 2 to 15 days with a mean of 6.3 days and a median survival after stent placement of 49–182 days with a mean of 86 days.

Another parameter to consider is stent patency, which is defined as the time period without need for re-intervention [43]. An important goal of palliative stent placement is that stent patency exceeds patient survival. The current literature reports median stent patency to range from 190 to 385 days, with an adequate resolution of GOO symptoms until death in the majority of patients [15, 19, 21, 22, 41]. Interestingly, Kim et al. showed that despite a significant increase in migration rate, chemotherapy after enteral stent placement was associated with a significant increase in maintenance of stent patency [22]. This was attributed to the reducing effect of chemotherapy on the tumor burden, which likely decreased the chance of tumor overgrowth or stent collapse by tumor compression. Furthermore, the authors noticed that chemotherapy may prevent or delay disease progression and subsequently may cause prolonged patient survival.

## Quality of Life

Although improvement of the quality of life (QoL) is considered an important goal in palliative cancer treatment, only a small number of studies did assess this outcome measure with regard to enteral stent placement in patients with malignant GOO [43].

Older publications used the Karnofsky performance status (KPS), an indicator for patients' general well-being, to evaluate the QoL [12, 32, 36]. A significant improvement of this measure was seen in two of these studies [12, 32], while the other study showed a nonsignificant improvement [36]. The KPS however only addresses physical functioning and might be too confined to adequately evaluate the QoL. More recent studies used more extensive QoL scoring questionnaires like the European Organisation for Research and

Treatment of Cancer [EORTC] QLQ-C30 version 3 and QLQ-PAN26, the Short Form-36 Physical Health score, and the 5 health dimensions of the EuroQol (EQ-5D) including the EuroQol visual analog scale [EQ-VAS] [7, 15, 19, 27]. These data revealed a significant improvement of the QoL in two [15, 27] out of four series while the other two [7, 19] revealed stable QoL scores until death. Though there are no data on the development of the QoL in case no enteral stent has been placed, it seems credible that enteral stenting has a positive influence on the QoL.

## Complications

### Stent Obstruction

The most frequently observed complication, often requiring re-intervention, is stent obstruction (Table 18.3). It is observed in the majority of studies with rates ranging from 3% to 44% (Table 18.3) [9, 11, 13, 15, 17, 19, 20, 22, 38, 39]. Stent obstruction may be caused by tumor ingrowth

(Fig. 18.1), tumor overgrowth (Fig. 18.2), tissue hyperplasia (Fig. 18.3), food impaction, or stent collapse (Fig. 18.4). In- and overgrowth, tissue hyperplasia, and stent collapse can be successfully treated with coaxial stent placement [15, 17, 19, 38], while impacted food can be removed endoscopically [22].

### Stent Migration

Stent migration is another frequently observed stent-related complication with rates ranging from 0% to 32% (Table 18.3). Stents can migrate completely or partially and either proximally or distally. Insertion of an additional stent is often sufficient in case obstructive symptoms reoccur after (partial) stent migration [19, 22, 39]. Proximally migrated stents can be retrieved endoscopically [9]. Distally migrated stents may be completely asymptomatic and sometimes pass out through the rectum, but may also get stranded in the intestine and lead to obstruction, bleeding, or perforation, requiring surgical intervention [11, 22, 38, 39].

**Table 18.3** Summary of complication data from the systematic review of Dormann et al. and prospective studies with a patient population of $n \geq 30$ and a follow-up until death, published between October 2003 and May 2011

| Complication | Frequency (%) |
|---|---|
| 30-day mortality [15, 19] | 22–23 |
| Perforation [9, 11, 13, 15, 17, 19, 20, 22, 38, 39] | 0–4 |
| Bleeding [9, 11, 13, 15, 17, 19, 20, 22, 38, 39] | 0–4 |
| Obstruction [9, 11, 13, 15, 17, 19, 20, 22, 38, 39] | 3–44 |
|   Covered stents [9, 11] | 3–7 |
|   Uncovered stents [9, 11, 15, 17, 19, 20] | 4–44 |
| Migration [9, 11, 13, 15, 17, 19, 20, 22, 38, 39] | 0–32 |
|   Covered stents [9, 11] | 17–32 |
|   Uncovered stents [9, 11, 15, 17, 19, 20] | 0–8 |
| Biliary obstruction [9, 11, 13, 15, 17, 19, 20, 22, 38] | 0–2 |
| Cholangitis [9, 11, 13, 15, 17, 19, 20, 22, 38] | 0–6 |
| Abdominal pain [9, 11, 13, 15, 17, 19, 20, 22, 38, 39] | 0–8 |
| Other[a] [9, 11, 13, 15, 17, 19, 20, 22, 38] | 0–4 |

[a]Consists of stent fracture, cardiac failure, anemia, pneumonia, ascites, gastroenteritis, peritonitis carcinomatosa, and bacteremia

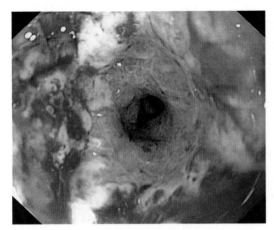

**Fig. 18.1** Endoscopic image of tumor ingrowth through the meshes of an uncovered enteral stent in the duodenum

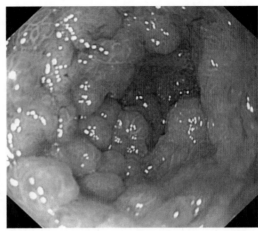

**Fig. 18.3** Endoscopic image of hyperplasia of the duodenal mucosa prolapsing through the meshes of an uncovered enteral stent

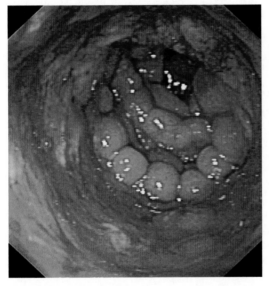

**Fig. 18.2** Endoscopic image of tumor overgrowth at the distal part of an uncovered enteral stent in the duodenum

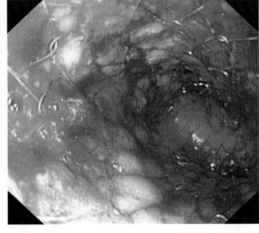

**Fig. 18.4** Endoscopic image of stent collapse due to tumor compression at the distal part of an uncovered enteral stent

## Influence of Stent Design on Obstruction and Migration Rates

Different types of stents have been tried in order to reduce obstruction and migration rates, with the most important features being an uncovered or a covered design. Both designs have their advantages and disadvantages.

The mesh-like framework of uncovered stents prevents migration by providing an anchoring function, which is achieved by embedding (tumor) tissue within the meshes after expansion. The disadvantage of this design is logically a higher obstruction rate due to tumor ingrowth through the stent mesh (Table 18.3). Covered stents on the other hand prevent obstruction from tumor ingrowth with a covering membrane. Unfortunately, this membrane causes a loss of the anchoring feature as described above, and subsequently, covered stents have a higher migration rate [9, 11]. Furthermore, covered stents do not prevent against re-obstruction by other causes than tumor ingrowth [11] and sometimes tumor ingrowth still occurs due to traumatic damage or chemical degradation of the covering membrane [44, 45].

The randomized prospective trial of Kim et al. found statistical significant differences between uncovered and covered stents regarding obstruction and migration rates, with an obstruction rate of 44.4% and 3.2% and migration rates of 8.3% and 32.2%, respectively [9]. These results are consistent with the nonrandomized prospective study of Lee et al. which revealed an obstruction rate of 19% and 7%, respectively, for uncovered and covered stents and migration rates of 0% and 17% [11]. In both publications, the negative features of the two types of stents compensated each other which resulted in similar stent patency times.

In order to overcome the shortcomings of the uncovered and covered stent designs, investigators are aiming to combine the best features of both in one design. For example, a dual expandable nitinol stent, consisting of an inner uncovered and an outer partially covered part that was placed fluoroscopically in a large prospective series, showed promising results with a migration rate of 4% and an obstruction rate of 14% [22].

## Perforation

Perforation of the intestinal wall is rare, with rates ranging from 0% to 4% (Table 18.3) and the majority of articles report no cases of perforation or a frequency of ≤1% [9, 11, 13, 15, 17, 19, 22, 38, 39] and only one publication has shown a percentage of 4% [20]. Perforation can occur intraprocedural as well as postprocedural. Intraprocedural perforation can be caused by balloon dilatation or by manipulation of the intestinal wall by the guide wire, endoscope, or stent [20]. Pressure erosion of the bowel wall by the bare metal ends of the stent or stent migration can cause late-onset perforation [9, 13] and sometimes fistula formation to surrounding structures [13].

## Bleeding

The occurrence of gastrointestinal bleeding during or after enteral stent placement mainly has the same causes as perforation and has comparable rates (Table 18.3) [9, 11, 13, 15, 17, 19, 20, 22, 38, 39]. In most cases, conservative treatment is adequate [17, 22]; however, some bleedings require endoscopic or radiologic intervention [19].

## Biliary Problems

Biliary obstruction after enteral stent placement develops in 0–2% of previously asymptomatic patients and cholangitis in 0–6% of cases [9, 11, 13, 15, 17, 19, 20, 22, 38]. Dormann et al. lumped together biliary obstruction and cholangitis under the title "biliary problems" in their systematic review and found a frequency of 1.3% after enteral stent placement [39]. It is hard to distinguish whether biliary complications are caused by stent placement across the papilla of Vater or by progression of the underlying disease.

Whether or not biliary drainage should be carried out prior to enteral stenting remains a topic for debate. In the majority of patients, biliary obstruction will occur either before or concomitant to GOO: In those cases, there is a sound reason to drain the biliary tree. But the question remains if in patients with GOO but no signs of obstruction of the biliary tree, biliary stents should be placed prophylactically [40]. An argument for the proactive approach has always been the expected difficulty to place a biliary (metal) stent through the meshes of an enteral stent placed across the papilla [40, 46]. More recent data from Mutignani et al. however revealed that biliary stents can successfully be placed through the meshes of the enteral stents either endoscopically or percutaneously [47]. After achieving biliary cannulation, they either widened the meshes of the enteral stent with a pneumatic balloon or removed those covering the papilla with a rat-tooth foreign body forceps or argon plasma coagulation. Besides the technical feasibility, one should take into consideration that most of the patients will not develop biliary problems after stent placement [39] and might be unnecessarily exposed to the risks linked with biliary stent insertion in case of a prophylactic approach. We therefore suggest to only treat patients with objective signs of biliary obstruction by inserting a metal biliary stent prior to enteral stenting. The minority of patients who develop biliary obstruction after enteral stenting can be treated with endoscopic or percutaneous transhepatic biliary decompression depending on the local expertise [40, 47].

## Abdominal Pain

Abdominal pain is reported to occur in 0–4% of the patients after enteral stent placement and normally lasts for 24–72 h postprocedure [9, 11, 13, 15, 17, 19, 20, 22, 38, 39]. In the majority of cases, it resolves spontaneously without any need for treatment with analgesics [39].

## Thirty-Day Mortality

The 30-day mortality rate is an important outcome measure after surgical procedures. However, there are only a small number of publications on enteral stent placement which assess this parameter.

The 30-day mortality rates were 22% and 23%, respectively, in two prospective multicenter studies from Europe [15, 19]. The vast majority of these patients, however, died from progressive malignant disease, and only one patient died from unsuccessfully treated cholangitis. Therefore, it is very difficult to interpret the 30-day mortality as an outcome parameter of enteral stent placement. In addition, there are no intraprocedural or directly procedure-related deaths reported in the literature. Based on these data, it seems that enteral stent placement is not likely to cause the death of a patient.

## Stent Placement Versus Surgery

Before stent placement came into the picture, the traditional palliative treatment of malignant unresectable GOO was a surgical gastrojejunostomy.

In this setting, however, gastrojejunostomy is associated with relatively high morbidity rates ranging from 31.6% to 61% [31, 36, 48–50] and 30-day mortality rates up to 30% [31] due to a poor general condition of the patients. Moreover, in many instances, the patient is too ill to undergo surgery and supportive treatment would be the only option [31, 51]. Stent placement therefore is considered an attractive alternative because of its less invasive character.

At present, there are two systematic reviews, one meta-analysis and one recent randomized controlled trial (RCT), which compared the results of enteral stent placement and gastrojejunostomy as a treatment for GOO [2–4, 7]. Only the systematic review from Jeurnink et al. specifically compared the technical success rates of both treatment modalities [2]. This article included all randomized and comparative studies published between January 1996 and December 2005 and calculated the odds ratio for technical success, which showed no statistical significant difference between enteral stent placement (96%) and gastrojejunostomy (99%) (OR: 0.22, CI: 0.02–2.1, p=0.2). The clinical success rate however seemed higher after stent placement in this review (89% vs. 72%, OR: 3.39, CI: 08–14.3, p=0.1) [2]. This result is in accordance to the other review and meta-analysis [3, 4]. Moreover, these publications and the RCT showed that oral intake was restored faster following stent placement [3, 4, 7] though the RCT from Jeurnink et al. showed that food intake sustains longer after gastrojejunostomy [7].

Procedure-related hospital stay is significantly shorter after stent placement, while there is no difference in survival [3, 4, 7]. Two prospective randomized studies assessed the QoL after both treatments [7, 27]. One study found that the QoL was significantly higher 1 month after stent placement in comparison to laparoscopic gastrojejunostomy [27], while the other revealed no difference in QoL after both treatments, although pain scores decreased more rapidly after stent placement [7].

Stent placement is associated with lower medical costs (Table 18.4) [35, 52–54]. This is mostly caused by lower initial costs resulting from a

**Table 18.4** Overview of articles comparing costs of enteral stent placement and gastrojejunostomy

| Publication | Stent[a] | GJJ[a] |
|---|---|---|
| Jeurnink et al. [52] | 8,819 | 12,433 |
| Johnsson et al. [35] | 7,215 | 10,190 |
| Mittal et al. [53] | 8,680 | 20,060 |
| Yim et al. [54] | 9,921 | 28,173 |

[a]All costs are noted in US dollars

shorter procedure time and a shorter hospital stay. One might expect that follow-up costs are higher after stent placement due to the higher re-intervention rate. However, Jeurnink et al. calculated all costs from randomization until death and found that follow-up costs were equal after both procedures [52]. The authors attribute this balance to the fact that patients needed additional hospital days and/or medical procedures, for reasons other than (recurrent or persistent) obstructive problems, after gastrojejunostomy (Table 18.4).

With regard to complications, the majority of the literature report no differences in morbidity and 30-day mortality rates [2–4]. However, there are some interesting data to mention. It seems that patients who underwent gastrojejunostomy were more likely to develop "medical complications" like respiratory tract infections, myocardial infarction, and acute renal failure, while stent placement seems more associated with "stent-related" complications like stent migration and obstruction [3]. Moreover delayed gastric emptying develops more frequently after gastrojejunostomy [4]. On the other hand, some studies show a shorter time to re-intervention and a higher number of re-interventions in comparison to surgery [6, 7].

In conclusion, there is evidence that stent placement is superior over surgical bypass in terms of rapid improvement of food intake, a shorter hospital stay, less severe complications, and lower medical costs. On the contrary, there is a higher recurrence rate of obstruction after stent placement, subsequently causing declines in food intake on the long term and more re-interventions. Based on this information, it seems reasonable to suggest stent placement in patients with a poor prognosis and gastrojejunostomy in patients with a longer life expectancy. Therefore, accurate prognostication is of major importance for an advice on which treatment modality to choose in each individual patient. Data on accurate and easy-to-use tools for prognostication in patients with malignant GOO have recently been published [55, 56].

## Miscellaneous

### Enteral Stenting for Benign Strictures

Enteral stenting has been tried in patients with GOO due to benign strictures who were not amenable to surgery and in whom the stenosis was refractory to balloon dilation [57–59]. However, the literature on this topic is extremely sparse, with only one publication reporting on a study population of more than two patients. In this study, Kim et al. reported on seven patients who underwent enteral stent placement for resistant benign anastomotic strictures after gastric surgery [59]. Fully covered retrievable stents were placed in four patients for temporary purpose while partially covered dual stents were inserted in three patients for permanent use. A clinical success rate of 71% was achieved (temporary n = 2, permanent n = 3). Stent migration was the only reported complication after a mean follow-up of 12 months and occurred in three out of four patients who received a covered stent.

Though the results of this small study are promising, more data, especially long-term results, are needed to clarify whether enteral stenting might be an attractive alternative to surgical revision for benign anastomotic strictures refractory to balloon dilatation. Furthermore, there is a lack of data concerning results of enteral stent placement for benign strictures due to other causes like post-ulcer scar tissue or corrosive injury.

### Magnetic Gastroenteral Anastomosis

Endoscopic creation of a gastroenteral anastomosis by using magnetic compression in the palliative treatment of GOO has been invented with the purpose to combine the safety of enteral stent placement with the long-term efficacy of a surgical bypass. There are two studies describing this relatively new minimally invasive technique; in both studies, a stent was inserted through the anastomosis to warrant its patency [60, 61].

The first study, a prospective single center study by Chopita et al., showed the procedure to be successful in 13 out of 15 patients (88.7%); in all technical successfully treated patients, the oral intake of solids was maintained until their death [60]. The mean survival was 5.2 months (range 1–10 months). Four complications (30.8%) occurred during the follow-up period: two instances of distal migration of the stent (the patients found them in their stools), one proximal migration, and one obstruction of the stent by solid food. The latter two complications were resolved endoscopically. Encouraged by these data, a European prospective multicenter study was conducted [61]. This study, however, was terminated prematurely because of serious adverse events. In total, 18 patients had been included; in 12 (66.7%), a gastroenteral anastomosis with concomitant placement of an enteral stent was achieved. The initially used specially designed fully covered *yo-yo*-shaped stent had a migration rate of 42.8%. Therefore, the investigators switched to an uncovered conventional duodenal stent which did not migrate. However, this stent led to a fatal perforation of the jejunal wall in one patient. The authors concluded that: "Endoscopic creation of a gastroenteral anastomosis by magnetic compression is feasible and safe; however, the necessity of a stent led to serious morbidity and even mortality in this study. The current system can therefore not be recommended for clinical use."

In conclusion, this new treatment option for GOO showed mixed results, with a fatal stent-related complication in one study and a relatively high stent migration rate in both studies. The creation of the gastroenteral anastomosis, however, appears to be safe. Therefore, further research on this interesting concept should focus on the creation of an anastomosis which does not need an enteral stent to keep it patent.

## Summary

Enteral stent placement as a palliative treatment in patients with nonresectable malignant GOO is technically feasible in the vast majority of cases. Moreover, clinical success is achieved in a large number of patients. These two important outcome parameters seem not to be influenced by tumor characteristics, the type of procedure, or the type of stent. Furthermore, the small number of publications which assessed the QoL showed stable or improved results after enteral stent placement.

Regarding complications, enteral stenting is generally safe with low rates of severe complications and no reported direct procedure- or stent-related mortality. However, migration and obstruction of enteral stents occur frequently, with both of these complications strongly influencing stent patency. Uncovered stents are associated with a high obstruction rate, while covered stents tend to migrate more regularly. New stent designs have been developed with the aim to overcome these shortcomings, and recent trials with these stents show promising results.

There is evidence that stent placement is superior over surgical bypass in terms of rapid improvement of food intake, a shorter hospital stay, less severe complications, and lower medical costs. In contrast, there is a higher recurrence rate of obstruction after stent placement, subsequently causing more re-interventions. At this moment, we, in general, recommend stent placement, and the option of a surgical bypass has to be considered only in fit patients with a life expectancy of more than 2 months.

## References

1. Truong S, Bohndorf V, Geller H, Schumpelick V, Gunther RW. Self-expanding metal stents for palliation of malignant gastric outlet obstruction. Endoscopy. 1992;24:433–5.
2. Jeurnink SM, van Eijck CH, Steyerberg EW, Kuipers EJ, Siersema PD. Stent versus gastrojejunostomy for the palliation of gastric outlet obstruction: a systematic review. BMC Gastroenterol. 2007;7:18.
3. Ly J, O'Grady G, Mittal A, Plank L, Windsor JA. A systematic review of methods to palliate malignant

gastric outlet obstruction. Surg Endosc. 2010;24:290–7.

4. Hosono S, Ohtani H, Arimoto Y, Kanamiya Y. Endoscopic stenting versus surgical gastroenterostomy for palliation of malignant gastroduodenal obstruction: a meta-analysis. J Gastroenterol. 2007;42:283–90.

5. Adler DG, Baron TH. Endoscopic palliation of malignant gastric outlet obstruction using self-expanding metal stents: experience in 36 patients. Am J Gastroenterol. 2002;97:72–8.

6. Jeurnink SM, Steyerberg EW, Hof G, van Eijck CH, Kuipers EJ, Siersema PD. Gastrojejunostomy versus stent placement in patients with malignant gastric outlet obstruction: a comparison in 95 patients. J Surg Oncol. 2007;96:389–96.

7. Jeurnink SM, Steyerberg EW, van Hooft JE, van Eijck CH, Schwartz MP, Vleggaar FP, Kuipers EJ, Siersema PD. Surgical gastrojejunostomy or endoscopic stent placement for the palliation of malignant gastric outlet obstruction (SUSTENT study): a multicenter randomized trial. Gastrointest Endosc. 2010;71:490–9.

8. Kim TO, Kang DH, Kim GH, Heo J, Song GA, Cho M, Kim DH, Sim MS. Self-expandable metallic stents for palliation of patients with malignant gastric outlet obstruction caused by stomach cancer. World J Gastroenterol. 2007;13:916–20.

9. Kim CG, Choi IJ, Lee JY, Cho SJ, Park SR, Lee JH, Ryu KW, Kim YW, Park YI. Covered versus uncovered self-expandable metallic stents for palliation of malignant pyloric obstruction in gastric cancer patients: a randomized, prospective study. Gastrointest Endosc. 2010;72:25–32.

10. Kim GH, Kang DH, Lee DH, Heo J, Song GA, Cho M, Yang US. Which types of stent, uncovered or covered, should be used in gastric outlet obstructions? Scand J Gastroenterol. 2004;39:1010–4.

11. Lee KM, Choi SJ, Shin SJ, Hwang JC, Lim SG, Jung JY, Yoo BM, Cho SW, Kim JH. Palliative treatment of malignant gastroduodenal obstruction with metallic stent: prospective comparison of covered and uncovered stents. Scand J Gastroenterol. 2009;44:846–52.

12. Lowe AS, Beckett CG, Jowett S, May J, Stephenson S, Scally A, Tam E, Kay CL. Self-expandable metal stent placement for the palliation of malignant gastroduodenal obstruction: experience in a large, single, UK centre. Clin Radiol. 2007;62:738–44.

13. Phillips MS, Gosain S, Bonatti H, Friel CM, Ellen K, Northup PG, Kahaleh M. Enteral stents for malignancy: a report of 46 consecutive cases over 10 years, with critical review of complications. J Gastrointest Surg. 2008;12:2045–50.

14. Maetani I, Ukita T, Nambu T, Shigoka H, Omuta S, Endo T, Takahashi K. Comparison of ultraflex and niti-s stents for palliation of unresectable malignant gastroduodenal obstruction. Dig Endosc. 2010;22: 83–9.

15. van Hooft JE, van Montfoort ML, Jeurnink SM, Bruno MJ, Dijkgraaf MG, Siersema PD, Fockens P. Safety and efficacy of a new non-foreshortening nitinol stent in malignant gastric outlet obstruction (DUONITI study): a prospective, multicenter study. Endoscopy. 2011;43:671–5.

16. Shi D, Liao SH, Geng JP. A newly designed big cup nitinol stent for gastric outlet obstruction. World J Gastroenterol. 2010;16:4206–9.

17. Shaw JM, Bornman PC, Krige JE, Stupart DA, Panieri E. Self-expanding metal stents as an alternative to surgical bypass for malignant gastric outlet obstruction. Br J Surg. 2010;97:872–6.

18. Kim ID, Kang DH, Choi CW, Kim HW, Jung WJ, Lee DH, Chung CW, Yoo JJ, Ryu JH. Prevention of covered enteral stent migration in patients with malignant gastric outlet obstruction: a pilot study of anchoring with endoscopic clips. Scand J Gastroenterol. 2010;45: 100–5.

19. van Hooft JE, Uitdehaag MJ, Bruno MJ, Timmer R, Siersema PD, Dijkgraaf MG, Fockens P. Efficacy and safety of the new WallFlex enteral stent in palliative treatment of malignant gastric outlet obstruction (DUOFLEX study): a prospective multicenter study. Gastrointest Endosc. 2009;69:1059–66.

20. Havemann MC, Adamsen S, Wojdemann M. Malignant gastric outlet obstruction managed by endoscopic stenting: a prospective single-centre study. Scand J Gastroenterol. 2009;44:248–51.

21. Gutzeit A, Binkert CA, Schoch E, Sautter T, Jost R, Zollikofer CL. Malignant gastroduodenal obstruction: treatment with self-expanding uncovered wallstent. Cardiovasc Intervent Radiol. 2009;32:97–105.

22. Kim JH, Song HY, Shin JH, Choi E, Kim TW, Jung HY, Lee GH, Lee SK, Kim MH, Ryu MH, Kang YK, Kim BS, Yook JH. Metallic stent placement in the palliative treatment of malignant gastroduodenal obstructions: prospective evaluation of results and factors influencing outcome in 213 patients. Gastrointest Endosc. 2007;66:256–64.

23. Lee SM, Kang DH, Kim GH, Park WI, Kim HW, Park JH. Self-expanding metallic stents for gastric outlet obstruction resulting from stomach cancer: a preliminary study with a newly designed double-layered pyloric stent. Gastrointest Endosc. 2007;66: 1206–10.

24. Maetani I, Isayama H, Mizumoto Y. Palliation in patients with malignant gastric outlet obstruction with a newly designed enteral stent: a multicenter study. Gastrointest Endosc. 2007;66:355–60.

25. Huang Q, Dai DK, Qian XJ, Zhai RY. Treatment of gastric outlet and duodenal obstructions with uncovered expandable metal stents. World J Gastroenterol. 2007;13:5376–9.

26. van Hooft J, Mutignani M, Repici A, Messmann H, Neuhaus H, Fockens P. First data on the palliative treatment of patients with malignant gastric outlet obstruction using the WallFlex enteral stent: a retrospective multicenter study. Endoscopy. 2007;39:434–9.

27. Mehta S, Hindmarsh A, Cheong E, Cockburn J, Saada J, Tighe R, Lewis MP, Rhodes M. Prospective randomized trial of laparoscopic gastrojejunostomy versus duodenal stenting for malignant gastric outflow obstruction. Surg Endosc. 2006;20:239–42.

28. Espinel J, Sanz O, Vivas S, Jorquera F, Munoz F, Olcoz JL, Pinedo E. Malignant gastrointestinal obstruction: endoscopic stenting versus surgical palliation. Surg Endosc. 2006;20:1083–7.
29. Kazi HA, O'Reilly DA, Satchidanand RY, Zeiderman MR. Endoscopic stent insertion for the palliation of malignant gastric outlet obstruction. Dig Surg. 2006;23:28–31.
30. Maire F, Hammel P, Ponsot P, Aubert A, O'Toole D, Hentic O, Levy P, Ruszniewski P. Long-term outcome of biliary and duodenal stents in palliative treatment of patients with unresectable adenocarcinoma of the head of pancreas. Am J Gastroenterol. 2006;101:735–42.
31. Del Piano M, Ballare M, Montino F, Todesco A, Orsello M, Magnani C, Garello E. Endoscopy or surgery for malignant GI outlet obstruction? Gastrointest Endosc. 2005;61:421–6.
32. Maetani I, Akatsuka S, Ikeda M, Tada T, Ukita T, Nakamura Y, Nagao J, Sakai Y. Self-expandable metallic stent placement for palliation in gastric outlet obstructions caused by gastric cancer: a comparison with surgical gastrojejunostomy. J Gastroenterol. 2005;40:932–7.
33. Mosler P, Mergener KD, Brandabur JJ, Schembre DB, Kozarek RA. Palliation of gastric outlet obstruction and proximal small bowel obstruction with self-expandable metal stents: a single center series. J Clin Gastroenterol. 2005;39:124–8.
34. Bessoud B, de Baere T, Denys A, Kuoch V, Ducreux M, Precetti S, Roche A, Menu Y. Malignant gastroduodenal obstruction: palliation with self-expanding metallic stents. J Vasc Interv Radiol. 2005;16:247–53.
35. Johnsson E, Thune A, Liedman B. Palliation of malignant gastroduodenal obstruction with open surgical bypass or endoscopic stenting: clinical outcome and health economic evaluation. World J Surg. 2004;28:812–7.
36. Maetani I, Tada T, Ukita T, Inoue H, Sakai Y, Nagao J. Comparison of duodenal stent placement with surgical gastrojejunostomy for palliation in patients with duodenal obstructions caused by pancreaticobiliary malignancies. Endoscopy. 2004;36:73–8.
37. Lindsay JO, Andreyev HJ, Vlavianos P, Westaby D. Self-expanding metal stents for the palliation of malignant gastroduodenal obstruction in patients unsuitable for surgical bypass. Aliment Pharmacol Ther. 2004;19:901–5.
38. Song HY, Shin JH, Yoon CJ, Lee GH, Kim TW, Lee SK, Yook JH, Kim BS. A dual expandable nitinol stent: experience in 102 patients with malignant gastroduodenal strictures. J Vasc Interv Radiol. 2004;15:1443–9.
39. Dormann A, Meisner S, Verin N, Wenk LA. Self-expanding metal stents for gastroduodenal malignancies: systematic review of their clinical effectiveness. Endoscopy. 2004;36:543–50.
40. Baron TH, Harewood GC. Enteral self-expandable stents. Gastrointest Endosc. 2003;58:421–33.
41. Kim JH, Song HY, Shin JH, Hu HT, Lee SK, Jung HY, Yook JH. Metallic stent placement in the palliative treatment of malignant gastric outlet obstructions: primary gastric carcinoma versus pancreatic carcinoma. AJR Am J Roentgenol. 2009;193:241–7.
42. Sabharwal T, Irani FG, Adam A. Quality assurance guidelines for placement of gastroduodenal stents. Cardiovasc Intervent Radiol. 2007;30:1–5.
43. Larssen L, Medhus AW, Hauge T. Treatment of malignant gastric outlet obstruction with stents: an evaluation of the reported variables for clinical outcome. BMC Gastroenterol. 2009;9:45.
44. Jung GS, Song HY, Seo TS, Park SJ, Koo JY, Huh JD, Cho YD. Malignant gastric outlet obstructions: treatment by means of coaxial placement of uncovered and covered expandable nitinol stents. J Vasc Interv Radiol. 2002;13:275–83.
45. Kim JH, Song HY, Shin JH, Jung HY, Kim SB, Kim JH, Park SI. Membrane degradation of covered stents in the upper gastrointestinal tract: frequency and clinical significance. J Vasc Interv Radiol. 2008;19:220–4.
46. Vanbiervliet G, Demarquay JF, Dumas R, Caroli-Bosc FX, Piche T, Tran A. Endoscopic insertion of biliary stents in 18 patients with metallic duodenal stents who developed secondary malignant obstructive jaundice. Gastroenterol Clin Biol. 2004;28:1209–13.
47. Mutignani M, Tringali A, Shah SG, Perri V, Familiari P, Iacopini F, Spada C, Costamagna G. Combined endoscopic stent insertion in malignant biliary and duodenal obstruction. Endoscopy. 2007;39:440–7.
48. Lillemoe KD, Cameron JL, Hardacre JM, Sohn TA, Sauter PK, Coleman J, Pitt HA, Yeo CJ. Is prophylactic gastrojejunostomy indicated for unresectable periampullary cancer? A prospective randomized trial. Ann Surg. 1999;230:322–8.
49. Wong YT, Brams DM, Munson L, Sanders L, Heiss F, Chase M, Birkett DH. Gastric outlet obstruction secondary to pancreatic cancer: surgical vs. endoscopic palliation. Surg Endosc. 2002;16:310–2.
50. van Wagensveld BA, Coene PP, van Gulik TM, Rauws EA, Obertop H, Gouma DJ. Outcome of palliative biliary and gastric bypass surgery for pancreatic head carcinoma in 126 patients. Br J Surg. 1997;84:1402–6.
51. Lopera JE, Brazzini A, Gonzales A, Castaneda-Zuniga WR. Gastroduodenal stent placement: current status. Radiographics. 2004;24:1561–73.
52. Jeurnink SM, Polinder S, Steyerberg EW, Kuipers EJ, Siersema PD. Cost comparison of gastrojejunostomy versus duodenal stent placement for malignant gastric outlet obstruction. J Gastroenterol. 2010;45:537–43.
53. Mittal A, Windsor J, Woodfield J, Casey P, Lane M. Matched study of three methods for palliation of malignant pyloroduodenal obstruction. Br J Surg. 2004;91:205–9.
54. Yim HB, Jacobson BC, Saltzman JR, Johannes RS, Bounds BC, Lee JH, Shields SJ, Ruymann FW, Van Dam J, Carr-Locke DL. Clinical outcome of the use of enteral stents for palliation of patients with malignant upper GI obstruction. Gastrointest Endosc. 2001;53:329–32.

55. van Hooft JE, Dijkgraaf MG, Timmer R, Siersema PD, Fockens P. Independent predictors of survival in patients with incurable malignant gastric outlet obstruction: a multicenter prospective observational study. Scand J Gastroenterol. 2010;45:1217–22.

56. Jeurnink SM, Steyerberg EW, Vleggaar FP, van Eijck CH, van Hooft JE, Schwartz MP, Kuipers EJ, Siersema PD. Predictors of survival in patients with malignant gastric outlet obstruction: a patient-oriented decision approach for palliative treatment. Dig Liver Dis. 2011;43:548–52.

57. Profili S, Meloni GB, Bifulco V, Conti M, Feo CF, Canalis GC. Self-expandable metal stents in the treatment of antro-pyloric and/or duodenal strictures. Acta Radiol. 2001;42:176–80.

58. Binkert CA, Jost R, Steiner A, Zollikofer CL. Benign and malignant stenoses of the stomach and duodenum: treatment with self-expanding metallic endoprostheses. Radiology. 1996;199:335–8.

59. Kim JH, Song HY, Park SW, Yoon CJ, Shin JH, Yook JH, Kim BS. Early symptomatic strictures after gastric surgery: palliation with balloon dilation and stent placement. J Vasc Interv Radiol. 2008;19:565–70.

60. Chopita N, Vaillaverde A, Cope C, Bernedo A, Martinez H, Landoni N, Jmelnitzky A, Burgos H. Endoscopic gastroenteral anastomosis using magnets. Endoscopy. 2005;37:313–7.

61. van Hooft JE, Vleggaar FP, Le MO, Bizzotto A, Voermans RP, Costamagna G, Deviere J, Siersema PD, Fockens P. Endoscopic magnetic gastroenteral anastomosis for palliation of malignant gastric outlet obstruction: a prospective multicenter study. Gastrointest Endosc. 2010;72:530–5.

Alessandro Repici and Daniel de Paula
Pessoa Ferreira

## Introduction and General Principles of Colonic Stenting

Despite the advent of screening colonoscopy for providing an early diagnosis of colorectal neoplasia, most patients still present with advanced disease and approximately 8–29% will develop partial or complete large bowel obstruction [1–3]. Traditionally acute malignant colonic obstruction has been considered a surgical emergency; however, the morbidity and mortality rates are higher (40–50% and 10–20%, respectively), when compared to elective surgery which has a much lower mortality (0.9–6%) [4, 5]. Because of this, placement of self-expandable metal stents (SEMS) in the management of colonic obstruction has gained popularity, becoming an alternative to surgery either as a palliative treatment for patients with advanced colorectal cancer (CRC) or as bridge to surgery in patients who are potential candidates for curative resection [6, 7]. Although these different indications have specific nuances and have been evaluated in dedicated clinical studies, most of the clinical outcomes of colorectal

stent placement are the same regardless of the stent indication [8].

Outcomes are evaluated primarily based on safety, technical, and clinical success. Safety is determined by the complication risk including the mortality rate. Technical success rate is determined by accurate stent placement across the lesion, while the definition of clinical success is extremely variable, though is most commonly defined as relief of obstructive symptoms within 48–72 h after stent placement and maintained without need for reintervention or stent-related complications. The average technical success rate which is not dependent on the indication is 96.2%, ranging from 66.6% to 100% [9–11]. Data from a recent systematic review of more than 80 studies shows a median rate of clinical success of 92%, ranging from 46% to 100% [9] (Table 19.1) [12–24]. In the following sections, the different indications and related outcome following colorectal SEMS placement are analyzed.

## Benign Strictures

Benign colorectal strictures are common complications of colorectal surgery and radiation therapy, and more rarely develop as a consequence of diverticulitis and inflammatory bowel disease. Traditionally, the most common and less invasive treatment option for benign colorectal strictures is endoscopic dilation [25, 26]. Repeated procedures are often necessary due to restenosis,

A. Repici, M.D. (✉)
Digestive Endoscopy Unit, IRCCS Istituto Clinico
Humanitas, Via Manzoni 56, Rozzano (Milano),
20089, Italy
e-mail: alessandro.repici@humanitas.it

D. de Paula Pessoa Ferreira
Instituto Clinico Humanitas, Rozzano, Milan,
Lombardia, Italy

R. Kozarek et al. (eds.), *Self-Expandable Stents in the Gastrointestinal Tract*,
DOI 10.1007/978-1-4614-3746-8_19, © Springer Science+Business Media New York 2013

**Table 19.1** Technical and clinical success following colonic stent placement

| Author | Year | Placement for bridge/palliation (n) | Technical/clinical success (%) |
|---|---|---|---|
| Branger [12] | 2002–2009 | 27/66 | 93/86 |
| West [13] | 2003–2008 | 6/21 | 96/92 |
| Small [14] | 1999–2008 | 65/168 | 96/99 |
| Kim [15] | 2003–2007 | 18/27 | 100/98 |
| Pommergaard [16] | 2002–2007 | 20/25 | 97/97 |
| Olubaniyi [17] | 2001–2006 | 3/28 | 83/78 |
| Dionigi [18] | 2000–2006 | 123/219 | 95/89 |
| Al Samarae [19] | 2001–2005 | 12/26 | 92/71 |
| Athreya [20] | 1998–2004 | 11/90 | 86/86 |
| Soto [21] | 1999–2003 | 22/36 | 94/97 |
| Meisner [22] | 1997–2003 | 38/51 | 92/82 |
| Sebastian [11] | 1990–2003 | 407/791 | 92/78 |
| Choi [23] | 1997–2002 | 37/37 | 89/88 |
| Khot [24] | 1990–2000 | 223/375 | 92/88 |

From Feo and Schaffzin [6], with kind permission from Springer Science + Business Media

and surgery remains the traditional treatment in recurrent cases [27]. A reoperation is generally complicated by adhesions and anatomical changes, frequently resulting in permanent colostomy [28]. In recent years, to overcome surgical limitations, stent placement has been proposed as a potential option for the treatment of benign colorectal strictures (Fig. 19.1) that fail to respond to endoscopic dilation attempts [22, 29, 30].

Experience using SEMS for benign colonic strictures is limited, and outcomes have been disappointing. Meisner et al. reported a 63% failure rate in eight patients; stent migration occurred in two patients and perforation in one [22]. Small et al. analyzed 23 patients undergoing colorectal stent placement for obstruction due to benign colorectal strictures [31]. A high technical success rate was found, but major complications occurred, including two perforations and four reobstructions. Stent migration was observed in two patients (9%).

Geiger et al. performed an extensive literature review from 1950 to 2007 and included 26 original articles totaling 63 patients who underwent stent placement for a benign colorectal strictures, including postoperative anastomotic (41%), diverticular (35%), undefined disease (13%), Crohn's disease (6%), and radiation induced (5%) [32]. There were 53 uncovered metallic stents placed, six covered polyester (plastic) stents, and four covered metallic stents. The overall patency rate at a mean follow-up of 18 months was 71% (41/58), with an overall migration rate of 43%. Mean time to migration was 82 days, with the earliest migrations (mean of 8 days) seen when covered polyester stents were used. Major complications were seen in 12 patients (21%) treated with uncovered metal stents, including severe pain, stent fracture, bladder perforation, enteral fistulization, significant bleeding, and stent occlusion.

Unfortunately, consistent data on long-term efficacy and safety are still lacking and do not support the use of expandable stents in the management of benign colorectal disease. Recently, Dai et al. reported a retrospective series of 14 patients with benign colorectal anastomotic stenosis who underwent stent placement with a mean follow-up of 41.2 months [28]. Only five patients (36%) had successful long-term results, although in all patients, bowel decompression and significant clinical improvement occurred immediately after stent placement. Furthermore, reoperation was necessary in 50% of patients because of stricture relapse.

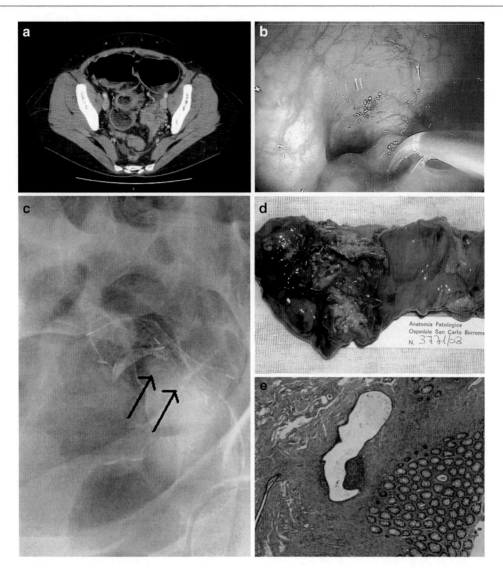

**Fig. 19.1** (**a**) CT scan shows large bowel obstruction secondary to an extrinsic mass involving the sigmoid colon. (**b**) A through-the-scope stent is inserted across the stricture. (**c**) Fluoroscopic image of the stent deployed with relief of acute obstruction. (**d**) Gross appearance of the resected specimen with the stent still retained in the stricture after preoperative stent placement and tumor resection. (**e**) Histopathology of typical findings of endometriosis, which caused obstruction of the sigmoid colon

## Extrinsic Obstruction

Malignant colorectal obstruction may also be caused by advanced extracolonic malignancy. In these cases, extrinsic compression, direct invasion into the colon, or a motility problem caused by the dissemination of the primary cancer may lead to bowel occlusion [33–35]. These patients often have complex strictures, potentially at more than one location, related to the underlying malignancy. They may also have adhesions due to prior surgery and/or chemoradiotherapy [35]. Considering the poor prognosis, short life expectancy, and high mortality and morbidity rate of palliative surgery, stent insertion is a reasonable nonsurgical palliative option [36, 37]. However, little data exist on the use of colorectal stents in patients with bowel occlusion caused by extrinsic lesions.

Caceres et al. reported their experience of colorectal stents in 35 patients with bowel occlusion due to advanced gynecologic cancer; 77% of patients experienced immediate relief of obstruction [33]. However, 33% of patients who had successful stent placement underwent additional procedures to relieve obstruction including gastrotomy [3], colostomy [4], or stent revision [2].

One study reported the outcome of colonic stenting in 15 patients with extracolonic malignancy compared to a group of 34 patients with colorectal cancer treated in the same period of time and at the same institution [36]. Patients with CRC were significantly more likely to have clinical success after endoscopic stent placement (94.1%) than those with extracolonic disease (20.0%) (P < .0001). Surgical diversion to relieve persistent obstructive symptoms after stent placement was required in 60% of patients with extracolonic tumors, compared to only 6% of patients with colorectal lesions. Furthermore, there was a significant increase in complications, including death, in patients with extracolonic lesions who underwent stent placement.

Patients with extracolonic and colonic cancers who did not experience relief of obstruction had carcinomatosis, which can lead to bowel immobilization, contributing to the decreased success and increased complication rate of colon stent placement. Multivariate analysis found that extracolonic malignancy was the sole predictor of failed endoscopic therapy.

In a recent small retrospective study that analyzed 12 procedures in 11 patients with colorectal obstruction from extracolonic malignancies, the technical and clinical success rates were 42% and 25%, respectively; the subsequent colostomy requirement rate was 45%, and the 30-day mortality rate was 36% [38]. The median survival time was 2 months. None of the five patients with ovarian cancer had a successful relief of obstructive symptoms after stent placement. Only two patients with a stent placed survived more than a month without a colostomy.

In 2008, a South Korean group reported a more favorable outcome and higher technical success

rate of SEMS in treating colorectal obstruction caused by extracolonic malignancy [39]. However, there was a high rate of complications (38.6%) such as perforation and bleeding. Unique to this study was that almost 80% of colonic obstruction was caused by advanced gastric cancer directly infiltrating the transverse colon. Given these relatively poor results, we believe that the endoscopic colonic stent placement for obstruction from extracolonic malignancy should only be attempted if decompressive surgery is not feasible. Patients and their family should be made aware of the limited success rate and potential for serious complications [35]. Further evaluation of the role of endoscopic stenting for large bowel obstruction from extracolonic malignancies should be performed in a randomized, prospective manner to further clarify the role of stents for palliation in this patient population [35].

## Palliation

Since Dohmoto first described colonic SEMS placement, their use for palliation of patients with locally advanced or metastatic disease has been extensively investigated, and systematic reviews have been published [8]. In 2002, British researchers systematically reviewed the data published from January 1990 to December 2000 of colonic SEMS placement for treatment of colorectal obstruction [24]. A total of 58 studies were identified, and included 598 stent placement attempts. Technical success was achieved in 92% and clinical success in 88%. Palliation was achieved in 90% of 336 cases, while 85% of 262 insertions succeeded as a "bridge to surgery" (95% had a one-stage surgical procedure). Mortality rate was 1%, two cases due to perforation and one failure to decompress the colon.

Several years later, Sebastian et al. published a pooled analysis of the efficacy and safety of SEMS in relief of malignant colorectal obstruction for both palliation and as a bridge to surgery [11]. A total of 1,198 patients were included; 44% underwent stent placement as a bridge to surgery, with a one-stage surgery rate of 78.1%. The median technical success was 94% (ranging from 90% to 100%), and 91% (ranging from 84% to 94%) of patients achieved relief of obstructive symptoms. Major complications related to stent placement included perforation in 3.76%, stent migration in 11.81%, and reobstruction in 7.34%. Locally advanced tumors, inadequate preparation, perforation, and migration were associated with need for colostomy. Stent-related mortality was 0.58%, mostly occurring in the palliative group. Two deaths were secondary to sepsis and three due to known bowel perforation.

The most recent and largest systematic review collected outcomes of 1,785 patients, with 1,845 stents placed for relief of malignant colorectal obstruction [9]. SEMS were placed as a palliative treatment in 43% of patients, as a bridge to surgery in 20% and indeterminate in 37%. A total of 1,600 (90%) patients had SEMS placed to overcome left-sided obstructions. The median rate of technical success was 96.2%, ranging from 66.6% to 100%, and the median rate of clinical success was 92%, ranging from 46% to 100%. In the 14 studies that reported duration of patency, the mean duration was 106 days (range 68–288 days). In total, 90.7% (118 of 130) of patients with known follow-up either died or ended their follow-up without recurrent obstruction. Only 45 studies specifically reported the need for reintervention which was required in 20% of patients when SEMS were placed for palliation. The median rate of migration was 11%, ranging from 0% to 50%. Perforation, caused by either the guidewire or stent, was reported on in 50 studies with a median rate of perforation of 4.5% (range 0–83%). Reobstruction was reported in 12% (range 1–92%), mostly as a result of tumor ingrowth and/or overgrowth and occurred from 48 h to 480 days after placement. Based on the level of evidence of the reviewed articles, a definitive statement that SEMS are safe and efficacious should be interpreted with caution.

Few randomized controlled trials comparing colostomy and SEMS for palliation of malignant colonic obstruction have been reported. In 2004, Xinopoulos et al. randomized 30 patients with inoperable malignant colonic obstruction: 15 to undergo SEMS placement and 15 to colostomy [40]. Stents were placed successfully in 93.3%

(14/15) of patients with no stent-related mortality reported. Long-term luminal patency without obstructive symptoms until death was achieved in 8 of 14 patients (57%) in whom the stent was successfully placed. Mean survival was 21.4 months in the SEMS group and 20.9 months in the colostomy group. Mean hospital stay was high in both groups and significantly higher in patients receiving colostomy (days 60 days vs. 28 days). However, the small sample size and other limitations in study design might have masked differences between groups.

In 2007, The Dutch Colorectal Stent Group planned a multicenter, prospective, randomized clinical trial, called the Stent-in 1 study, to evaluate the effectiveness of endoscopic stent placement and surgery in patients with bowel obstruction and advanced disease [41, 42]. The study was terminated prematurely after enrolling 21 patients because of an unexpected high rate of adverse events in the stent arm. Eleven adverse events (six perforations) resulting in 3 deaths occurred in the stent arm versus one adverse event in the surgical arm ($P < 0.001$). Of the six perforations, two occurred at the proximal edge of the stent by erosion through a normal colon wall, one was located in the region of the proximal half of the stent, one was a colon blowout, and the last two were late tumor perforations in patients receiving chemotherapy. The investigators concluded that this poor outcome was related to the stent used (WallFlex, Boston Scientific Natick, MA) and/or stent-related perforations in patients receiving chemotherapy. This data has not been confirmed in previous and subsequent studies using the same stent for palliation of colonic obstruction where a perforation rate of about 5% was found, much lower than that in the Dutch study [43–46].

A recent retrospective study has compared the long-term outcomes of endoscopic stent placement ($n = 71$) with those of surgery ($n = 73$) for palliation of colonic obstruction in patients with advanced colorectal cancer [47]. Early success rates in the SEMS group and the surgical group were not significantly different (95.8% vs. 100%, $P = 0.12$). Although the patency duration of the stent placed initially was shorter than that of surgery, placement of a second stent within the first stent for recurrent obstruction prolonged the benefit of endoscopically treated patients with the median bowel patency comparable to that of the surgical group. The SEMS group had significantly fewer early complications (15.5% vs. 32.9%, $P = 0.015$) but more late complications ($P = 0.028$) when compared to the surgery group; however, the rates of major complications did not differ between the two groups. These results confirmed SEMS to be an effective and acceptable long-term therapy for palliation of malignant colorectal obstruction comparable with that of surgery.

In a recent retrospective study, Small and colleagues reported the largest published experience in long-term outcomes on SEMS placement for palliation of malignant colorectal obstruction in 168 patients who underwent SEMS placement [14]. Forty-one patients (24.4%) in the palliation group had complications including perforation (9%), occlusion (9%), migration (5%), and erosion/ulcer (2%). Mean stent patency was 145 days in the palliative group. One hundred eight of 122 patients (88.5%) remained free of obstruction from stent deployment until death. Intraluminal lesions, bevacizumab, and distal colon stent placement were associated with a higher complication rate. Bevacizumab therapy nearly tripled the risk of perforation.

The findings of few prospective trials and many recent retrospective series further demonstrate the usefulness of SEMS for definitive palliative treatment of malignant colorectal strictures [48–56]. SEMS can provide rapid and effective relief of obstructive symptoms, with acceptable morbidity and need for reintervention and extremely low mortality. Colonic SEMS placement is typically performed with the patient under moderate sedation and entails less acute debilitation, more rapid recovery, and a shorter hospital stay compared with surgery. Such benefits are of particular value in patients with limited life expectancy when surgical treatment may even be considered unethical and associated with significantly decreased quality of life [57].

## Bridge to Surgery

Since Tejero et al. described the use of stents as a bridge to surgery in 1994, SEMS placement for this indication has been increasingly accepted among gastroenterologists and surgeons [58, 59]. It is well recognized from the surgical literature that emergency surgery on an unprepared bowel is associated with high morbidity (10–36%) and high mortality (6–30%) compared with elective surgery (4–14% of morbidity, 1–7% of mortality) [60]. In patients with malignant colonic obstruction who are candidates for curative surgery, placement of a colonic SEMS allows bowel decompression before definitive surgical resection (Fig. 19.2). This strategy aims to provide sufficient time for resuscitation, rehydration, normalization of hydro-electrolyte balance, institution of nutritional therapy and bowel preparation before surgery, thorough cancer staging

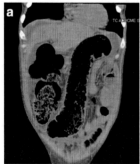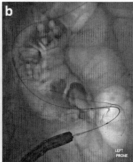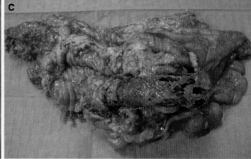

**Fig. 19.2** (a) CT scan of large bowel obstruction due a resectable sigmoid cancer. (b) Same patient with a SEMS deployed to decompress acute obstruction. (c) Resected specimen with the stent in place across the neoplastic stricture

(including complete colonoscopy), and the ability to provide neoadjuvant therapy in patients with rectal cancer [6, 11]. Furthermore, it avoids stoma formation, which is associated with adverse psychologic parameters. Moreover, SEMS placement may shorten hospital stay and may be more cost-effective than emergency surgery [61–64]. In these ways, colorectal stent deployment serves as a favorable bridge to surgery.

A large systematic review was published by a group of Swiss surgeons to evaluate different strategies for acute malignant left-sided colonic obstruction [65]. The study included 29 studies with 2,286 patients. The stent group had a lower mortality, lower complication rate, and a shorter hospital stay than the surgical group. The authors concluded that colonic SEMS placement is a promising nonsurgical option, allowing elective cancer resection. Nevertheless, the authors noted that the quality of the studies was limited, with only three randomized trials, and which limited the validity of the findings.

A number of different studies (mostly retrospective) have compared outcome of SEMS placement followed by elective open surgery with those of emergency surgery without prior stent placement. A greater proportion of patients in the stent group underwent successful resection with a primary anastomosis and a decrease in stoma formation [45].

Martinez-Santos et al. studied 72 consecutive patients with malignant left-sided colorectal obstruction [66]. After SEMS placement, obstruction was relieved in 95% (41/45) of patients. Of 26 patients who underwent elective surgery after stenting, primary anastomosis was possible in 22 ((84.6%) vs. 41.4% in the emergency surgery group, $P=0.0025$), with a reduction in need for colostomy (15.4% vs. 58.6% in the emergency surgery group). The anastomotic failure rate was similar while the reintervention rate was lower (0 vs. 17%, $P=0.014$) in the stent group. The total hospital stay (14.23 vs. 18.52 days; $P=0.047$), intensive care unit stay (0.3 vs. 2.9 days; $P=0.015$), and the number of patients with severe complications (11.6% vs. 41.2%; $P=0.008$) were significantly lower in the stenting as a bridge to surgery group.

The strategy of stent placement as a bridge to surgery is even less invasive if followed by elective laparoscopic resection. This inspired Morino and colleagues to present data on a small series of patients treated by SEMS placement for decompression of malignant obstruction followed by laparoscopic one-stage resection [67]. The investigators concluded that the strategy of SEMS followed by laparoscopy resulted in patient comfort, rapid postoperative recovery, and short hospital stay. Studies in a larger cohort of patients confirmed that colonic stenting followed by laparoscopic resection provides a safe and effective minimally invasive approach to the management of malignant colonic obstruction [68, 69].

Three randomized controlled trials assessing outcomes of colonic stent placement as a bridge to surgery were recently published with conflicting results [70–72]. In 2009, Cheung et al. published the first randomized controlled trial comparing an endo-laparoscopic approach (24 patients) with conventional open surgery (24 patients) in the treatment of obstructing left-sided colon cancer [70]. SEMS were successfully implanted in 20 patients with clinical success rates of 83%. In four patients, endoscopists failed to cannulate the obstruction. Patients in the endo-laparoscopic group had significantly less cumulative blood loss and pain in addition to a lower incidence of anastomotic leakage and wound infection. Significantly more patients in the endo-laparoscopic group had a successful one-stage operation performed (16% vs. 9%, $p=0.04$), and none had a permanent stoma compared to six patients in the emergency open surgery group ($p=0.03$). No stent-related complications occurred [70].

The following year, a French multicenter randomized controlled trial showed contradictory results [71]. Sixty patients were randomized and included for the final analysis, 30 patients underwent emergency surgery, and 30 underwent SEMS as a bridge to elective one-stage surgical resection without stoma (the primary outcome). Seventeen patients in the surgery group underwent stoma placement versus 13 patients in the SEMS group ($p=0.30$). No statistically significant difference was noted concerning secondary outcomes. Sixteen (53.3%) SEMS placement attempts were technical failures. Two colonic perforations directly related to the stent placement occurred among the 30 randomized patients, leading to premature closure of the study.

The third RTC is a Dutch multicenter study, called the Dutch Stent-in II study, and included 98 patients assigned to receive colonic stenting ($n=47$ patients) or emergency surgery ($n=51$) [72]. No difference was recorded between treatment groups in 30-day mortality, overall mortality, morbidity, and stoma rates at latest follow-up. The most common serious adverse events were abscess (3 in the colonic stenting group vs. 4 in the emergency surgery group), perforations (6 vs. none), and anastomotic leakage (5 vs. 1). The study was prematurely closed because two successive interim analyses showed increased 30-day mortality in the colonic stent group primarily due to a higher rate of post-stent placement complications. The conflicting data call for further evidence-based studies of stent placement as a bridge to surgery before it can be routinely recommended [8].

Subclinical perforation may occur during stent placement, which may consequently spread tumor cells into the peripheral circulation [73]. The impact of such events on long-term oncologic outcome is still unknown and deserves further investigation. Currently, only few studies have evaluated long-term outcome in patients with potentially curable colorectal cancer after stent placement as a bridge to surgery compared to emergency surgery alone. One study published in abstract form reported no difference in 3-year survival between patients treated with SEMS insertion followed by surgical resection and patients who underwent emergency surgery (48% vs. 50%) [74]. A subsequent study noted a 3-year survival rate of 80% in patients who had SEMS insertion as a bridge to potentially curative resection compared with 74% in patients who underwent emergency resection [75].

## Covered Versus Uncovered SEMS

SEMS can be classified as covered or uncovered according to the presence or absence of a covering membrane on the surface of the metal mesh.

Covering of the stents was developed to reduce or prevent tumor ingrowth, an important cause of early uncovered stent occlusion [76–79]. However, covered stents migrate more often, since integration of the wire mesh into the tumor and surrounding tissue, which anchor the stent, does not occur [78]. Nevertheless, there have been few randomized studies, comparing outcomes of these two different kinds of stents in the treatment of large bowel obstruction.

Initially, covered stents were designed in cylindrical form, but they proved to be ineffective because of high rates of migration [63, 76, 78, 80, 81]. Subsequently, manufacturers developed covered stents in the shape of a dumbbell or funnel with uncovered ends designed to prevent migration.

Lee et al. studied 80 patients with malignant colorectal obstruction [82]. Thirty-nine (20 bridge to surgery and 19 palliative) patients were treated with uncovered stents, while dumbbell covered stents were inserted in 41 (23 bridge to surgery and 18 palliative) patients. Technical and clinical success rates were not significantly different [82]. Early migration (within 7 days) occurred equally in both groups. However, the late stent migration was much more common in the covered stent group than the uncovered stent group (0% vs. 40%, respectively, $p=0.005$). Loss of stent function during the long-term follow-up period was more frequent in the covered stent group than in the uncovered stent group (18.8% vs. 60%, respectively, $p=0.018$) [82].

A pooled analysis of the efficacy of SEMS in malignant colorectal obstruction confirmed a significantly higher migration rate in the covered stent group (30.58%) than in the uncovered group (6.8%) and a stent occlusion rate in the covered stent group significantly lower than in the uncovered group (4.7% vs. 7.81%) [1].

However, other studies also demonstrated lower occlusion rates in uncovered stents with larger diameters [44, 51, 54, 82, 83]. A Korean group retrospectively studied the outcomes of uncovered stent insertion in 73 patients and covered stent insertion in 30 patients with malignant colonic obstruction [84]. Stent occlusion due to tumor ingrowth occurred in 12.3% of uncovered stents and tumor overgrowth in 3.3% of covered stents. The stent migration rate was higher but not significantly different in the covered stent group than uncovered stent group (16.7% vs. 13.7%).

A recent randomized prospective study analyzed a total of 151 patients with malignant colorectal obstruction who underwent stent placement and found a mean duration of patency of 6.0 months (range 3.6–8.4 months) in the uncovered group and 7.3 months (range 4.3–10.3 months) in the covered group [35]. There was no statistically significant difference between the two groups.

A recent systematic review analyzed a total of 124 covered stents and 171 uncovered stent placements [9]. Only minor differences were seen between the technical and clinical success rates. The type of stent used did not impact the risk of perforation. The authors concluded that the benefit of the covered stents is related to their ability to resist tumor ingrowth, reflected in lower reobstruction rates compared with uncovered stents, although covered stents appeared more prone to migration than uncovered stents.

In theory, covered stents should be preferred for palliation, while uncovered stents should be used for preoperative decompression as a bridge to surgery [23]. In addition, results from a recent study suggest that uncovered SEMS be used in colorectal obstruction due to unresectable extrinsic tumors, considering the lower migration rate and shorter remaining life expectancy of these patients [39].

## Quality of Life

It is known that emergency surgical decompression is associated with high morbidity and mortality rates and often results in temporary or permanent colostomy, which has a significant impact on quality of life [49, 85]. Unfortunately, comparative data concerning quality of life among patients who underwent surgery or stent placement for relief of malignant bowel obstruction are lacking.

Patients with advanced or metastatic colorectal cancer have multiple health-related factors affecting their quality of life, and inevitably, the declining physical status dominates the clinical presentation of these patients. So it is quite difficult to measure the benefit of a specific palliative procedure by means of quality of life that a significant improvement on the individual's physical, emotional, functional, and social well-being is not expected [86].

Studies have shown that patients who undergo stent placement tolerate an oral diet earlier (5 days on average) and have return of bowel function significantly earlier, which contributes to an early improvement in quality of life [87, 88]. Recently, the first prospective study was published that evaluated quality of life after palliation of malignant colorectal obstruction in 44 patients (30 treated with SEMS placement and 14 with surgical diversion) [86]. The high mortality from advanced malignancy resulted in a substantial patient dropout rate and limited statistical conclusions, especially at later time points (8, 12, and 24 weeks). Both SEMS placement and surgical diversion provided durable improvement in symptoms of large bowel obstruction. Stent placement was associated with improved quality of life related to gastrointestinal function and overall quality of life for patients with a longer lifespan. As the study progressed, fewer patients were willing to consider surgical diversion.

## Cost-Effectiveness

The cost-effectiveness of SEMS is another important issue to be evaluated. SEMS are expensive, but the shorter initial hospital stay and lower rate of colostomy formation may offset their costs [8]. A retrospective study compared hospital costs and clinical outcomes between endoscopic stent placement and colostomy in the palliation of malignant colonic obstruction [89]. The median hospital stay (8 vs. 12 days; P < .0001) and the median cost ($15,071 vs. $24,695; P < .001) were significantly lower after stent placement. The authors concluded that, although the technical and clinical outcomes for colostomy and stent placement appeared comparable, stent placement was less costly and associated with shorter hospital stay and fewer complications.

The cost-effectiveness of two competing strategies (stenting followed by elective surgery vs. emergency primary resection) was analyzed by American and Canadian investigators [90, 91]. Both analyses concluded that colonic stent placement followed by elective surgery is significantly more effective and cost-effective than emergency surgery as a result of shorter hospitalization and a lower complication rate.

In late 1990s, a British retrospective study of a small group of patients showed that palliative stenting compared with surgical decompression was associated with a mean cost of £1769, whereas stent placement as a bridge surgery versus emergency Hartman resection followed by elective reversal saved a mean of £685 [87]. Similar results were obtained in a Swiss prospective study that observed a cost reduction of 19.7% in the stent group [63].

In the previously mentioned randomized study by Xinopoulos et al. of palliative colonic SEMS placement and colostomy, a cost-effectiveness analysis was also performed, including the cost of post-interventional care [40]. The cost-effectiveness analysis showed that although colostomy was less expensive, the total difference in average costs for the two methods was 6.9% (132 Euros) in favor of colonic stenting.

In summarizing these studies, although SEMS seem to be cost-effective, results are difficult to compare because cost calculations vary significantly between different health care systems, and differ when SEMS are placed for palliation compared to bridge to surgery, and the cost of stents is decreasing [8].

## Complications

Colonic stent placement is generally considered a low-risk procedure with a mortality rate of less than 1% [14, 44, 51, 57]. Complications are usually divided into early (within 30 days), including perforation, bleeding, and misplacement, and late, including mainly stent migration, reobstruction, tenesmus, and rarely, perforation.

Stent migration may be asymptomatic or result in recurrence of obstructive symptoms, bleeding, or tenesmus if the stent passed into the anorectum.

Migrated stents may pass spontaneously through the anus but in the majority of the cases are removed endoscopically or digitally if impacted in the distal rectum [92]. The migration rates of uncovered stents range from 3% to 12%, compared to that of covered stents which migration occurs in up to 30–50% of patients [93].

Migration occurs more frequently within the first week and may be due to technical factors such as small stent diameter, colonic angulation, insufficient length of the stent to allow stent flaring, and postoperative chemotherapy or radiation therapy which may induce tumor shrinkage [24, 76, 94, 95]. Other factors that may predispose to stent migration include fecal impaction, placement within partially obstructed lesions and strictures caused by benign disease or extrinsic compression [92]. Stent migration occurs 3 times more frequently with stents placed in the distal rectum compared with the left colon [96]. Repeat stent placement can usually be successfully performed, and the use of larger diameter stents should be considered [76, 97].

Reobstruction is one of the most frequently reported complications of stent placement. Tumor overgrowth is the commonest cause, with stent migration, tumor ingrowth through the stent mesh, and fecal obstruction occurring less frequently [11]. Stent fracture and disintegration are quite uncommon but a possible cause of reobstruction. The likelihood of stent occlusion by tumor growth increases with the time elapsed after stent placement because of the natural tendency of neoplasms to invade the colonic lumen, thus making this complication more frequent in the setting of palliation of malignant strictures [51]. A systemic review of the published data on stent placement for the treatment of colorectal obstruction showed a rate of stent occlusion of 16% (49/302) in patients with a stent inserted for palliation [98]. In the past, tumor ingrowth was treated with endoscopic laser ablation, but more recently, insertion of an additional stent is becoming the standard and preferred treatment of tumor ingrowth and overgrowth [10]. Careful sizing to allow a 2-cm extension of the stent on either ends into normal colonic mucosa is advised to reduce the incidence of tumor overgrowth [92]. In a recent study, stent occlusion because of tumor ingrowth or overgrowth occurred in 8 patients (15.4%) at a mean time of 127 days [93] and was successfully treated with additional overlapping stent placement in the majority of cases. After the second stent deployment, reocclusion did not develop until the end of the follow-up period or patient death, confirming the clinical value of additional stent placement to manage occluded stents [14, 47].

Perforation is considered the most dangerous complication of colonic stent placement for the patient and most frightening for the physician. The overall risk of perforation has been estimated to be ≤5% [9, 10, 14, 38]. A notable article on stent-related perforation collected data on cause, timing, treatment, and mortality related to perforation in a total of 2,287 patients [99]. More than 80% of perforations occurred within 30 days of stent placement (half within 1 day of the procedure). Mortality related to perforation was 0.8% per stented patient, but the mortality of patients experiencing perforation was 16.2%. Concomitant chemotherapy, corticosteroid medications, and radiotherapy were significantly associated with perforation. The overall perforation-related mortality was far less than that of patients undergoing emergency surgery for bowel obstruction. Khot et al. reported a perforation rate of 2% in patients in who balloon dilation of the stricture or stent was performed during placement compared to 10% in of patients who had balloon dilatation [24]. Aggressive guidewire manipulation is another potential cause of perforation [63, 74, 100]. Pre-stenting perforation (the so-called procedure-related perforation) accounts for 15% to 20% of cases and is usually related to guidewire or catheter misplacement or to stricture dilation [8]. Overinflation of air in an already dilated proximal bowel may result in a closed-loop perforation far away from the site of the lesion usually cecal perforation due to overdistension. Stent-related perforation may also occur because of tumor fracture caused by the radial force of the stent or due to overpressure of the stent ends on the healthy mucosa. In some recent prospective trials, an unexpected high rate of perforation has led to premature study closure [41, 71, 72]. Bevacizumab-based chemotherapy is emerging as a major risk factor for post-stent placement perforation [14]. Several studies have found that bevacizumab therapy nearly triples the risk of perforation and significantly shortens the mean time to delayed perforation [2, 41, 57]. The anti-angiogenic effect may weaken the bowel wall and predispose to perforation at the point of SEMS pressure. This risk may be independent from the stent itself, since a recent review has demonstrated that the addition of bevacizumab to cancer therapy significantly increases the risk of spontaneous gastrointestinal perforation compared with controls in the absence of stent placement [101].

Some factors may be associated with a favorable following colonic stent placement. In a Korean study, patients with shorter length stents (<10 cm) had better outcomes than those with longer length stents (>10 cm) ($P=0.008$) [56]. Furthermore, patients with a distal colorectal obstruction had better clinical results than those with a proximal colorectal obstruction ($P=0.015$). The largest reported study of complications of SEMS from a single center with proven experience reveals several clinical predictors for complications [10]. Two of the most important risk factors were characteristics of the patients: gender and degree of occlusion. For unclear reasons, male gender increased susceptibility to an adverse event. The completely occluded bowel may result in friable, microperforated tissue and is associated with a severely tight stricture that makes SEMS deployment technically challenging. Other risk factors were related to procedural/endoscopic technique. The perforation rate was significantly lower when stents were placed by expert endoscopists with proven expertise in pancreaticobiliary therapy. This is probably related to the basic skill set of endoscopists who perform therapeutic ERCP and who are familiar with guidewire manipulation, ability to traverse complex strictures, fluoroscopy images, and proper stent advancement and deployment.

## References

1. Deans GT, Krukowski ZH, Irwin ST. Malignant obstruction of the left colon. Br J Surg. 1994;81: 1270–6.
2. Cennamo V, Fuccio L, Mutri V, et al. Does stent placement for advanced colon cancer increase the

risk of perforation during bevacizumab based therapy? Clin Gastroenterol Hepatol. 2009;7:1174–6.

3. Baque P, Chevallier P, Karimdjee Solihi F, et al. Colostomy vs self-expanding metallic stents: comparison of the two techniques in acute tumoral left colonic obstruction. Ann Chir. 2004;129:353–8.

4. Leitman IM, Sullivan JD, Brams D, et al. Multivariate analysis of the morbidity and mortality from initial surgical management of obstructing carcinoma of the colon. Surg Gynaecol Obstet. 1992;174:513–8.

5. Mulcahy HE, Skelly MM, Hussain A, et al. Long-term outcome following curative surgery for malignant large bowel obstruction. Br J Surg. 1996;83:707–10.

6. Feo L, Schaffzin DM. Colonic stents: the modern treatment of colonic obstruction. Adv Ther. 2011; 28:73–86.

7. Adler DG. Management of malignant colonic obstruction. Curr Treat Options Gastroenterol. 2005; 8:231–7.

8. Repici A, Ferreira DPP. Expandable metal stents for malignant colorectal strictures. Gastrointest Endosc Clin N Am. 2011;21:511–33.

9. Watt AM, Faragher IG, Griffin TT, Rieger NA, Maddern GJ. Self-expanding metallic stents for relieving malignant colorectal obstruction: a systematic review. Ann Surg. 2007;246:24–30.

10. Baron TH. Colonic stenting: technique, technology, and outcomes for malignant and benign disease. Gastrointest Endosc Clin N Am. 2005;15:757–71.

11. Sebastian S, Johnston S, Geoghegan T, Torreggiani W, Buckley M. Pooled analysis of the efficacy and safety of self-expanding metal stenting in malignant colorectal obstruction. Am J Gastroenterol. 2004;99: 2051–7.

12. Branger F, Thibaudeau E, Mucci-Hennekinne S, et al. Management of acute malignant large-bowel obstruction with self-expanding metal stent. Int J Colorectal Dis. 2010;25:1481–5.

13. West M, Kiff R. Stenting of the colon in patients with malignant large bowel obstruction: a local experience. J Gastrointest Cancer. 2011;42:155–9.

14. Small AJ, Coelho-Prabhu N, Baron TH. Endoscopic placement of self-expandable metal stents for malignant colonic obstruction: long-term outcomes and complication factors. Gastrointest Endosc. 2010;71: 560–72.

15. Kim H, Kim SH, Choi SY, et al. Fluoroscopically guide placement of self-expanding metallic stents and stent graft in the treatment of acute malignant colorectal obstruction. J Vasc Interv Radiol. 2008;19: 1709–16.

16. Pommergaard HC, Vilmann P, Jakobsen HL, Achiam MP. A clinical evaluation of endoscopically placed self-expanding metallic stent in patients with acute large bowel obstruction. Scand J Surg. 2009; 98:143–7.

17. Olubaniyi BO, Mcfaul CD, Yip VS, Abbott G, Johnson M. Stenting for large bowel obstruction – evolution of a service in a general district hospital. Ann R Coll Surg Engl. 2009;91:55–8.

18. Dionigi G, Villa F, Rovera F, et al. Colonic stenting for malignant disease: review of literature. Surg Oncol. 2007;16:153–5.

19. Al Samaraee A, Fasih T, Hayat M. Use of self-expandable stents for obstructive distal and proximal large bowel cancer: a retrospective study in a single centre. J Gastrointest Cancer. 2010;41:43–6.

20. Athreya S, Moss J, Urquhart G. Colorectal stenting for colonic obstruction: indications, complications, effectiveness and outcome 5 year review. Eur J Radiol. 2006;60:91–4.

21. Soto S, Lopez-Roses L, Gonzalez-Ramirez A. Endoscopic treatment of acute colorectal obstruction with self expandable metallic stent: experience in a community hospital. Surg Endosc. 2006;20:1072–6.

22. Meisner S, Hensler M, Knop FK. Self expanding metal stent for colonic obstruction: experiences from 104 procedures in a single center. Dis Colon Rectum. 2004;47:444–50.

23. Choi JS, Choo SW, Park KB, et al. Interventional management of malignant colorectal obstruction: use of covered and uncovered stents. Korean J Radiol. 2007;8:57–63.

24. Khot U, Lang AW, Murali K, Parker MC. Systematic review of efficacy and safety of colorectal stents. Br J Surg. 2002;89:1096–102.

25. Werre A, Mulder C, van Heteren C, Bilgen ES. Dilation of benign strictures following low anterior resection using Savary-Gilliard bougies. Endoscopy. 2000;32:385–8.

26. Johansson C. Endoscopic dilation of rectal strictures: a prospective study of 18 cases. Dis Colon Rectum. 1996;39:423–8.

27. Suchan KL, Muldner A, Manegold BC. Endoscopic treatment of postoperative colorectal anastomotic strictures. Surg Endosc. 2003;17:1110–3.

28. Dai Y, Chopra SS, Wysocki WM, Hünerbein M. Treatment of benign colorectal strictures by temporary stenting with self-expanding stents. Int J Colorectal Dis. 2010;25:1475–9.

29. Paul L, Pinto I, Gomez H, et al. Metallic stents in the treatment of benign diseases of the colon: preliminary experience in 10 cases. Radiology. 2002;223: 715–22.

30. Dormann AJ, Deppe H, Wigginghaus B. Self-expanding metallic stents for continuous dilatation of benign stenoses in gastrointestinal tract: first results of long-term follow-up in interim stent application in pyloric and colonic obstructions. Gastroenterology. 2001;39:957–60.

31. Small AJ, Young-Fadok TM, Baron TH. Expandable metal stent placement for benign colorectal obstruction: outcomes for 23 cases. Surg Endosc. 2008; 22:454–62.

32. Geiger TM, Miedema BW, Tsereteli Z, et al. Stent placement for benign colonic stenosis: case report, review of the literature, and animal pilot data. Int J Colorectal Dis. 2008;23:1007–12.

33. Caceres A, Zhou Q, Iasonos A, et al. Colorectal stents for palliation of large-bowel obstructions in

recurrent gynecologic cancer: an updated series. Gynecol Oncol. 2008;108:482–5.

34. Keswani RN, Azar RR, Edmundowicz SA, et al. Stenting for malignant colonic obstruction: a comparison of efficacy and complications in colonic versus extracolonic malignancy. Gastrointest Endosc. 2009;69(3 Pt 2):675–80.

35. Park S, Cheon JH, Park JJ, et al. Comparison of efficacies between stents for malignant colorectal obstruction: a randomized, prospective study. Gastrointest Endosc. 2010;72:304–10.

36. Miyayama S, Matsui O, Kifune K, et al. Malignant colonic obstruction due to extrinsic tumor: palliative treatment with a self-expanding nitinol stent. AJR Am J Roentgenol. 2000;175:1631–7.

37. Pothuri B, Guirguis A, Gerdes H, et al. The use of colorectal stents for palliation of large bowel obstruction due to recurrent gynecologic cancer. Gynecol Oncol. 2004;95:513–7.

38. Trompetas V, Saunders M, Gossage J, Anderson H. Shortcomings in colonic stenting to palliate large bowel obstruction from extracolonic malignancies. Int J Colorectal Dis. 2010;25:851–4.

39. Shin SJ, Kim TI, Kim BC, et al. Clinical application of self-expandable metallic stent for treatment of colorectal obstruction caused by extrinsic invasive tumors. Dis Colon Rectum. 2008;51:578–83.

40. Xinopoulos D, Dimitroulopoulos D, Theodosopoulos T, et al. Stenting or stoma creation for patients with inoperable malignant colonic obstructions? Results of a study and cost-effectiveness analysis. Surg Endosc. 2004;18:421–6.

41. Van Hooft JE, Fockens P, Marinelli AW, et al. Early closure of a multicenter randomized clinical trial of endoscopic stenting versus surgery for stage IV left-sided colorectal cancer. Endoscopy. 2008;40: 184–91.

42. Van Hooft JE, Fockens P, Marinelli AW, et al. Premature closure of the Dutch Stent-in I study. Lancet. 2006;368(9547):1573–4.

43. Dronamraju SS, Ramamurthy S, Kelly SB, Hayat M. Role of self-expanding metallic stents in the management of malignant obstruction of the proximal colon. Dis Colon Rectum. 2009;52:1657–61.

44. Repici A, De Caro G, Luigiano C, et al. WallFlex colonic stent placement for management of malignant colonic obstruction: a prospective study at two centers. Gastrointest Endosc. 2008;67:77–84.

45. Brehant O, Fuks D, Bartoli E, et al. Elective (planned) colectomy in patients with colorectal obstruction after placement of a self-expanding metallic stent as a bridge to surgery: the results of a prospective study. Colorectal Dis. 2009;11:178–83.

46. Repici A, Adler DG, Gibbs CM, et al. Stenting of the proximal colon in patients with malignant large bowel obstruction: techniques and outcomes. Gastrointest Endosc. 2007;66:940–4.

47. Lee HJ, Hong SP, Cheon JH, et al. Long-term outcome of palliative therapy for malignant colorectal obstruction in patients with unresectable metastatic colorectal cancers: endoscopic stenting versus surgery. Gastrointest Endosc. 2011;73:535–42.

48. Baraza W, Lee F, Brown S, Hurlstone DP. Combination endo-radiological colorectal stenting: a prospective 5-year clinical evaluation. Colorectal Dis. 2008;10:901–6.

49. Law WL, Choi HK, Chu KW. Comparison of stenting with emergency surgery as palliative treatment for obstructing primary left-sided colorectal cancer. Br J Surg. 2003;90:1429–33.

50. Im JP, Kim SG, Kang HW, et al. Clinical outcomes and patency of self-expanding metal stents in patients with malignant colorectal obstruction: a prospective single center study. Int J Colorectal Dis. 2008;23:789–94.

51. Repici A, Fregonese D, Costamagna G, et al. Ultraflex precision colonic stent placement for palliation of malignant colonic obstruction: a prospective multicenter study. Gastrointest Endosc. 2007;66:920–7.

52. Karoui M, Charachon A, Delbaldo C, et al. Stents for palliation of obstructive metastatic colon cancer: impact on management and chemotherapy administration. Arch Surg. 2007;142:619–23. discussion 623.

53. Faragher IG, Chaitowitz IM, Stupart DA. Long-term results of palliative stenting or surgery for incurable obstructing colon cancer. Colorectal Dis. 2008;10: 668–72.

54. Small AJ, Baron TH. Comparison of Wallstent and Ultraflex stents for palliation of malignant left-sided colon obstruction: a retrospective, case-matched analysis. Gastrointest Endosc. 2008;67:478–88.

55. Vemulapalli R, Lara LF, Sreenarasimhaiah J, et al. A comparison of palliative stenting or emergent surgery for obstructing incurable colon cancer. Dig Dis Sci. 2010;55:1732–7.

56. Jung MK, Park SY, Jeon SW. Factors associated with the long-term outcome of a self-expandable colon stent used for palliation of malignant colorectal obstruction. Surg Endosc. 2010;24:525–30.

57. Manes G, de Bellis M, Fuccio L, et al. Endoscopic palliation of patients with incurable malignant colorectal obstruction by means of a self-expanding metal stent: analysis of results and predictors of outcome in a large multicenter series. Arch Surg. 2011; 146:1157–62.

58. Baron TH, Kozarek RA. Endoscopic stenting of colonic tumours. Best Pract Res Clin Gastroenterol. 2004;18:209–29.

59. Tejero E, Mainar A, Fernández L, et al. New procedure for the treatment of colorectal neoplastic obstructions. Dis Colon Rectum. 1994;37:1158–9.

60. Riedl S, Wiebelt H, Bergmann U, Hermanek Jr P. Postoperative Komplikationen und Leralität in der chirurgischen Therapie des Coloncarcinomas. Chirurg. 1995;66:597–606.

61. Cole SJ, Boorman P, Osman H, et al. Endoluminal stenting for relief of colonic obstruction is safe and effective. Colorectal Dis. 2000;2:282–7.

62. Carne PW, Frye JN, Robertson GM, Frizelle FA. Stents or open surgery for palliation of colorectal cancer: a retrospective, cohort study of perioperative

outcome and long-term survival. Dis Colon Rectum. 2004;47:1455–61.

63. Binkert CA, Ledermann H, Jost R, et al. Acute colonic obstruction: clinical aspects and cost-effectiveness of preoperative and palliative treatment with self-expanding metallic stents: a preliminary report. Radiology. 1998;198:199–204.

64. Osman HS, Rashid HI, Sathananthan N, Parker MC. The cost effectiveness of self-expanding metal stents in the management of malignant left-sided large bowel obstruction. Colorectal Dis. 2000;2:233–7.

65. Breitenstein S, Rickenbacher A, Berdajs D, et al. Systematic evaluation of surgical strategies for acute malignant left-sided colonic obstruction. Br J Surg. 2007;94:1451–60.

66. Martinez-Santos C, Lobato RF, Fradejas JM, et al. Self-expandable stent before elective surgery versus emergency surgery for the treatment of malignant colorectal obstructions: comparison of primary anastomosis and morbidity rates. Dis Colon Rectum. 2002;45:401–6.

67. Morino M, Bertello A, Garbarini A, et al. Malignant colonic obstruction managed by endoscopic stent decompression followed by laparoscopic resections. Surg Endosc. 2002;16:1483–7.

68. Stipa F, Pigazzi A, Bascone B, et al. Management of obstructive colorectal cancer with endoscopic stenting followed by single-stage surgery: open or laparoscopic resection? Surg Endosc. 2008;22:1477–81.

69. Olmi S, Scaini A, Cesana G, et al. Acute colonic obstruction: endoscopic stenting and laparoscopic resection. Surg Endosc. 2007;21:2100–4.

70. Cheung HY, Chung CC, Tsang WW, et al. Endo-laparoscopic approach vs conventional open surgery in the treatment of obstructing left-sided colon cancer: a randomized controlled trial. Arch Surg. 2009; 144:1127–32.

71. Pirlet IA, Slim K, Kwiatkowski F, et al. Emergency preoperative stenting versus surgery for acute left-sided malignant colonic obstruction: a multicenter randomized controlled trial. Surg Endosc. 2010; 10:1471–6.

72. Van Hooft JE, Bemelman WA, Oldenburg B, et al. Colonic stenting versus emergency surgery for acute left-sided malignant colonic obstruction: a multi-centre randomised trial. Lancet Oncol. 2011;12:344–52. Erratum in: Lancet Oncol. 2011; 12:418.

73. Maruthachalam K, Lash GE, Shenton BK, Horgan AF. Tumour cell dissemination following endoscopic stent insertion. Br J Surg. 2007;94:1151–4.

74. Saida Y, Sumiyama Y, Nagao J, Uramatsu M. Long-term prognosis of preoperative "bridge to surgery" expandable metallic stent insertion for obstructive colorectal cancer: comparison with emergency operation. Dis Colon Rectum. 2003;46(10 Suppl):S44–9.

75. Dastur JK, Forshaw MJ, Modarai B, et al. Comparison of short-and long-term outcomes following either insertion of self-expanding metallic stents or emergency surgery in malignant large bowel obstruction. Tech Coloproctol. 2008;12:51–5.

76. Baron TH, Dean PA, Yates III MR, et al. Expandable metal stents for the treatment of colonic obstruction: techniques and outcome. Gastrointest Endosc. 1998; 47:277–85.

77. Tack J, Gevers AM, Rutgeerts P. Self-expandable metallic stents in the palliation of rectosigmoid carcinoma: a follow-up study. Gastrointest Endosc. 1998;48:267–71.

78. Choo IW, Do YS, Suh SW, et al. Malignant colorectal obstruction: treatment with a flexible covered stent. Radiology. 1998;206:415–21.

79. Rey JF, Romanczyk T, Greff M. Metal stents for palliation of rectal carcinoma: a preliminary report on 12 patients. Endoscopy. 1995;27:501–4.

80. Diaz LP, Pabon IP, Lobato RF, et al. Palliative treatment of malignant colorectal strictures with metallic stents. Cardiovasc Intervent Radiol. 1999;22:29–36.

81. Saida Y, Sumiyama Y, Nagao J, et al. Stent endoprosthesis for obstructing colorectal cancers. Dis Colon Rectum. 1996;39:552–5.

82. Lee KM, Shin SJ, Hwang JC, et al. Comparison of uncovered stent with covered stent for treatment of malignant colorectal obstruction. Gastrointest Endosc. 2007;66:931–6.

83. Repici A, Reggio D, De Angelis C, et al. Covered metal stents for the management of inoperable malignant colorectal strictures. Gastrointest Endosc. 2000;52:735–40.

84. Park JK, Lee MS, Ko BM, et al. Outcome of palliative self-expanding metal stent placement in malignant colorectal obstruction according to stent type and manufacturer. Surg Endosc. 2011;25:1293–9.

85. Tilney HS, Lovegrove RE, Purkayastha S, et al. Comparison of colonic stenting and open surgery for malignant large bowel obstruction. Surg Endosc. 2007;21:225–33.

86. Nagula S, Ishill N, Nash C, et al. Quality of life and symptom control after stent placement or surgical palliation of malignant colorectal obstruction. J Am Coll Surg. 2010;210:45–53.

87. Tomiki Y, Watanabe T, Ishibiki Y, et al. Comparison of stent placement and colostomy as palliative treatment for inoperable malignant colorectal obstruction. Surg Endosc. 2004;18:1572–7.

88. Fiori E, Lamazza A, Volpino P, et al. Palliative management of malignant antro-pyloric strictures. Gastroenterostomy vs. endoscopic stenting. A randomized prospective trial. Anticancer Res. 2004;24: 269–71.

89. Varadarajulu S, Roy A, Lopes T, et al. Endoscopic stenting versus surgical colostomy for the management of malignant colonic obstruction: comparison of hospital costs and clinical outcomes. Surg Endosc. 2011;25:2203–9.

90. Targownik LE, Spiegel BM, Sack J, et al. Colonic stent vs. emergency surgery for management of acute left-sided malignant colonic obstruction: a decision analysis. Gastrointest Endosc. 2004;60:865–74.

91. Singh H, Latosinsky S, Spiegel BM, Targownik LE. The cost-effectiveness of colonic stenting as a bridge

to curative surgery in patients with acute left-sided malignant colonic obstruction: a Canadian perspective. Can J Gastroenterol. 2006;20:779–85.

92. Dharmadhikari R, Nice C. Complications of colonic stenting: a pictorial review. Abdom Imaging. 2008; 33:278–84.

93. Suh JP, Kim SW, Cho YK, et al. Effectiveness of stent placement for palliative treatment in malignant colorectal obstruction and predictive factors for stent occlusion. Surg Endosc. 2010;24:400–6.

94. De Gregorio MA, Mainar A, Tejero E, et al. Acute colorectal obstruction: stent placement for palliative treatment-results of a multicenter study. Radiology. 1998;209:117–20.

95. Shim CS, Cho JY, Jung IS, et al. Through-the-scope double colonic stenting in the management of inoperable proximal malignant colonic obstruction: a pilot study. Endoscopy. 2004;36:426–31.

96. Alcantara M, Serra X, Bombardó J, et al. Colorectal stenting as an effective therapy for preoperative and palliative treatment of large bowel obstruction: 9 years' experience. Tech Coloproctol. 2007;11: 316–22.

97. Tejero E, Fernandez-Lobato R, Mainar A, et al. Initial results of a new procedure for treatment of malignant obstruction of the left colon. Dis Colon Rectum. 1997;40:432–6.

98. Goyal A, Schein M. Current practices in left-sided colonic emergencies: a survey of US gastrointestinal surgeons. Dig Surg. 2001;18:399–402.

99. Datye A, Hersh J. Colonic perforation after stent placement for malignant colorectal obstruction-causes and contributing factors. Minim Invasive Ther Allied Technol. 2011;20:133–40.

100. Camunez F, Echenagusia A, Simo G, et al. Malignant colorectal obstruction treated by means of self-expanding metallic stents: effectiveness before surgery and in palliation. Radiology. 2000;216: 492–7.

101. Hapani S, Chu D, Wu S. Risk of gastrointestinal perforation in patients with cancer treated with bevacizumab: a meta-analysis. Lancet Oncol. 2009;10:559–68.

# Part 6

## Future

# Self-Expandable Metal Stents: Transluminal Stents

# 20

## Kenneth F. Binmoeller

The relief of luminal obstruction, whether due to malignant or benign disease, is a major goal of therapeutic endoscopy. The expandable metal stent has significantly contributed to this goal. Insertion of an expandable metal stent exemplifies the ideal flexible endoscopic procedure. The stent is a remarkably simple tool that is easy to deliver through the endoscope working channel. The procedure can be performed quickly and safely without specialized skills. The relief of lumen obstruction is immediate and lasting.

Flexible endoscopic interventions have historically been limited to the lumen of the gastrointestinal tract. The linear array echoendoscope, which enables real-time ultrasound visualization of a tool pushed out of the accessory channel, extends the reach of endoscopic intervention to targets outside of the gut wall. In contrast to Natural Orifice Transluminal Endoscopic Surgery (NOTES), endoscopic ultrasonography (EUS) enables transmural interventions with the echoendoscope remaining within the gastrointestinal lumen. EUS-guidance intervention creates a platform to perform various transluminal treatments using coaxial tools already familiar to the flexible endoscopist. One of these tools is the self-expandable metal stent (SEMS). This chapter reviews recent applications of SEMS for transluminal therapy.

K.F. Binmoeller, M.D. (✉)
Paul May and Frank Stein Interventional Endoscopy Center, California Pacific Medical Center,
2351 Clay Street, Suite 600, San Francisco,
CA 94115, USA
e-mail: kbinmoeller@endovision.com

## Pseudocyst Drainage (Cystenterostomy)

First reported in the mid-1980s [1], transmural drainage of pancreatic pseudocysts (PC) represents the first endoscopic application of a transluminal stent. Pseudocysts producing a prominent visible bulge into the lumen of the stomach or duodenum can be entered with a diathermic catheter device such as a needle knife [2]. After removal of the inner needle, a guidewire is advanced through the catheter to facilitate insertion of a stent to drain the cyst. The advent of EUS-guided fine needle aspiration (FNA) and interventional EUS in the early 1990s significantly extended the reach of endoscopic drainage to include cysts that did not produce a visible bulge in the enteric lumen [3]. In addition, EUS made pseudocyst access theoretically safer and less *blind* because it enables the endoscopist to identify and avoid interposed vessels and gastric varices.

The placement of multiple double-pigtail plastic stents to drain pseudocysts is widely practiced [4]. Although there are no studies to document the superiority of two or more stents over a single stent, multiple stents are thought to enable drainage both alongside as well as through the stents. Nonetheless, reinterventions for stent exchange are needed in 17.7–27% of cases [4–6]. In theory, a covered SEMS with a substantially large lumen diameter should improve drainage and thus the need for reintervention (Fig. 20.1). A covered SEMS may also reduce the risk of

R. Kozarek et al. (eds.), *Self-Expandable Stents in the Gastrointestinal Tract*,
DOI 10.1007/978-1-4614-3746-8_20, © Springer Science+Business Media New York 2013

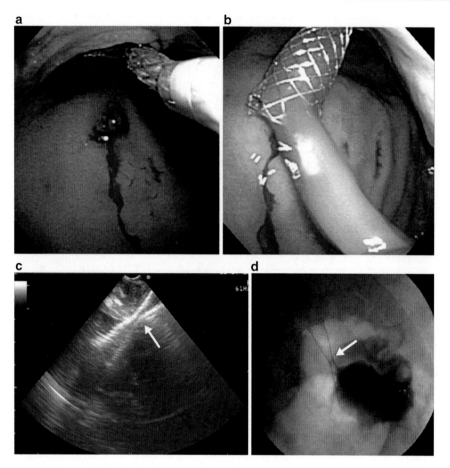

**Fig. 20.1** Transgastric pseudocyst drainage with a covered tubular SEMS (10 mm Wallflex, Boston Scientific). (**a**) Endoscopic view of delivery catheter prior to stent deployment. (**b**) Pseudocyst contents draining after stent deployment. (**c**) Endosonographic view of stent after deployment. (**d**) Fluoroscopic view of stent after deployment. *Arrow* shows waist where stent straddles wall

leakage between the cyst and enteric lumens when these are inadequately adherent and the risk of bleeding from the cystenterostomy due to the stent's tamponade effect.

The concept of using a SEMS to drain a pseudocyst was introduced by Maisin et al. in 1994 in a case report of a patient who had failed several attempts at nasocystic drainage of an infected pseudocyst [7]. As covered SEMS were not available at the time, a 10 mm × 4.5 cm uncovered SEMS was placed. The stent was then left in place permanently. In 2008, Talreja et al. reported the placement of covered SEMS in 18 patients with pancreatic fluid collections [8]. The patients had not undergone previous treatment attempts. The authors inserted a 10 mm × 60 mm biliary SEMS (Viabil; Conmed, Utica, NY) as well as a 10-F plastic stent either alongside (n = 4) or through (n = 14) the SEMS lumen to prevent migration. The authors reported a 95% technical success rate with a 75% complete resolution of fluid collections. However, there was a high complication rate of over 40%, including one internal stent migration. Tarantino et al. reported the use of a 10-mm covered biliary SEMS (Wallstent, Boston Scientific Corps) in a patient with an abscess that failed double-pigtail stent and irrigation through a nasocystic catheter [9]. The stent was placed transduodenally and the abscess resolved. The stent was easily removed with a snare 4 weeks later.

Esophageal SEMS with larger lumen diameters have also been used to treat pseudocysts that are refractory to conventional endoscopic drainage with pigtail stents. Antillon et al. used a 22-mm covered esophageal SEMS (Alimaxx-E, Endochoice) with a 27-mm flare to drain walled-off pancreatic necrosis that had failed four prior necrosectomy sessions with plastic stenting [10]. The larger SEMS was placed alongside a previously inserted plastic stent and Foley irrigation catheter. The SEMS was removed 2 weeks after placement and the pseudocyst subsequently resolved. Belle et al. described the use of partially covered SEMS with diameters of 20–25 mm inserted through the scope (Leufen, Achen, Germany) for drainage of walled-off pancreatic necrosis [11]. In all three of the treated patients, it was possible to enter the cyst through the SEMS with an upper endoscope to perform additional endoscopic necrosectomy. In addition, the cysts resolved in all patients.

## Gallbladder Drainage (Cholecystenterostomy)

Percutaneous cholecystostomy is well established as an alternative to surgical cholecystostomy in patients with acute cholecystitis who are at high risk for surgery. Limitations of percutaneous cholecystostomy include procedural risks related to an external puncture such as pneumothorax and drawbacks of a percutaneous drain such as discomfort, skin infection, and tube dislodgement. Transpapillary drainage of the gallbladder with either a naso-gallbladder drainage tube or plastic stent is a further option, but intubation of the cystic duct can be technically demanding [12].

With endoscopic ultrasound, the gallbladder can usually be visualized immediately adjacent to the duodenum or stomach. In the setting of acute cholecystitis, the gallbladder becomes adherent to the bowel wall and therefore more akin to a pseudocyst. Thus, EUS-guided transmural

gallbladder drainage is possible using the same technique as that for pseudocyst drainage.

Baron and Topazian reported the first case of transmural gallbladder drainage in a patient with hilar cholangiocarcinoma who developed cholecystitis after intraductal SEMS placement [13]. A prior attempt at transpapillary decompression of the cystic duct was hindered by the presence of the bile duct stents. A curved linear array echoendoscope was used to visualize the enlarged gallbladder from the duodenal bulb. In this patient, the distance between the gallbladder lumen and duodenal lumen was only 6 mm. The gallbladder neck was punctured with a 19-G FNA needle and a guidewire inserted into the gallbladder through the needle. The tract was dilated over the wire with a 4-mm balloon followed by placement of a 7 F by 4 cm double-pigtail stent. Acute cholecystitis resolved and an additional double-pigtail stent was placed alongside the first stent a few weeks later to augment drainage of gallbladder contents.

Kwan et al. reported a case series of cholecystoduodenostomy in three patients with acute cholecystitis [14]. The authors used a cystenterotome to apply cautery over a guidewire to enlarge the puncture tract, rather than a dilation balloon. The authors argued for cautery over balloon dilation based on the theory that cautery induces tissue desiccation and inflammation that may contribute to fusion of tissue planes, thereby reducing the risk of bile leakage and promoting the formation of a fistula tract. As an additional measure to reduce the risk of bile leakage, the authors placed a nasocystic catheter in all patients to enable active aspiration of bile from the gallbladder. The transnasal catheter was subsequently replaced with a double-pigtail stent. A small bile leak in one patient resolved with conservative management.

Lee et al. reported EUS-guided drainage of the gallbladder in nine patients who were elderly or at high surgical risk and required emergency cholecystenterostomy [15]. Four patients underwent gallbladder drainage into the stomach antrum (cholecystogastrostomy) rather than the duodenum (cholecystoduodenostomy). The authors gave preference to transgastric drainage of the

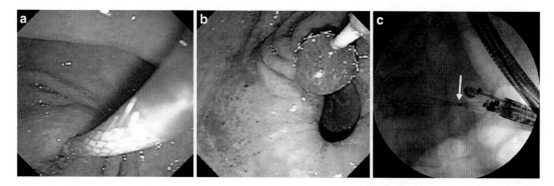

**Fig. 20.2** Transduodenal gallbladder drainage with a covered tubular SEMS (10 mm Wallstent, Boston Scientific). (**a**) Endoscopic view of delivery catheter prior to stent deployment. (**b**) Gallbladder contents draining after stent deployment. (**c**) Fluoroscopic view of stent after deployment. *Arrow* shows waist where stent straddles wall

gallbladder in those patients likely to undergo cholecystectomy later, based on the argument that the gallbladder will be easier to remove when adhesions form around the antrum compared to the duodenum, where the cystic and common bile ducts may be affected. The authors placed 5-F nasocystic catheters in all patients and did not witness any bile leakage. There were no immediate complications apart from one pneumoperitoneum, which did not adversely impact the clinical course.

Use of a covered SEMS may seal the gap between stent and fistula tract to prevent bile leakage (Fig. 20.2). Jang et al. reported on the use of a modified covered SEMS with flared ends (Bonastent, Standard Sci Tech, Seoul Korea) to drain the gallbladder in 15 patients with acute cholecystitis who were unsuitable for cholecystectomy, either through the stomach (n = 10) or duodenum (n = 5) [16]. Functional success was achieved in all patients within 3 days after placement of the covered SEMS. Two patients experienced pneumoperitoneum and both responded to conservative management. During a median follow-up of 145 days, no patient experienced recurrent cholecystitis.

The published experience with EUS-guided cholecystenterostomy is small, and it is important to note that only patients with acute cholecystitis and likely adherence of the gallbladder to the bowel wall have been treated. The gallbladder is normally a mobile intraperitoneal organ, and even transmural puncture of a normal gallbladder

with a 22-gauge FNA needle carries a substantial risk of bile leakage. In a study of EUS-guided puncture of the gallbladder to sample bile for microlithiasis in patients with idiopathic pancreatitis, Jacobson et al. reported symptomatic bile leakage in two of three patients, prompting the authors to discontinue further recruitment for the study [17].

Drainage of a nonadherent gallbladder will require initial securement of the gallbladder to the enteric wall to reduce the risk of bile leakage. In animal studies (porcine model), Fritscher-Ravens et al. deployed T-anchors into the gallbladder (n = 7) under real-time EUS guidance to affix the gallbladder to the bowel wall to allow traction for subsequent passage of 7-F catheters and plastic stents [18]. Single sutures were held with a pin and cylinder stitch locking mechanism.

## Bile Duct Drainage (Bilioenterostomy)

Transpapillary stent placement by endoscopic retrograde cholangiopancreatography (ERCP) is the established modality of choice for bile duct drainage in patients with obstruction due to malignant biliary strictures. However, ERCP may not be possible due to tumor infiltration of the duodenum, failed biliary cannulation, or an inaccessible papilla. In such cases, percutaneous transhepatic cholangiography and drainage (PTCD) is usually performed as an alternative route to decompress

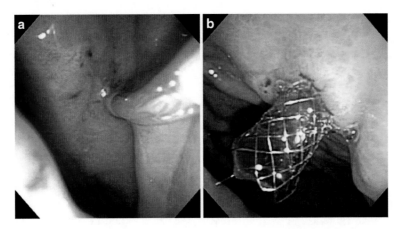

**Fig. 20.3** Transgastric transhepatic bile duct drainage with a covered tubular SEMS (8 mm Wallflex, Boston Scientific). (**a**) Endoscopic view of delivery catheter prior to stent deployment. (**b**) Bile duct contents draining after stent deployment

the bile duct and palliate obstructive symptoms. However, PTCD has a complication rate of up to 32% that includes bilio-cutaneous fistula formation, cholangitis, peritonitis, empyema, hematoma, and liver abscesses [19]. Additionally, the quality of life in patients with PTCD is impaired by the percutaneous drain that requires maintenance and, in some cases, exchanges.

EUS-guided transluminal drainage of the bile duct has recently emerged as an alternative to PTCD when transpapillary drainage is unsuccessful. In contrast to the retrograde approach of ERCP, EUS-guided drainage is antegrade [20]. The left hepatic bile duct can be accessed from the stomach to perform a hepaticogastrostomy, or the extrahepatic bile duct can be accessed from the duodenum to perform a choledochoduodenostomy (Fig. 20.3). Transluminal drainage has a number of theoretical advantages over PTCD. Similar to transpapillary drainage by ERCP, transluminal drainage is internal, which eliminates the drawbacks of external percutaneous drainage, such as local skin pain, infection, drain care, and bile loss. Transluminal drainage is not limited by obesity and less limited by ascites than PTCD. Transluminal access to the bile duct is performed under color Doppler guidance, which may be safer than standard fluoroscopic guidance of PTCD. A practical advantage of transluminal drainage is the ability to perform this procedure in the same session as a failed ERCP, potentially

by the same operator if they are skilled in both ERCP and EUS [21].

Technical success rates for transluminal bile duct drainage using plastic stents have been high; however, bile leak has been a significant risk, occurring in 19% of patients [22, 23]. The use of a covered SEMS rather than a plastic stent has been advocated to seal off the fistula tract [23]. However, the use of a covered SEMS may result in stent migration. At least one fatality from covered SEMS migration has been reported [24]. In a case series of hepaticogastrostomy, Bories et al. reported two cases of upstream intraductal stent migration, resulting in a biloma in one patient and cholangitis in the other [25]. In a series of eight patients undergoing transduodenal placement of a fully covered SEMS for palliative biliary drainage, one upstream stent migration 12 h after implantation resulted in duodenal perforation that required surgery [23].

SEMS with a modified design to prevent migration have been reported for bilio-enterostomy. Park et al. [26] reported a prospective study using a fully covered SEMS with flared ends (Bonastent, Standard Sci Tech) to prevent distal or proximal migration [26]. Fourteen patients with malignant biliary obstruction underwent hepaticogastrostomy (n=9) or choledochoduodenostomy (n=5). Stent placement was successful in all patients, but despite the anti-migration design, downstream stent migration into the bowel occurred in one patient. In a case report, Ito et al. used a SEMS designed with a *wavy* contour and uneven outer surface (Zeostent, Zeon Medical Inc., Tokyo, Japan) to prevent stent migration [27].

An advantage of using a SEMS is that it creates a larger diameter fistula that may allow subsequent passage of an endoscope for cholangioscopy and various intraductal interventions such as biopsy and tumor ablation. This is analogous to passing an endoscope across the cystenterostomy for debridement of walled-off pancreatic necroses. Eum et al. reported direct endoscopic ablative treatments with photodynamic therapy and argon plasma coagulation in three patients who had previously undergone placement of a 10-mm SEMS [28].

An alternative approach to create a choledochoduodenostomy is the use of mating magnets. Jamidar et al. used a novel, hinged device comprising a 7-F stent with a central ferrous metallic component [29]. The metalloplastic device was inserted into the bile duct of pigs using a standard ERCP technique over a 0.035-in. guidewire. A second magnet was then endoscopically positioned in the duodenum to mate with the bile duct magnet and exert compressive ischemic force. Anastomoses ranging from 5 to 10 mm were successfully accomplished in all survival animals. What is unknown is whether a transluminal stent will be required to maintain drainage across the anastomosis. At the time of this publication, no clinical experience using this device has been reported.

There are theoretical advantages of transluminal drainage of the bile duct by hepaticogastrostomy or choledochoduodenostomy over conventional transpapillary drainage by ERCP. With transluminal drainage, the fistula is upstream from the obstructing stricture, and therefore, the stent is not subject to tumor ingrowth or overgrowth, and the pancreas is avoided, eliminating any risk of pancreatitis. Transluminal drainage avoids the ampulla and accidental cannulation or injection of the pancreatic duct. The problem of *difficult bile duct cannulation* and instrumentation across the stricture (wire passage, dilation, and stenting) is also eliminated.

## Gastrojejunostomy: Gastric Bypass

Surgical gastrojejunostomy has long been the standard palliative therapy for malignant gastric outlet obstruction (GOO) caused by carcinoma of the stomach, duodenum, or pancreas. More recently, the growth in gastric bypass operations for obesity has markedly increased the performance of gastrojejunostomies.

Endoscopic placement of an enteric (intraluminal) SEMS is an alternative treatment option (see Chaps. 7 and 11). This endoscopic procedure leads to resumption of oral intake in about 90% of the patients; however, it may be complicated by recurrent obstruction, caused by either stent migration or tumor infiltration [30, 31]. A randomized, controlled trial showed a significantly higher incidence of recurrent obstructive symptoms in patients treated with enteric stents compared to surgery [32].

The creation of a transluminal anastomosis between the stomach and small bowel using an expandable metal stent was first reported in dog studies by Cope et al. in 1999 [33]. The authors used bare or partially covered flared 10-mm or 12-mm Z stents (Cook Medical). The gastroenteric anastomosis (GEA) was created by introducing rare earth magnets perorally into the stomach and jejunum under endoscopic and fluoroscopic guidance and mating these across the gastric and jejunal walls. The magnet pairs were excreted in 5–7 days, and the partially covered stents significantly extended the patency rate of the GEA to 7 weeks or more. Use of a fully covered "Yo-Yo" stent design (Cook Medical) with 12-mm diameter and strongly flared ends was reported in dogs and found to be patent at 6 months in four of five animals [34].

Chopita et al. reported the first clinical trial using the Yo-Yo stent in 15 patients with malignant biliary and duodenal obstruction [35]. Magnets were 12–14 mm in diameter with an attractive force of 1,000 g. The success rate was 86.6% (13 of 15 patients). One perforation occurred and was attributed to manipulation of the recently formed fistula. Three stents migrated (two distal, one proximal) without further complication. In a multicenter European study, Van Hooft et al. evaluated the Yo-Yo stent in 18 patients with malignant obstruction [31]. Migration of the Yo-Yo stent occurred in three of seven patients (42.8%); subsequently, the authors switched to a conventional 6-cm uncovered tubular duodenal stent design (duodenal Evolution stent, Cook Medical). Subsequent stenting using this design caused fatal perforation in one patient, after which the study was terminated.

The use of endoscopic ultrasonography to gain access to the jejunum for creation of a gastroenteric anastomosis was reported by Cope et al. in dogs [36]. The investigators filled the jejunum with water to improve sonographic targeting of the small bowel adjacent to the stomach. After puncturing the jejunum from the gastric lumen with a standard 22-G FNA needle, a 0.018-in. wire was inserted into the jejunum and captured with a previously inserted snare. A sheath was railroaded over the wire to deploy double T-anchors. The tract was dilated to 12 mm and immediately bridged with a fully covered SEMS.

Fritscher-Ravens et al. described creation of a compression gastroenterostomy wholly under EUS guidance [18]. The jejunum was punctured from the stomach with a modified 19-G FNA needle that enabled placement of a T-tag anchor to keep the jejunum in apposition with the stomach wall. A guidewire was then inserted through the FNA needle for coaxial insertion of an anastomotic device formed from two 7-F catheter segments. After removal of the guidewire, the catheter segments formed a cross on the jejunal side that was compressed against a spring plate on the stomach side. In 4–7 days, an anastomosis ranging from 3 to 9 mm was formed. The authors were able to dilate the anastomoses for 10 Fr stent placement and/or passage of an endoscope into the duodenum.

## Lumen Apposing Transluminal Stent

Tubular stents, conceived for lumen recanalization, have several limitations when applied to transluminal drainage. First, they do not impart lumen-to-lumen anchorage. This may result in leakage of contents if there is physical separation of lumens. Second, stent migration may occur, due to the absence of a stricture to hold it in place. Third, the length of tubular stents exceeds the anatomical requirement of a short transluminal anastomosis. The exposed stent ends may cause tissue trauma, resulting in bleeding or perforation. Finally, the longer the stent length, the more prone the stent is to clogging.

A lumen apposing, dual anchor stent (AXIOS, Xlumena Inc., Mountain View, California USA) was recently developed for transluminal drainage. The stent is designed to provide robust anchorage across nonadherent luminal structures. Made of braided wire, the self-expandable stent has bilateral lumen apposing anchors to impart luminal apposition (Fig. 20.4a). Fully expanded, the stent anchor diameter is approximately twice that of the stent lumen. The stent anchors are designed to distribute pressure evenly on the luminal wall. The stent is fully covered to prevent tissue ingrowth and tract leakage, as well as enable removability.

The AXIOS stent is delivered through a 10.5-F catheter and is 138 cm in working length. A tapered "nose cone" at the catheter tip facilitates passage across tissue planes into the target structure or lumen. Two radiopaque markers on the catheter indicate each end of the preloaded stent to enable fluoroscopic control of stent position. An endoscopically visible marker identifies the point at which the proximal stent anchor should be released.

The handle of the AXIOS delivery system is Luer-locked onto the echoendoscope instrumentation channel inlet port, analogous to a standard FNA needle (Fig. 20.4b). This gives the operator full control of stent deployment with the right hand, while the left hand holds the echoendoscope. The handle consists of a distal portion for catheter control and a proximal portion for stent control. The catheter portion positions and locks the catheter in preparation for stent deployment. Advancement of the "catheter control hub" advances the catheter into the target lumen, and the "catheter lock" retains the desired catheter position. The stent portion releases each stent anchor independent of one another in two sequential

a                                          b

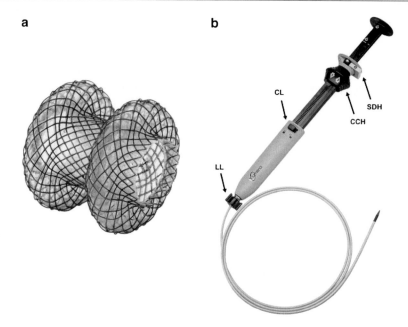

**Fig. 20.4** AXIOS stent and delivery system (Xlumena, Mountain View, CA). (**a**) Fully covered nitinol braided stent with bilateral flanges consisting of handle and catheter. (**b**) The handle Luer locks (*LL*) to the inlet port of the working channel and has a distal portion for catheter control and a proximal portion for stent control. The "catheter control hub" (*CCH*) advances and retracts the catheter. The "stent deployment hub" (*SDH*) retracts the catheter sheath to release each stent anchor independent of one another in two sequential steps. *CL* = Catheter Lock

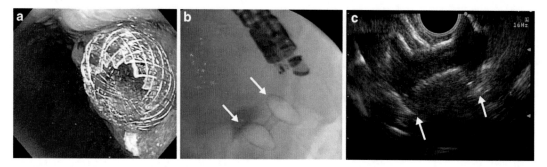

**Fig. 20.5** Transluminal drainage using the AXIOS stent. (**a**) Endoscopic view. (**b**) Fluoroscopic view. (**c**) Endosonographic view. *Arrow* shows proximal and distal flanges of stent

steps, with a full "stop" after the release of the distal anchor to prevent premature deployment of the proximal anchor. Retraction of the "stent deployment hub" to the halfway mark retracts the catheter sheath to deploy the distal anchor in the target lumen. The "catheter lock" can then be released to retract the "catheter control hub" to engage the distal anchor against the wall of the target lumen. Complete retraction of the "stent deployment hub" deploys the proximal anchor in the bowel lumen.

The AXIOS stent has been evaluated in animal studies for various transluminal applications (Fig. 20.5). A cholecystenterostomy was created under EUS guidance in four survival pigs [37]. The stents retained their position without inducing pressure injury or a hyperplastic tissue reaction over a 1-month animal survival period. Contrast injection after stent deployment showed no leakage of contrast outside of the fistula tract. The stent covering prevented ingrowth through the mesh, making removal easy using a snare

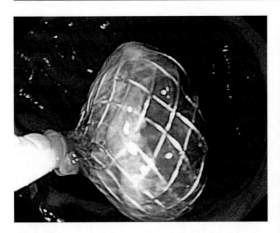

**Fig. 20.6** Endoscopic view of AXIOS stent removal using a snare

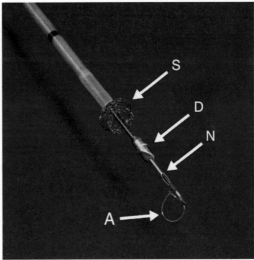

**Fig. 20.8** Prototype *all-in-one* device (AXT, Xlumena) consisting of needle (*N*), dilator (*D*), anchor (*A*), and stent (*S*)

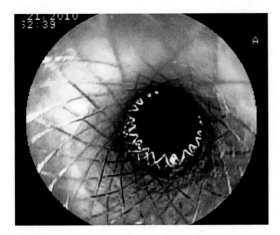

**Fig. 20.7** Transluminal passage of endoscope through the AXIOS stent to access target lumen

tightened over the saddle portion. Necropsy showed fusion of the gallbladder and stomach walls at the site of the cholecystogastrostomy and a leak-free fistula tract. A gastrojejunostomy was created in five animals (one acute and four survival). The stents remained fully patent in all animals throughout the implantation period (up to 4.5 weeks) and were easily removed (Fig. 20.6).

A transluminal stent can facilitate passage of an endoscope into the target lumen (Fig. 20.7). This extends the gamut of potential endoluminal interventions such as biopsy, tumor resection, and tumor ablation. In the gallbladder, biliary interventions for stone disease such as mechanical and electrohydraulic lithotripsy for stone

removal are possible. In the above animal studies, the AXIOS stent lumen was found to be easily intubated with the endoscope and to stabilize the endoscope during manipulation, including retroflexion, without dislodgement.

## Exchange-Free Platform for Transluminal Stenting

Future developments in transluminal stenting include a catheter-based system that delivers multiple tools in a coaxial fashion without the need for device exchange (Fig. 20.8). This will reduce the risk of leak into the intermural space and streamline the procedure. A prototype *all-in-one* device (AXT, Xlumena) was evaluated in porcine survival studies with technical success in creation of a cholecystogastrostomy in three animals [38]. The AXT device Luer locks to the echoendoscope and is designed for single operator, single-hand deployment. The exchange-free system is composed of a unique anchor needle that punctures the walls of the GI tract and bile duct and maintains continuous apposition of the two lumens to prevent leakage of contents during instrumentation. The AXIOS stent is then delivered and deployed directly over the anchor needle.

# References

1. Kozarek RA, Brayko CM, Harlan J, et al. Endoscopic drainage of pancreatic pseudocysts. Gastrointest Endosc. 1985;31:322–7.

2. Binmoeller KF, Seifert H, Walter A, et al. Transpapillary and transmural drainage of pancreatic pseudocysts. Gastrointest Endosc. 1995;42:219–24.

3. Grimm H, Binmoeller KF, Soehendra N. Endosonography-guided drainage of a pancreatic pseudocyst. Gastrointest Endosc. 1992;38:170–1.

4. Seewald S, Ang TL, Kida M, et al. EUS 2008 Working Group document: evaluation of EUS-guided drainage of pancreatic-fluid collections (with video). Gastrointest Endosc. 2009;69:S13–21.

5. Kruger M, Schneider AS, Manns MP, et al. Endoscopic management of pancreatic pseudocysts or abscesses after an EUS-guided 1-step procedure for initial access. Gastrointest Endosc. 2006;63:409–16.

6. Lopes CV, Pesenti C, Bories E, et al. Endoscopic-ultrasound-guided endoscopic transmural drainage of pancreatic pseudocysts and abscesses. Scand J Gastroenterol. 2007;42:524–9.

7. Maisin JM, Bradette M, Buscail L, et al. Patency of endoscopic cystoduodenostomy maintained by a Z stent. Gastrointest Endosc. 1994;40:765–8.

8. Talreja JP, Shami VM, Ku J, et al. Transenteric drainage of pancreatic-fluid collections with fully covered self-expanding metallic stents (with video). Gastrointest Endosc. 2008;68:1199–203.

9. Tarantino I, Traina M, Barresi L, et al. Transgastric plus transduodenal necrosectomy with temporary metal stents placement for treatment of large pancreatic necrosis. Pancreas. 2010;39:269–70.

10. Antillon MR, Bechtold ML, Bartalos CR, et al. Transgastric endoscopic necrosectomy with temporary metallic esophageal stent placement for the treatment of infected pancreatic necrosis (with video). Gastrointest Endosc. 2009;69:178–80.

11. Belle S, Collet P, Post S, et al. Temporary cystogastrostomy with self-expanding metallic stents for pancreatic necrosis. Endoscopy. 2010;42:493–5.

12. Kozarek RA. Selective cannulation of the cystic duct at time of ERCP. J Clin Gastroenterol. 1984;6:37–40.

13. Baron TH, Topazian MD. Endoscopic transduodenal drainage of the gallbladder: implications for endoluminal treatment of gallbladder disease. Gastrointest Endosc. 2007;65:735–7.

14. Kwan V, Eisendrath P, Antaki F, et al. EUS-guided cholecystenterostomy: a new technique (with videos). Gastrointest Endosc. 2007;66:582–6.

15. Lee SS, Park DH, Hwang CY, et al. EUS-guided transmural cholecystostomy as rescue management for acute cholecystitis in elderly or high-risk patients: a prospective feasibility study. Gastrointest Endosc. 2007;66:1008–12.

16. Jang JW, Lee SS, Park DH, et al. Feasibility and safety of EUS-guided transgastric/transduodenal gallbladder drainage with single-step placement of a modified covered self-expandable metal stent in patients unsuitable for cholecystectomy. Gastrointest Endosc. 2011;74:176–81.

17. Jacobson BC, Waxman I, Parmar K, et al. Endoscopic ultrasound-guided gallbladder bile aspiration in idiopathic pancreatitis carries a significant risk of bile peritonitis. Pancreatology. 2002;2:26–9.

18. Fritscher-Ravens A, Mosse CA, Mills TN, et al. A through-the-scope device for suturing and tissue approximation under EUS control. Gastrointest Endosc. 2002;56:737–42.

19. Lameris JS, Stoker J, Nijs HG, et al. Malignant biliary obstruction: percutaneous use of self-expandable stents. Radiology. 1991;179:703–7.

20. Binmoeller KF, Nguyen-Tang T. Endoscopic ultrasound-guided anterograde cholangiopancreatography. J Hepatobiliary Pancreat Sci. 2011;18:319–31.

21. Cabansag CN, Binmoeller KF, Shah J. Single-Operator, Single-Session EUS-based ERCP for pancreaticobiliary disease. Gastrointest Endosc. 2009;69:AB155.

22. Itoi T, Itokawa F, Sofuni A, et al. Endoscopic ultrasound-guided choledochoduodenostomy in patients with failed endoscopic retrograde cholangiopancreatography. World J Gastroenterol. 2008;14: 6078–82.

23. Siddiqui AA, Sreenarasimhaiah J, Lara LF, et al. Endoscopic ultrasound-guided transduodenal placement of a fully covered metal stent for palliative biliary drainage in patients with malignant biliary obstruction. Surg Endosc. 2011;25:549–55.

24. Martins FP, Rossini LG, Ferrari AP. Migration of a covered metallic stent following endoscopic ultrasound-guided hepaticogastrostomy: fatal complication. Endoscopy. 2010;42(Suppl 2):E126–7.

25. Bories E, Pesenti C, Caillol F, et al. Transgastric endoscopic ultrasonography-guided biliary drainage: results of a pilot study. Endoscopy. 2007;39:287–91.

26. Park DH, Koo JE, Oh J, et al. EUS-guided biliary drainage with one-step placement of a fully covered metal stent for malignant biliary obstruction: a prospective feasibility study. Am J Gastroenterol. 2009; 104:2168–74.

27. Ito K, Fujita N, Noda Y, et al. Endosonography-guided biliary drainage with one-step placement of a newly developed fully covered metal stent followed by duodenal stenting for pancreatic head cancer. Diagn Ther Endosc. 2010;2010:426534.

28. Eum J, Park DH, Ryu CH, et al. EUS-guided biliary drainage with a fully covered metal stent as a novel route for natural orifice transluminal endoscopic biliary interventions: a pilot study (with videos). Gastrointest Endosc. 2010;72:1279–84.

29. Jamidar P, Cadeddu M, Mosse A, et al. A hinged metalloplastic anastomotic device: a novel method for choledochoduodenostomy. Gastrointest Endosc. 2009;69:1333–8.

30. Dormann A, Meisner S, Verin N, et al. Self-expanding metal stents for gastroduodenal malignancies: systematic review of their clinical effectiveness. Endoscopy. 2004;36:543–50.

31. van Hooft JE, Uitdehaag MJ, Bruno MJ, et al. Efficacy and safety of the new WallFlex enteral stent in palliative treatment of malignant gastric outlet obstruction (DUOFLEX study): a prospective multicenter study. Gastrointest Endosc. 2009;69:1059–66.

32. Jeurnink SM, Steyerberg EW, van Hooft JE, et al. Surgical gastrojejunostomy or endoscopic stent placement for the palliation of malignant gastric outlet obstruction (SUSTENT study): a multicenter randomized trial. Gastrointest Endosc. 2010;71: 490–9.

33. Cope C, Clark TW, Ginsberg G, et al. Stent placement of gastroenteric anastomoses formed by magnetic compression. J Vasc Interv Radiol. 1999;10: 1379–86.

34. Cope C, Ginsberg GG. Long-term patency of experimental magnetic compression gastroenteric anastomoses achieved with covered stents. Gastrointest Endosc. 2001;53:780–4.

35. Chopita N, Vaillaverde A, Cope C, et al. Endoscopic gastroenteric anastomosis using magnets. Endoscopy. 2005;37:313–7.

36. Cope C, Faigel DO, Ginsberg GG, et al. Creation of a gastroenteric anastomosis with endoscopy and percutaneous gastrostomy in pigs. J Vasc Interv Radiol. 2008;19:124–8.

37. Binmoeller KF, Shah J. A novel lumen-apposing stent for transluminal drainage of nonadherent extraintestinal fluid collections. Endoscopy. 2011;43: 337–42.

38. Binmoeller KF, De La Mora-Levy JG. An exchange-free device for advanced translumenal therapy. Gastrointest Endosc. 2010;71:AB349.

# Index